Concepts and Activities

Nursing Health Assessment

D1368732

Concepts and Activities

Nursing
Health Assessment

Margaret A. Fitzgerald, RN,C, MS
Assistant Professor, Graduate Nursing
Simmons College
Boston
Family Nurse Practitioner
Family Health Center
Lawrence, Massachusetts

Springhouse Corporation
Springhouse, Pennsylvania

Staff

Executive Director, Editorial
Stanley Loeb

Senior Publisher, Trade and Textbooks
Minnie B. Rose, RN,BSN,MEd

Art Director
John Hubbard

Editors
Diane Labus, David Moreau, Kathy Goldberg, Nancy Priff

Copy Editors
Diane M. Armento, Pamela Wingrod

Clinical Consultant
Maryann Foley, RN,BSN

Designers
Stephanie Peters (associate art director), Mary Stangl (book designer), Donald G. Knauss, Laurie Mirijanian, Janice Nawn, Susan Hopkins Rodzewich, Anita Curry (cover design)

Typography
Diane Paluba (manager), Elizabeth Bergman, Joyce Rossi Biletz, Phyllis Marron, Robin Mayer, Valerie L. Rosenberger

Manufacturing
Deborah Meiris (director), Anna Brindisi, Kate Davis, T.A. Landis

Editorial Assistants
Caroline Lemoine, Louise Quinn, Betsy K. Snyder

Authorization to photocopy items for internal or personal use, or the internal or personal use of specific patients, is granted by Springhouse Corporation for users registered with the Copyright Clearance Center (CCC) Transactional Reporting Service, provided that the base fee of $00.00 per copy, plus $.75 per page, is paid directly to CCC, 27 Congress St., Salem, MA 01970. For those organizations that have been granted a photocopy license by CCC, a separate system of payment has been arranged. The fee code for users of the Transactional Reporting Service is 0874345804/94 $00.00 + $.75.

CAHA-011293

Library of Congress Cataloging-in-Publication Data
Nursing Health Assessment / [edited by] Margaret A. Fitzgerald.
   p. cm. – (Concepts and activites)
   Includes bibliographical references and index.
   1. Nursing Assessment I. Fitzgerald, Margaret A. II. Series.
   [DNLM: 1. Nursing Assessment—programmed instruction. 2. Physical Examination—nursing—programmed instruction. 3. Medical History Taking—methods—programmed instruction. WY 18 N982 1994]
RT48.N8827 1994
610.73—dc20
DNLM/DLC   93-37148
ISBN 0-87434-580-4   CIP

Contents

Contributors

Elizabeth A. Blackington, RN,CS, MS, MEd, Adult Nurse Practitioner, Boston Primary Care; Adjunct Graduate Nursing Faculty, Simmons College, Boston

Deborah A. Brown, RN,CS, MSN, ANP, Nurse Practitioner, Ambulatory Care/Rheumatology, The Arthritis Center, Braintree Hospital Rehabilitation Network, Braintree, Mass.

Susan Dial Busch, RN,C, MS, Nurse Researcher, Beth Israel Hospital, Boston

Judith Smith Casey, RN,C, MS, Adult Nurse Practitioner, Brighton Marine Health Center, Brighton, Mass.

Rebecca K. Donohue, RN,C, MS, ANP, OGNP, Assistant Professor, Simmons College, Boston

Rosamunde G. Ebacher, RN,C, MS, OGNP, Nurse Practitioner, Women's Health, Greater Lawrence Family Health Center, Lawrence, Mass.

Margaret A. Fitzgerald, RN,C, MS, Assistant Professor, Graduate Nursing, Simmons College, Boston; Family Nurse Practitioner, Family Health Center, Lawrence, Mass.

Stacey A. Lerager, RN,C, MSN, Adult Nurse Practitioner, Primary Care, Brighton Marine Health Center, Brighton, Mass.

Maryellen Maguire-Eisen, RN, MSN, ANP, OCN, Dana Farber Cancer Institute, Boston

John R. Roberts, RN,CS, MSN, ANP, Adult Nurse Practitioner, Neponset Health Center, Boston

Marianne C. Tawa, RN,C, MSN, ANP, Adult Nurse Practitioner, Brigham and Women's Hospital, Boston

Acknowledgments

I would like to recognize all of the individuals who contributed to this book:

The chapter authors—thank you for sharing your talent and for handling deadlines, computer glitches, reviews, and rewrites with good humor and grace. It has been a privilege to work with each of you.

My husband, Marc Comstock—thank you for your ongoing, expert computer consultation.

The graduate students and graduating class of 1993, faculty, and staff of the Graduate Program in Primary Health Care Nursing at Simmons College—thank you for your support during this undertaking.

My family and friends—thank you for sharing this book with me during these many months.

Dedication
To my daughters, Kara and Melissa Levasseur, whose presence in my life is my greatest joy.

To my husband, Marc Comstock, whose love sustains me.

And to the memory of my parents, John and Margaret Fitzgerald, and my sister, Jean Fitzgerald, MS, RN, CS, PNP.

Preface

As one of the first books in a new series, *Concepts and Activities in Nursing Health Assessment* delivers a unique way for nursing students to study an important core subject. Each chapter provides a combination of key concepts that crystallize essential, need-to-know information, followed by various study activities designed to challenge the student and boost information retention.

This new series gives students basic information about core nursing subjects as well as a forum for testing and applying that knowledge. Each volume covers a separate nursing subject and provides sufficient information and clear graphics (numerous illustrations, charts, and diagrams) to be used as a free-standing reference. Although not as comprehensive as a textbook, each book provides sufficient detail for students to understand the subject's essential concepts and complete all of the book's study activities.

Concepts and Activities in Nursing Health Assessment is written for student nurses in BSN, AD, diploma, and LPN programs who need to master the basics of conducting a comprehensive and accurate patient health assessment. It is especially useful in curricula that do not require a large core text. In other curricula, it can serve as a supplement to a major text or as a study guide.

This book is organized to provide the reader with a holistic overview of the principles, tools, and skills necessary for performing a complete assessment. Early chapters focus on explaining the role of assessment in the nursing process and on helping the reader to master the skills needed to conduct a health history and a detailed physical examination. Later chapters, which are arranged by body system, offer a comprehensive view of pertinent history-taking and physical examination procedures used in a head-to-toe assessment.

All chapters are formatted for easy access and use. Each begins with a list of objectives to focus the reader's attention, followed by an overview of concepts that clearly presents core information and establishes the data base from which the reader can complete the study activities. Activities may include multiple-choice questions, true-or-false statements, carefully selected fill-in-the blank statements, matching exercises, and short-answer questions. Each chapter concludes with a list of study activities answers, including rationales whenever the answer is not immediately apparent.

To provide the most current, accurate, and clinically appropriate information, *Concepts and Activities in Nursing Health Assessment* was prepared by practicing clinicians and academicians and reviewed extensively by nurses from appropriate specialty areas. Their combined efforts have produced a valuable information source and a ready-reference for years to come.

CHAPTER 1

Assessment and the nursing process

OBJECTIVES

After studying this chapter, the reader should be able to:
1. Identify the steps in the nursing process.
2. Describe the nurse's role in the nursing process.
3. Explain how the subjective and objective data gathered during assessment relate to the nursing process.
4. Identify methods of collecting and organizing assessment data.
5. Discuss the relationship of assessment to the other steps of the nursing process.

OVERVIEW OF CONCEPTS

To help the nurse meet diverse roles and responsibilities, the nursing profession has developed the nursing process. A system derived from the scientific method of problem solving, the nursing process considers all the factors that affect a patient's care. Using the nursing process as a guide, the nurse can formulate strategies to respond to a patient's current and potential needs. The process involves interactive problem solving between the nurse and patient and forms the basis for nursing actions and decisions. The nursing process includes five steps: assessment, nursing diagnosis, planning, implementation, and evaluation.

Assessment is the foundation for the other four steps. In nursing, assessment means the ongoing, systematic collection of data from many sources. Besides data related to the patient's physical status, assessment includes data on the patient's socioeconomic, cultural, developmental, and emotional status as well as spiritual beliefs. Systematic collection and review of these data allow identification of problems that nursing care can address and permits assignment of nursing diagnoses. Effectiveness of the remaining steps of the nursing process relies heavily on the accuracy and thoroughness of assessment.

Nursing process steps

The nursing process helps determine which health problems the nurse can help alleviate, which potential problems the nurse can help prevent, what kind of and how much assistance the patient requires, who can best provide such assistance, and which desired outcomes are realistic.

It is a dynamic activity that begins when the nurse compiles subjective data (information reported by the patient during the health history) and objective data (information collected through physical assessment techniques and diagnostic studies). The data base grows as the nurse uses the nursing process. New data are added to the subjective and objective data base if the patient's condition changes, additional diagnostic testing results become available, or the patient reveals more information. The process may be goal-directed and individual- or patient-centered. Ideally, it does not force the patient to conform to established solutions. The nursing process invites patient participation by respecting individuality and identifying the patient's unique characteristics that will direct the way problems are defined and solved.

Assessment

The initial phase of the nursing process, assessment takes place during the nurse's first encounter with a new patient and continues throughout the nurse-patient association. Simply stated, assessment is the collection of relevant data from various sources (such as the patient, patient's spouse or significant other, medical records, and diagnostic test results) to form a complete picture about the patient's health.

Data generally are categorized in two ways, based on the collection method. *Subjective data* come directly from the patient during the health history interview. Experts estimate that roughly 90% of health care problems can be accurately assessed from information revealed by the health history interview. (For more information on the health history, see Chapter 2, The health history.)

Objective data are identified through physical assessment techniques and diagnostic studies. These data reflect findings that are not interpreted. Examples are "cool, moist skin; pulse, 150 beats/minute; blood pressure, 70/40 mm Hg." Such statements as "patient is in shock" or "patient is hypovolemic" are not objective because they interpret the data and reflect an opinion rather than state verifiable facts.

The patient is the primary source of assessment data. However, the patient's condition, age, or developmental level may necessitate gathering information from secondary sources, such as family members, friends, coworkers, community service groups, and other members of the health care team. Data from secondary sources may be valuable because they supply alternative viewpoints to the patient's and sometimes add data unknown to the patient. If possible, the nurse should obtain the patient's consent before obtaining information from secondary sources. Information obtained through a secondary source may be sensitive and must be handled accordingly.

Interview. For the assessment that begins the nursing process, the structured interview is the most common way to collect patient data. This interview is goal-directed, aimed at developing a data base for the nursing assessment. The interview also allows the patient to ask questions or voice concerns. (For details, see Chapter 2, The health history.)

Observation. By looking at the patient, the nurse collects valuable data about the patient's emotional state, immediate comfort level, and general physical condition. Observing tone of voice and body language may help isolate patient stress that might require further investigation. (For details, see Chapter 3, Physical assessment skills.)

Physical assessment. The nurse performs a physical assessment to collect objective data after the interview. The nursing process, as an ongoing method of problem identification and intervention, requires the nurse to establish a baseline for all assessment. (For details, see Chapter 3, Physical assessment skills.)

Recording the data. Data recording, or documentation, follows the baseline assessment and can be accomplished in several ways. Many health care facilities have standardized admission forms with assessment categories arranged in a checklist. This format saves time and energy by requiring the nurse to write only the information that cannot be checked off.

The nurse should organize the data into body systems (such as respiratory or cardiovascular) or into assessment patterns (such as communicating or valuing), conforming to the currently accepted list of nursing diagnoses. Whatever the organizational pattern, the nurse should record the data systematically, overlook no details, use appropriate terminology, and refer regularly to the baseline assessment. Also, the nurse must make sure the documentation is accessible, understandable, complete, and easy to read by all appropriate staff. Legally, these assessment data become a permanent part of the patient's medical record, so accuracy and completeness are essential.

Although the primary interview and physical assessment usually are performed as initial admission activities, assessment is ongoing. The nurse collects and records additional information regularly. Assessment can be a deliberate activity, or it can occur incidentally while the nurse administers medications or helps the patient with activities of daily living in the home.

Nursing diagnosis

Assigning one or more appropriate nursing diagnoses to a patient's situation is the nursing process step that follows assessment. A nursing diagnosis is a statement of actual or potential health problems that can be resolved, diminished, or otherwise changed by nursing interventions. The problem areas can be identified by the patient, significant others, the nurse, or any combination of the three.

The labels assigned to specific nursing diagnoses are becoming standardized so all nurses will use the same terminology. The current list of nursing diagnoses (clinically tested and accepted for general use) is published every other year by the North American Nursing Diagnosis Association (NANDA). All nursing diagnoses are grouped into func-

---

Functional patterns for grouping nursing diagnoses

Nursing interventions are based on human responses which are described by Marjorie Gordon as functional health patterns. These patterns represent the phenomena that the nurse detects through assessment. Nursing diagnoses serve as labels that describe patient responses and provide the basis for planning appropriate interventions that the nurse can implement and evaluate.

Today, every nursing diagnosis falls into one of these functional patterns:

- Health-perception–health-management pattern
- Nutritional-metabolic pattern
- Elimination pattern
- Activity-exercise pattern
- Sleep-rest pattern
- Cognitive-perceptual pattern
- Self-perception–self-concept pattern
- Role-relationship pattern
- Sexuality-reproductive pattern
- Coping–stress-tolerance pattern
- Value-belief pattern

Adapted with permission from Gordon, M. *Manual of Nursing Diagnosis, 1993-1994.* St. Louis: Mosby, Inc., 1993.

---

tional patterns. (For details, see *Functional patterns for grouping nursing diagnoses*.)

The complete nursing diagnosis statement has three parts: a problem, an etiology, and the signs and symptoms. The first part identifies the problem, for example, "Constipation." The second part states the etiology (causal or contributing factors), individualizing a particular nursing diagnosis to a specific patient. "Constipation" could be related to such causes as dietary disturbances, immobility, or adverse drug reactions. The third part of the statement records the signs and symptoms and other subjective and objective data that are essential cues for assigning the diagnosis. In this example, the third part of the statement might be "as exhibited by lack of bowel movement for 3 days."

Planning

Once the nursing diagnosis is formulated, the nurse can proceed to the planning step of the nursing process, determining the nursing plan of care for the patient. This consists of two major components: outcome criteria (patient goals) and nursing interventions.

Outcome criteria. Outcome criteria represent patient goals and state the desired patient behaviors or responses that should result from the nursing care. Each criterion should be measurable and objective, concise, realistic for the patient, and attainable by nursing management. Each criterion should include only one behavior, express that behavior in terms of patient expectations, and indicate a time frame.

All outcome criteria should have three major components:

- *content area,* which describes the subject that the patient will focus on or the physiologic or psychological response to be elicited

- *action verb,* which describes how the patient will achieve the goal of the content area
- *time frame,* which is a target date for completion of the expected outcome criterion.

Each criterion also may have criterion modifiers, which add significant details that delineate specified limits for a specific action.

Nursing interventions. After developing the outcome criteria, the nurse determines the interventions needed to help the patient reach the desired goals. Interventions are the actions that the nurse implements to help the patient meet the identified outcome criteria.

After compiling the interventions, the nurse, the patient, and other people involved can review them. The nurse evaluates with the patient the potential effects of each strategy and its probable outcomes, anticipating risks as well as benefits to prevent problems.

Each intervention must provide for patient safety, take into account available resources (including supplies and personnel), agree with the patient's stated value system, and complement other health care activities required for the patient's welfare. Next, the nurse considers the rules governing nursing actions and patient behaviors in the health care facility. This ensures that the nursing interventions are legally sound and defensible. Finally, the nurse makes sure the interventions are appropriate for the patient's age, condition, developmental level, and environment.

Then, the nurse chooses plans, goals, and interventions and document them in the patient's record. Called the nursing care plan, this written guide directs the patient's nursing care from admission to discharge. It can be updated and revised as needed.

Implementation

As soon as the nursing care plan is established and recorded, the nurse implements the plan by working with the patient and other people to perform the designated interventions. Interventions usually fall into three categories: interdependent, dependent, and independent.

Interdependent interventions are those the nurse performs in collaboration with other health care professionals to improve the patient's knowledge and skills. For example, if a patient's communication goals require a speech pathologist's intervention, the nurse acts interdependently by supporting the speech pathologist's strategies. This type of collaboration helps the patient achieve goals.

Dependent interventions are activities the nurse performs at the direct request of a physician to help fulfill the medical regimen. These activities may include performing an invasive procedure, such as venipuncture or bladder catheterization.

Independent interventions do not require a physician's direction for implementation because their execution is suited to the nurse's education and knowledge. Such activities are reflected in and broadly regulated by nurse practice acts in most states. For example, at a basic level, the community nurse can identify and monitor vital signs, provide skin and mouth care, and teach the patient how to care for a surgical wound after hospitalization.

Before implementing the care plan, the nurse should quickly reassess the patient to ensure that the planned interventions are appropriate. The care plan may call for ambulating the patient every 2 hours throughout the day. However, reassessment may reveal that the patient recently returned from a physical therapy session and is fatigued; therefore, ambulation would be inappropriate despite the established plan. In other words, the plan must be flexible and individualized.

Evaluation

Integral to the nursing process, evaluation is a formal and systematic procedure for determining the effectiveness of nursing care. Evaluation provides descriptive data that enable the nurse to understand the patient's status and thereby make better-informed decisions about what to change and what to maintain.

The nurse evaluates the care to determine whether the outcome criteria have been met. If criteria are unmet or partially met, the nurse can reapply the nursing process. In this way, evaluation enables the nurse to design and implement a revised nursing care plan, reevaluating outcome criteria continually and replanning until each nursing diagnosis is resolved.

The completed nursing process should fully portray the patient's situation as it relates to nursing practice. A complete assessment is the cornerstone of the nursing process and the structure on which all other nursing activities rely. The general assessment provides an overall picture of the patient's situation, whereas an in-depth assessment of the patient's physical signs and symptoms as well as the patient's situation offers more detail. The initial assessment supplies the foundation for the patient's care. Ongoing assessments keep the nursing process dynamic, current, and in step with the patient's situation.

STUDY ACTIVITIES

Short answer

1. How does the nurse gather subjective and objective assessment data?

_____

2. Describe the most common methods for organizing and recording assessment data.

_____

3. A home health nurse is caring for George Stein, age 60, who weighs 230 lb and has Type II diabetes mellitus. Mr. Stein recently was prescribed insulin. He tells the nurse his wife is administering his insulin injections because he does not know how to use insulin or a syringe. He also is unaware of which diet to follow, and states that he does not exercise even though he knows he should. Based on Gordon's description of human responses, Mr. Stein exhibits problems in which functional health patterns?

Matching related elements

Match the nursing process step on the left with the corresponding nursing activity on the right.

4. _D_ Assessment   **A.** Performing nursing interventions

5. _B_ Nursing diagnoses   **B.** Stating the patient's health problem

6. _E_ Planning   **C.** Determining effectiveness of nursing care

7. _A_ Implementation   **D.** Collecting data

8. _C_ Evaluation   **E.** Developing outcome criteria and nursing interventions

ANSWERS

Short answer

1. The nurse gathers subjective data directly from the patient through the health history interview. Objective data are obtained through physical assessment techniques and diagnostic studies.

2. Assessment data commonly are organized into body systems or assessment patterns as presented by the NANDA list of nursing diagnoses.

3. Mr. Stein exhibits problems in the nutritional-metabolic pattern, related to his obesity and lack of dietary knowledge; activity-exercise pattern, related to his lack of exercise; and health perception–health management pattern, related to lack of knowledge of insulin use and dependence on his wife for insulin administration.

Matching related elements

4. D
5. B
6. E
7. A
8. C.

CHAPTER 2

The health history

OBJECTIVES

After studying this chapter, the reader should be able to:
1. Identify the purpose and components of the health history.
2. Describe the necessary steps in obtaining an accurate health history.
3. Discuss effective and ineffective interviewing techniques.
4. Gather appropriate information for each health history component.
5. Describe health history modifications for specific patients.
6. Document a health history correctly.

OVERVIEW OF CONCEPTS

The health history is the major subjective data source about a patient's health status. Besides organizing physiologic, psychological, cultural, and psychosocial information, it sets the stage for the physical assessment by providing insights into actual or potential health problems.

The health history format provides a logical sequence for the interview and an organized record of the patient's responses. It has five major sections: biographic data, health and illness patterns, health promotion and protection patterns, role and relationship patterns, and a summary of health history data. (For a list, see *Nursing health history*.) The nursing health history interview gives the nurse essential data for developing an individualized care plan.

Developing interviewing skills

To obtain an accurate health history, the nurse needs a basic knowledge of interpersonal and communication skills and of the "therapeutic use of self." The following paragraphs provide guidelines for a successful interview.

Nurse–patient communication

The interview is a nurse–patient dialogue, not a simple question-and-answer session. The nurse should seek to develop an effective communication style, eliminating such barriers as the nurse's own cultural and emotional biases. Self-awareness—recognizing and accepting one's feelings, beliefs, and values, including personal biases, strengths, and weaknesses—allows the nurse to communicate more effectively with others who have different values and beliefs. This is important in obtaining accurate, unbiased information. The nurse's health experiences

Nursing health history

The nursing health history provides subjective data about the patient as a person. The list below includes all the components of a comprehensive nursing health history.

Biographic data
Name; address; telephone number; contact person; sex; age and birth date; birthplace; Social Security number; race, nationality, and cultural background; marital status and names of persons living with the patient; education; religion; occupation.

Health and illness patterns
- Reason for seeking health care
- Current health status
- Past health status
- Family health status
- Status of physiologic systems
- Developmental considerations

Health promotion and protection patterns
- Health beliefs
- Personal habits

- Sleep and wake patterns
- Exercise and activity patterns
- Recreational patterns
- Nutritional patterns
- Stress and coping patterns
- Socioeconomic patterns
- Environmental health patterns
- Occupational health patterns

Role and relationship patterns
- Self-concept
- Cultural, spiritual, and religious influences
- Family role and relationship patterns
- Sexuality and reproductive patterns
- Social support patterns
- Emotional health status

Summary of health history data
Highlights key areas of each component.

---

and life experiences also can influence the therapeutic effectiveness of the nurse–patient relationship.

Effective interview skills rely on nonverbal as well as verbal communication. The nurse must be aware of such nonverbal communications (body language) as eye movements, facial expressions, body gestures, and posture. Disparities between the patient's words and actions may provide important insights.

Therapeutic use of self

Using interpersonal skills in a healing way to help the patient is the "therapeutic use of self." Central to the concept is self-awareness, which permits approaching a patient with empathy and acceptance and establishes the open, nonthreatening environment needed to obtain a more accurate health history. Three important techniques enhance a nurse's therapeutic use of self: exhibiting empathy, demonstrating acceptance, and giving recognition.

Exhibiting empathy. Empathy, the capacity for understanding another's feelings, helps establish a relationship based on trust and encourages the patient to share personal information. To show empathy, use phrases that address the patient's feelings (for example, "That must have upset you").

Demonstrating acceptance. Accepting the patient's verbal and nonverbal communication is crucial to a successful interview. Acceptance does not signify agreement or disagreement with the patient; rather, it demonstrates an effort to remain neutral and nonjudgmental. Neutral statements ("I hear what you are saying" or "I see") show acceptance. Nonverbal behaviors, such as nodding or making momentary eye contact, also provide encouragement without indicating agreement or disagreement. However, the "right" words may be useless if the nurse's nonverbal communication, such as rigid posture or an uninterested look, reveals different feelings.

Giving recognition. Recognizing the patient's communication efforts puts the patient at ease during the interview. This involves listening actively to what the patient says and providing occasional verbal or nonverbal acknowledgment to encourage the patient to continue speaking.

Patient expectations

Personal values and previous experiences with the health care system can affect the patient's health history expectations. Many people seek health care only for illness or unfamiliar symptoms. Before they will provide reliable data, some patients may ask why the information is needed. Many do not understand why the nurse obtains the health history, believing this is the task of the physician. Explain that comprehensive health care starts with a health profile based on a broad range of information and that the health history identifies actual or potential health problems. Some patients will be reluctant to share personal information; reassure them that this information will remain confidential.

Behavioral considerations

Encounters with a hostile or angry patient occur occasionally. To maintain control of the interview, listen without showing disapproval and control any feeling of anger. Speak in a firm, quiet voice and use short sentences. A composed, unobtrusive, nonthreatening manner usually soothes the patient. If this approach fails, terminate the interview; inform the patient of the reason for the termination and, if possible, arrange to complete the interview later.

Cultural and ethnic considerations

A patient's cultural and ethnic background can have a subtle and complex effect on the health history interview. *Culture* refers to an integrated system of learned behavior patterns that are characteristic of members of a society and are not biologically inherited. *Ethnicity* is an affiliation with a group of people classified according to a common racial, national, religious, linguistic, or cultural origin or background.

Culture and ethnicity affect a person's beliefs, values, attitudes, and customs. They also help shape educational, occupational, and familial opportunities and expectations. Culture also affects the way a person experiences health and illness. The degree of these effects depends on whether the patient has undergone acculturation (modification caused by contact with another culture) or assimilation (loss of original cultural identity when an individual becomes part of a different, dominant culture).

Besides being aware of the patient's cultural orientation, seek to understand personal attitudes towards patients from different cultures. Try to develop an attitude of cultural relativism (acknowledgment of another person's cultural standards) and to judge the patient's actions by the patient's own cultural standards. Also, avoid stereotyping a patient based on cultural background. Remember that a patient may share certain characteristics with others of the same culture yet also exhibit individual differences.

Effective interviewing techniques

To obtain the most benefit from a health history interview, make the patient feel comfortable and respected. Using effective interviewing techniques helps the patient to identify resources and improve problem-solving abilities. Remember, however, that techniques that succeed in one situation may be ineffective in another. Examples of effective interviewing techniques follow.

Offering general leads. General questions give the patient a chance to speak freely. Such questions as "What brought you here today?" or "Are you concerned about any other things?" direct the patient to discuss the most significant concerns.

Restating. To help clarify what the patient means, restate the essence of the patient's comments.

Reflecting. Reflection gives the patient a chance to reconsider a response and add information.

Verbalizing the implied meaning. Stating what is implied or unspoken sometimes helps interpret a patient's statement accurately or yields additional insight into a patient's symptoms or concerns.

Clarification. Because many variables affect the interview and because interpretations of health behaviors or symptoms vary, the nurse may have to clarify meanings. If the patient has given confusing information, the nurse may have to seek clarification by admitting, for example, "I'm having some difficulty following your story. Could we try to clear this up?"

Using silence. Silence sometimes lets the patient reorganize thoughts and consider what to say next, while giving the nurse a chance to observe. Using silence effectively is a crucial skill; it can even convey empathy.

Summarizing. To help clarify information and ease the transition between health history sections, provide a brief summary after each major health history component, followed by a close-ended question.

Interviewing techniques to avoid

Some interviewing techniques create communication problems between the nurse and the patient. The following paragraphs discuss such techniques.

Asking why questions. A question that begins with "Why" may be perceived as a threat or a challenge because it forces the patient to justify feelings and thoughts. Some patients feel they should invent an answer if they do not have one. "Why" questions also may be difficult for patients who lack specific knowledge or are unaware of a crucial fact.

Using inappropriate language. Do not impede communication by using technical jargon or abstract terms that are inappropriate for the patient's developmental level, education, or background. Patients may perceive this as an unwillingness to share information or an attempt to hide something from them.

Giving false reassurances. False reassurances, such as "Everything will be fine," devalue a patient's feelings and communicate a lack of sensitivity.

Changing the subject or interrupting. These actions prevent the patient from completing a thought and shift the conversation's focus. Such behavior indicates a lack of empathy. Also, interrupting the patient's flow of words may confuse the patient. Wait until the patient completes a thought before clarifying a relevant point.

Using clichés or stereotyped responses. Avoid using such phrases as "You'll feel better in the morning" or "Where there's life there's hope." These phrases minimize the seriousness of the problem and may discourage the patient from expressing genuine feelings.

Jumping to conclusions. Premature interpretations and hasty conclusions invite inadequate or inaccurate information.

Using defensive responses. A patient may express anger and frustration about a treatment program or health care facility with a verbal attack. A defensive response will imply that the patient has no right to express such feelings, which may increase the patient's anger.

Asking leading questions. By its phrasing, a leading question suggests the "right" answer. Such a question may force the patient to supply a socially acceptable response rather than an honest one. For example, the question "You've never had a sexually transmitted disease, have you?" may force the patient to answer "No."

Conducting the interview

Physical surroundings, psychological atmosphere, the structure of the interview, time constraints, and questioning style can all affect the interview. To be an effective interviewer, the nurse should adapt a communication style to fit each patient's needs and situation. The following paragraphs provide guidelines for conducting the interview effectively.

Physical and psychological comfort

Physical surroundings can directly affect the patient's comfort and willingness to provide accurate information. A private room with a door helps ensure freedom from interruptions. An arrangement of comfortable chairs facing but slightly offset from each other creates a friendly feeling. Positioning the chairs 2′ to 4′ apart promotes eye contact and hearing and allows the nurse to observe the patient fully. If the patient is confined to bed or is a child, sit at eye level to minimize feelings of intimidation or powerlessness generated by standing over the patient.

The interview structure

Ideally, the interview includes an introductory phase, a working phase, and a termination phase. Each requires a different communication style to establish the proper tone and provide transition to the next phase.

In the *introductory phase,* the nurse explains the purpose and desired outcome of the health history. This phase starts with the nurse's introduction. Then the nurse shows the patient where to sit and establishes a time frame for the interview. During the *working phase,* the nurse obtains a detailed health history. Inform the patient that note-taking is necessary to ensure that information is recorded accurately. During the *termination phase,* the nurse summarizes the information gathered during the interview.

Constraints on the interview

A patient in pain may have difficulty completing the health history interview. The nurse may need to provide pain medication or other comfort measures before attempting to complete the interview. With a sedated patient, the nurse may need to wait until the medication's effect has dissipated before completing the interview.

For a patient who is well or not in discomfort, schedule the necessary time for the health history. A comprehensive history usually takes about 1 hour. However, the history may need to be modified for certain patients, possibly reducing the interview time to 15 or 20 minutes. When taking a focused history, prioritize the information. For an elderly patient with an extensive health history, the interview may take more than 1 hour.

Types of questions

Generally, the health history includes two types of questions: close-ended, which require only a yes or no response; and open-ended, which permit more subtle and flexible responses and elicit more information. In terms of quantity and quality, open-ended questions usually yield the most useful information. Such questions allow patients to give their perceptions of a problem and help them feel they are actively participating in and have some control over the interview.

An inexperienced nurse may tend to use close-ended questions until comfortable with various interview situations. Close-ended questions may help direct a rambling conversation. They also are useful when the interview requires brevity—for example, when a patient reports extreme pain or has life-threatening condition.

**Obtaining health
history data**

Modify the structure of the health history to meet the patient's current health status. For example, if the patient is moderately or acutely ill, collect pertinent medical information first and do the less-structured, more time-consuming interview parts last, or postpone them until the patient feels better. If the patient is unconscious or cannot provide health history data for any other reason, obtain information from secondary sources, such as the patient's family, friends, or old medical or nursing records. If possible, obtain the patient's permission to do this and verify the data with the patient at a later date.

Health history data include biographic data, health and illness patterns, health promotion and protection patterns, role and relationship patterns, and a summary of health history data.

Biographic data

The first information gathered in a complete health history, biographic data identify the patient and provide important sociocultural information. Record the following information:
• patient's full name
• current address
• home and business telephone numbers, if applicable
• contact person's name, address, and telephone number
• sex
• age and birth date
• place of birth
• race, nationality, and cultural background
• marital status and names of persons living with the patient
• education
• religion
• occupation.

Health and illness patterns

This section of the comprehensive health history includes the patient's reason for seeking health care; current, past, and family health status; status of physiologic systems; and developmental considerations.

Determine the reason for seeking health care by asking, "What brings you here today?" If the patient has specific symptoms, record that information in the patient's own words.

To assess current health status, ask the patient with a specific symptom or health concern to describe the problem in detail, including any suspected cause. Called a symptom or problem analysis, this technique promotes a systematic and thorough assessment. (For details, see *Symptom analysis.*)

To assess past health status, record childhood and other illnesses, injuries, previous hospitalizations, surgical procedures, immunizations, allergies, and medications taken regularly.

Information about family health status can unmask potential health problems. Determine the general health status of immediate

Symptom analysis

When assessing a patient with a symptom or health concern, the nurse uses a symptom analysis to help the patient describe the problem fully. A method for obtaining a systematic and thorough assessment, the symptom analysis is easy to remember with the mnemonic device, PQRST. The following questions serve as a guide to effective symptom analysis.

Provocative or palliative
What causes the symptom? What makes it better or worse?
- First occurrence. What were you doing when you first experienced or noticed the symptom?
- Recurrence. What seems to trigger the problem?

Quality or quantity
How does the symptom, feel, look, or sound? How much of it are you experiencing now?
- Quality. How would you describe the symptom—how it feels, looks, or sounds?
- Quantity. How much are you experiencing now? So much that it prevents you from performing any activities? Is it more or less than you experienced at any other time?

Region or radiation
Where is the symptom located? Does it spread?
- Region. Where does the symptom occur?
- Radiation. In the case of pain, does it travel to another part of your body?

Severity
How does the symptom rate on a severity scale of 1 to 10, with 10 being the most extreme?
- Severity. How bad is the symptom at its worst? Does it force you to lie down, sit down, or slow down?
- Course. Does the symptom seem to be getting better, getting worse, or staying about the same?

Timing
When did the symptom begin? How often does it occur? Is it sudden or gradual?
- Onset. On what date did the symptom first occur? What time did it begin?
- Type of onset. How did the symptom start: suddenly? gradually?
- Frequency. How often do you experience the symptom: hourly? daily? weekly? monthly? When do you usually experience it: during the day? at night? in the early morning? Does it awaken you? Does it occur before, during, or after meals? Does it occur seasonally?
- Duration. How long does an episode of the symptom last?

family members, including maternal and paternal grandparents, parents, siblings, aunts, uncles, and children. If any are deceased, note the year and cause of death.

Assessing the status of physiologic systems helps identify potential or undetected disorders. Before starting the review, prepare the patient for specific questions about the past and current function and maintenance of each body system. For most patients, conduct the physiologic systems review in head-to-toe sequence. (For guidelines on questions to ask about each body system, see *Assessing physiologic systems,* pages 16 to 18.)

Assessment of the patient's developmental status provides an overview of the patient's growth, physical abilities and limitations, and cognitive abilities. The length of this section of the health history will vary with the patient. In most cases, the developmental section of a child's health history will be more detailed than that of an adult. Focus on the patient's physical development assessment on activities of daily living and the physical capacity to perform them. This is particularly impor-

(Text continues on page 18.)

Assessing physiologic systems

When assessing a patient's health and illness patterns, the nurse asks selected questions about the function of each body system. Use the phrases below as guidelines for the questions.

General health status
- Unusual symptoms or problems
- Excessive fatigue
- Inability to tolerate exercise
- Number of colds or other minor illnesses per year
- Unexplained episodes of fever, weakness, or night sweats
- Impaired ability to carry out activities of daily living (ADLs)

Skin, hair, and nails
- Known skin disease (Note type, date of onset, and treatment.)
- Itching
- Skin reaction to hot or cold weather
- Presence and location of scars, sores, ulcers
- Presence and location of skin growths, such as warts, moles, tumors, or masses
- Color changes noted in any of the above lesions
- Changes in amount, texture, or character of hair
- Presence or development of baldness
- Excessive nail splitting, cracking, or breaking

Head and neck
- Lumps, bumps, or scars
- Headaches
- Recent head trauma, injury, or surgery
- Concussion or unconsciousness from head injury (Note the date.)
- Dizzy spells or fainting
- Interference with normal range of motion
- Pain or stiffness in neck
- Enlarged lymph nodes or glands

Nose and sinuses
- History of frequent nosebleeds
- History of allergies (Note type and treatment.)
- Postnasal drip
- Frequent sneezing
- Frequent nasal drainage (Note color, frequency, and amount.)
- Impaired ability to smell
- Pain over the sinuses
- History of nasal trauma or fracture
- Difficulty breathing through nostrils
- History of sinus infection and treatment received

Mouth and throat
- History of frequent sore throats–especially strep throat (Perform a symptom analysis.)
- Current or past mouth lesions, such as abscesses, ulcers, or sores
- History of oral herpes infections
- Date and results of last dental examination
- Overall description of dental health
- Use of dentures or bridges
- Bleeding gums
- History of hoarseness
- Changes in voice quality
- Difficulty chewing or swallowing
- Changes in ability to taste

Eyes
- Date and results of last vision examination
- Date and results of last glaucoma check (for patients over age 50 or with a family history of glaucoma)
- History of eye infections or eye trauma
- Use of eyeglasses or contact lenses
- Itching, tearing, or discharge (Perform a symptom analysis.)
- Eye pain; spots or floaters in visual field
- History of glaucoma or cataracts
- Blurred or double vision
- Unusual sensations, such as twitching
- Light sensitivity
- Swelling around eyes or eyelids
- Vision disturbances, such as rainbows around lights, blind spots, or flashing lights
- History of retinal detachment
- History of strabismus or amblyopia

Ears
- Date and results of last hearing evaluation
- Abnormal sensitivity to noise
- Ear pain
- Ringing or crackling in the ears
- Recent changes in hearing ability
- Use of hearing aids
- History of ear infection or vertigo
- Feeling of fullness in the ear
- Ear care habits
- Frequency of ear infections (Note treatments and outcomes.)

Assessing physiologic systems *(continued)*

Respiratory system
- History of breathing problem or dyspnea (Perform a symptom analysis.)
- Chronic cough, dyspnea
- Sputum production (Note color, odor, and amount.)
- Wheezing or noisy respirations
- History of pneumonia, bronchitis, or asthma

Cardiovascular system
- History of chest pain, palpitations, or heart murmur
- Hypertension (Note age at onset and treatment.)
- Need to sit up to breathe, especially at night
- Coldness or numbness in extremities
- Color changes in fingers or toes
- Swelling or edema in extremities
- Leg pain
- Hair loss on legs

Breasts
- Date and results of last breast examination (including last mammography)
- Breast self-examination habits
- Breast pain, tenderness, or swelling
- History of nipple changes or nipple discharge

Gastrointestinal system
- Indigestion, normal stool pattern, abdominal pain
- History of ulcers
- History of vomiting blood
- Nausea and vomiting
- History of liver disease or jaundice
- History of gallbladder disease
- Abdominal swelling or ascites
- Changes in bowel elimination pattern
- History of diarrhea or constipation
- History of hemorrhoids
- Use of digestive aids or laxatives
- Date and results of last rectal exam and stool for occult blood

Urinary system
- Painful urination
- Frequency and amount of urination
- Hesitancy in starting urine stream
- Changes in urine stream
- History of kidney stones
- Blood in urine
- History of decreased or excessive urine output
- Dribbling, incontinence, or stress incontinence
- Difficulty with toilet training (for children)
- Bed-wetting
- History of urinary tract infections (Note the number of episodes, date of last episode, and treatment.)

Female reproductive system
- Menstrual history, including age of onset, average duration, and amount of flow
- Date of last menstrual period
- Painful menstruation
- History of excessive menstrual bleeding
- History of missed periods
- History of bleeding between periods
- Vaginal discharge
- Date and results of last Papanicolaou test
- Obstetric history (for women of childbearing age), including problems during pregnancy and number of pregnancies, miscarriages, abortions, live births, and stillbirths
- Satisfaction with sexual performance
- History of painful intercourse
- Contraceptive practices
- History of sexually transmitted disease (Note the type and treatment.)
- Knowledge of how to prevent sexually transmitted disease, including AIDS
- Problems with infertility

Male reproductive system
- Presence of penile or scrotal lesions
- Prostate problems
- Testicular self-examination habits
- Satisfaction with sexual performance
- History of sexually transmitted disease (Note the type and treatment.)
- Contraceptive practices
- Knowledge of how to prevent sexually transmitted disease, including AIDS
- Problems with attaining and maintaining erection
- Problems with infertility

Nervous system
- History of fainting or loss of consciousness
- History of seizures or other nervous system problems; use of medication for seizure control
- History of cognitive disturbances, including recent or remote memory loss, hallucinations, disorientation, speech and language dysfunction, or inability to concentrate

(continued)

Assessing physiologic systems *(continued)*

Nervous system *(continued)*
- History of sensory disturbances, including tingling, numbness, or sensory loss
- History of motor problems, including problems with gait, balance, coordination; tremor; spasm; or paralysis
- Interference by cognitive, sensory, or motor symptoms with ADLs

Musculoskeletal system
- History of fractures (Note the date, affected bone, and treatment.)
- Muscle cramping, twitching, pain, or weakness
- Limitations on walking, running, or participating in sports
- Joint swelling, redness, or pain
- Joint deformity
- Joint stiffness, including time and duration
- Noise with joint movement
- Spinal deformity
- Acute or chronic back pain (Perform a symptom analysis.)
- Musculoskeletal-related interference with ADLs

Immune system and blood
- History of anemia (Note the type, date, and treatment.)
- History of bleeding tendencies
- History of easy bruising

- History of low platelet count
- History of blood transfusion
- History of allergies, including eczema, hives, and itching (Note the usual method for treating allergies.)
- Chronic, clear nasal discharge
- Frequent sneezing
- Conjunctivitis
- Interference of allergies with ADLs
- History of frequent, unexplained systemic infections
- Unexplained gland swelling

Endocrine system
- History of endocrine disease, such as thyroid problems, adrenal problems, or diabetes (Note the type, date, and treatment.)
- Unexplained changes in height or weight
- Increased thirst
- Increased urinary output
- Increased food intake
- Heat or cold intolerance
- History of goiter
- Unexplained weakness
- Previous hormone therapy
- Changes in hair distribution
- Changes in skin pigmentation (Perform a symptom analysis.)

tant for elderly patients. (For additional information, see Chapter 4, Activities of daily living and sleep patterns.) Focus the assessment of cognitive abilities on the patient's thought processes, perceptions, comprehension, and ability to reason.

Health promotion and protection patterns
What a patient does (or does not do) to stay healthy is affected by such factors as health beliefs, personal habits (including tobacco use, alcohol consumption, and prescription and nonprescription drug use), sleep and wake patterns, exercise and activity, recreation, nutrition, stress and coping, socioeconomic status, environmental health patterns, and occupational health patterns. To help assess health promotion and protection patterns, ask the patient to describe a typical day. The response can provide valuable data on health behaviors and lifestyle patterns. Actively listen for indications of stress at home or work, and determine whether the patient's schedule is reasonable. Although data will overlap, be sure to assess all (or most) elements, depending on the patient.

Role and relationship patterns

Role and relationship patterns reflect the patient's psychosocial (psychological, emotional, social, spiritual, and sexual) health. To assess role and relationship patterns, investigate the patient's self-concept, cultural influences, spiritual and religious influences, family role and relationship patterns, sexuality and reproductive patterns, social support patterns, and emotional health status. Each of these patterns can influence the patient's health. (For more information on evaluating family role and relationship patterns, see *Assessing the family*, page 20.)

Summary of health history data

Conclude the health history by summarizing all findings. For the well patient, list the patient's health promotion strengths and resources along with defined health education needs. If the interview points out a significant health problem, tell the patient what it is, what to expect, and what can be done about it.

Always conclude the interview by giving the patient the opportunity to have the last word: "Should we talk about anything else?" or "Do you have any information you want to add or questions you want to ask?"

Modifications for pediatric patients

Most modifications in the health history for children occur in the following sections: past health status, status of physiologic systems, developmental considerations, and nutritional assessment. Substitute questions about school for occupational information and assess safety hazards by concentrating on the parent's efforts to prevent accidents. If the child is age 8 or older, ask fewer questions about the perinatal history. If the patient is an adolescent, do not obtain data about specific developmental milestones that occurred during the first 2 years of life.

Although an older child can participate more fully during the health history, a young child can discuss symptoms to some degree and corroborate a parent's information. Therefore, direct as many questions as possible to the child, basing the questions on the child's developmental age so the child can understand and answer them. Sometimes having the child draw a picture and explain the image will provide information. During the assessment, take the opportunity to assess the parent–child relationship.

An adolescent can answer most health history questions, except, perhaps, those dealing with family history and specific details of serious childhood illnesses and hospitalizations. Because an adolescent may be reluctant to reveal thoughts and feelings, interactions can be challenging. A straightforward, noncondescending manner is usually the best approach. To respect the patient's right to privacy, ask if the adolescent wants a parent present during the interview. For an adolescent who may be sexually active, conduct the interview without a parent present and ensure the patient that the information given will re-

Assessing the family

Assessment of how and to what extent the patient's family fulfills its functions is an important part of the health history. Use this guide to assess how the patient perceives family functions. Because the questions target a nuclear family–that is, mother, father, and children–they may need modification for single-parent families, families that include grandparents, patients who live alone, or unrelated individuals who live as a family.

Affective function

Assessing how family members feel about, and get along with, each other provides important information. To assess affective function, ask the following questions:
- How do the members of your family treat each other?
- How do family members regard each other?
- How do family members regard each other's needs and wants?
- How are feelings expressed in your family?
- Can family members safely express both positive and negative feelings?
- What happens when family members disagree?
- How do family members deal with ccnflict?

Socialization and social placement

These questions provide information about the flexibility of family responsibilities, which is helpful for planning a patient's discharge. To assess socialization and social placement, ask the following questions:
- How satisfied are you with your role and your partner's role as a couple?
- Do you and your partner agree about how to bring up the children? If not, how do you work out differences?
- Who is responsible for taking care of the children? Is this mutually satisfactory?
- How well do you feel your children are growing up?
- Are family roles negotiable within the limits of age and ability?
- Do you share cultural values and beliefs with the children?
- How do you feel about being a parent?

Health care function

This assessment will uncover many cultural beliefs. Identify the family caregiver and use that information when planning care. To assess health care function, ask the following questions:
- Who takes care of family members when they are sick? Who makes medical appointments?
- Are your children learning skills, such as personal hygiene, healthful eating habits, and the importance of sleep and rest?
- How does your family adjust when a member is ill and unable to fulfill expected roles?

Family and social structures

The patient's view of the family and other social structures affects health care. To assess the importance of family and social structures, ask the following questions:
- How important is your family to you?
- Do you have any friends that you consider family?
- Does anyone other than your immediate family (for example, cousins) live with you?
- Are you involved in community affairs? Do you enjoy these activities?

Economic function

Financial problems frequently cause family conflict. Ask these questions to explore money issues and how they relate to roles within the family:
- Does your family income meet the family's basic needs?
- Does money allocation consider family needs in relation to individual needs?
- Who makes decisions about family money allocation?

main confidential. Be aware that the nurse may be legally obligated to keep confidential (including withholding from the parent) information given by a teen concerning sexual activity, contraception, and treatment of STDs.

Modifications for pregnant patients

Because pregnant patients are usually well, use the same health history format and interview process as for a young adult, but emphasize certain sections during different stages of pregnancy. On the initial prenatal visit, perform the comprehensive health history and note any obstetric and gynecologic history.

If the patient has experienced more pregnancies than live births, ask about abortions, miscarriages, and stillbirths. This information may be recorded using the *TPAL* system. The first element, *T,* represents the number of term neonates (born after 37 weeks' gestation). The second element, *P,* stands for the number of preterm neonates (born before 37 weeks' gestation). The third element, *A,* indicates the number of pregnancies ending in spontaneous abortion (miscarriage) or therapeutic abortion (induced abortion); occasionally, these are differentiated as *SAB* (spontaneous abortion) and *TAB* (therapeutic abortion). The last element, *L,* stands for the number of living children.

For example, suppose Ms. Ewing has had six pregnancies. Two pregnancies resulted in preterm infants, one of whom died at age 3 weeks. Two other pregnancies resulted in full-term infants. The patient also has had one miscarriage and one therapeutic abortion. The nurse would record this information as T2, P2, A2, L3 (or T2, P2, SAB1, TAB1, L3).

Other assessment questions involve infertility, STDs, and reproductive disorders, such as ovarian cysts. Also analyze the patient's family history for evidence of genetic diseases, such as cystic fibrosis, Tay-Sachs disease, and metabolic disorders. Be sure to explore the perinatal history of living children. Significant findings include a history of difficult labor or delivery (including cesarean delivery); induced labor; forceps delivery; fourth-degree perineal lacerations; precipitous or prolonged labor (over 24 hours); and delivery of infants with Apgar scores below 5 after 1 minute, who needed resuscitation, or who were small or large for gestational age.

Assess for perinatal factors that could put a pregnant patient at risk, such as a maternal history of blood group incompatibilities, diabetes, heart disease, hypertension, kidney disease, or eclampsia. Be sure to list all medications the patient has used before and during the pregnancy, including nonprescription drugs. Additional risk factors include exposure to environmental or occupational health hazards, such as radiation and toxic chemicals.

Alcohol, recreational drugs, and certain medications can adversely affect the fetus. Tobacco, caffeine, and STDs (such as genital herpes, gonorrhea, syphilis, and human immunodeficiency virus) are potential fetal health hazards. Viral infections, such as rubella and mononucleosis, in the first trimester can negatively affect fetal development even though maternal risk is minimal.

Determine whether the patient receives regular prenatal care. Ask if she has any problems that might interfere with adequate nutrition, such as nausea (in the first trimester) or heartburn (in the last trimester). Perform an in-depth nutritional assessment, noting whether the patient uses vitamin and mineral supplements and understands the need for increased caloric intake and a well-balanced diet.

Assessment of role and relationship patterns for a pregnant patient focuses on her psychological adjustment to the pregnancy. The following questions help assess these factors:
• Is this a planned pregnancy?
• How do you feel about being pregnant?

During the third trimester, assess the effect of the pregnancy on the sleep-wake cycle. The patient may experience considerable discomfort when she cannot change positions readily. Her ability to perform activities of daily living and to exercise adequately are other important concerns.

Modifications for elderly patients

Make health history modifications only if the patient shows age-related sensory impairment or a specific physiologic problem, such as aphasia resulting from a stroke. Most elderly people living in the community are well and can provide a comprehensive health history. If the patient tires easily or cannot concentrate, schedule two or more interview sessions to complete the comprehensive health history.

Although the format for an elderly patient remains practically the same as that used for a younger adult, the approach to the health history sections should change slightly. Because of increased age, an elderly patient is more likely to have chronic illnesses, causing various symptoms and requiring several medications. Therefore, focus on current problems instead of past ones. Also, ask the patient to bring in current medications to the interview.

Be sure to thoroughly assess an elderly patient's role and relationship patterns. The patient may experience feelings of loss and social isolation as the spouse and friends die or become disabled by illness. Because of changed social roles, an elderly patient may have difficulty maintaining a sense of achievement, productivity, and independence. Find out how the patient is dealing with changes in physical appearance or with performing activities of daily living. Ask the patient to describe a typical day. Inquire about the patient's financial status to determine if income is adequate to obtain food, shelter, and health care.

Initiate other modifications if the patient appears confused. In such cases, skip over most assessment areas and concentrate on specific current symptoms (such as pain, nausea, depression, or impaired sight). Ask a close friend or relative of the patient to supply missing information.

Modifications for patients with disabilities

Modifications for a disabled patient depend on the disability. If, for example, the patient is severely hearing-impaired or unable to speak, use a written health history questionnaire. After the patient completes the questionnaire, concentrate on the identified problem areas. Another approach is to write any additional questions that need to be answered, and pass notes back and forth with the patient. Ask a patient with severe vision and hearing impairments to bring a relative or friend to help. For a hearing-impaired or mute patient, the services of a sign language interpreter may be necessary.

Do not modify the health history format for a physically disabled patient unless the patient cannot tolerate the length of time required to complete the history. Remember to speak slowly and clearly; also do not become impatient while waiting for an answer. For a patient with mild or moderate intellectual impairment, use simple phrases and schedule brief sessions to accommodate a short attention span. A close relative or friend usually is needed to provide information about a severely impaired or intellectually disabled patient.

Documenting the health history

The system used to document the health history and other parts of the assessment varies with each health care facility. A facility may use computerized records, which provide standardized formats for documentation; source-oriented records, in which each professional group documents separate data on each patient; or a problem-oriented record (POR), also called a problem-oriented medical record (POMR). The POR system focuses on the patient's problems and documents data according to the SOAPIE format, which closely follows the nursing process steps:

- *S* stands for *subjective* data (what the patient reports)
- *O* represents *objective* data (what the nurse observes, inspects, palpates, percusses, and auscultates)
- *A* indicates *assessment* (nursing diagnosis and a statement of the patient's progress or lack of progress)
- *P* stands for *plan* (plan of patient care)
- *I* represents *implementation* (nursing interventions that carry out the plan)
- *E* stands for *evaluation* (review of the results of the implemented plan).

Regardless of the system used to record the health history, the nurse must document data according to the following legal guidelines:

- Use the appropriate form and write in ink.
- Be sure the patient's name and identification number are on each page.
- Record the date and time of each entry.
- Use standard, accepted abbreviations only.
- Document symptoms in the patient's own words.
- Be specific; avoid generalizations and vague expressions.
- Write on every line. Do not leave blank spaces.
- If a certain space does not apply to the patient, write NA (*not applicable*) in the space.
- Do not backdate or squeeze writing into a previously documented entry. Do not use "white out."

• Document only work done personally; never document for someone else.
• Do not document value judgments and opinions.
• Sign every entry with your first and last name and title.

The patient's record is used by other health care professionals to determine subsequent health needs. Before recording the health history, analyze notes and recollections to formulate a careful assessment of the patient-supplied subjective data. Follow the guidelines discussed below when documenting the health history.

Write the history clearly and concisely, omitting biases. If a particular section of the health history has no significant data, note that fact. This is called *recording pertinent negatives*; for example, "Patient denies family history of diabetes, heart disease, or cancer." Usually, pertinent positives in the history are recorded before pertinent negatives; for example, "Patient has a positive history of ulcer and a negative family history of colon cancer." Include a written summary of significant health history data at the end. The summary is particularly important as a source for the nursing diagnoses derived from subjective data.

STUDY ACTIVITIES

Short answer

1. John Thomas, age 65, has a history of lung disease and complains of dyspnea. Give an example of an appropriate open-ended question and an appropriate close-ended question the nurse might ask this patient to assess his complaint.

_____

2. Mr. Thomas tells the nurse he's felt lonely since his wife died 10 months ago. What would be an appropriate empathic response to his statement? What would be an inappropriate response?

_____

3. Marie Harrison, age 54, is unconscious after sustaining a major head injury. The nurse needs to obtain her health history but must use secondary sources of information because Ms. Harrison cannot communicate. Which sources would be acceptable?

_____

4. Jill Thompson, age 3, arrives in the emergency department complaining of abdominal pain. Which method could the nurse use to perform a complete symptom analysis of her complaint?

_____

5. Rosalie Jacobson, age 32, has been pregnant four times. One pregnancy ended in miscarriage and another in a therapeutic abortion. She has two living children—one born at 36 weeks' gestation and another at 40 weeks' gestation. How should the nurse document Ms. Jacobson's pregnancy history?

Matching related elements

Match the data in the left column with the appropriate component of the health history in the right column.

6. ___ Status of physiologic systems   **A.** Biographical data

7. ___ Stress and coping patterns   **B.** Health and illness patters

8. ___ Contact person   **C.** Health promotion and protection patterns

9. ___ Self-concept   **D.** Role and relationship patterns

10. ___ Synopsis of health problem or health promotion strengths   **E.** Summary of health history data

Fill in the blanks

11. The nurse demonstrates therapeutic use of self by exhibiting

_____, demonstrating _____, and giving _____.

12. Ideally, the health history begins with an _____ phase,

moves into a _____ phase, and concludes with a _____ phase.

13. ~~CLOSED-ENDED~~ questions require a yes or no answer. ~~OPEN-ENDED~~ questions elicit more information.

14. In the SOAPIE format of documentation, the *S* stands for

~~SUBJECTIVE~~ data, the *O* stands for ~~OBJECTIVE~~ data, and the *A* indicates ~~ASSESSMENT~~.

ANSWERS   Short answer

1. To assess Mr. Thomas's complaint, the nurse might ask open-ended questions such as, "Can you tell me more about the shortness of breath you've been having?" "What actions relieve the problem?" or "What actions exacerbate the problem?" Appropriate close-ended questions would be, "Are you always short of breath?" or "Is it more difficult to breathe at night?"

2. "This must be a difficult time for you" is an appropriate empathic response because it does not belittle or judge the patient's reaction to his loss. "Why do you feel this way?" would be an inappropriate response because it challenges Mr. Thomas to explain his grief rather than showing that the nurse accepts his feelings as valid.

3. Acceptable secondary information sources (those other than the patient) for health history data include family members, close friends, and old medical and nursing records.

4. The nurse could use the *PQRST* method to analyze the patient's symptoms. In this method, the nurse asks questions that explore five major aspects of the symptom, represented by the letters of the PQRST mnemonic. *P* stands for provocative or palliative; *Q* stands for quality or quantity; *R* represents region or radiation; *S* stands for severity; and *T* indicates timing.

5. The nurse should document Ms. Jacobson's pregnancy history, using the TPAL system, as follows: T1, P1, A2 (or SAB1, TAB1), L2. This represents one term infant (born after 37 weeks' gestation); one preterm infant (born before 37 weeks' gestation); one miscarriage and one therapeutic abortion; and two living children.

Matching related elements
6. B
7. C
8. A
9. D
10. E

Fill in the blank
11. empathy; acceptance; recognition
12. introductory; working; termination
13. Close-ended; Open-ended
14. subjective; objective; assessment

CHAPTER 3

Physical assessment skills

OBJECTIVES After studying this chapter, the reader should be able to:
1. Discuss the purpose and components of the physical assessment.
2. Identify the equipment required in the physical assessment.
3. Describe the purposes and demonstrate the techniques of inspection, palpation, percussion, and auscultation.
4. Explain how to approach the physical assessment, including ways to put the patient at ease.
5. Describe how to perform and document a general survey.
6. Identify normal vital sign ranges.
7. Demonstrate how to assess and document vital signs.
8. Demonstrate how to measure height and weight properly.

OVERVIEW OF CONCEPTS The physical assessment is the second step in an overall assessment. Typically, it follows the gathering of subjective findings, including the health history and review of body systems. During the physical assessment, the nurse obtains and documents objective data about the patient.

An accurate physical assessment requires an intelligent, systematic approach. The nurse must develop expertise in using special equipment and in performing the four basic assessment techniques: inspection (observing), palpation (feeling body surfaces with the fingers), percussion (tapping the fingers against body surfaces to elicit sound), and auscultation (listening to body sounds).

Assessment equipment For much of the physical assessment, the nurse relies directly on the senses as basic tools. However, to complete certain assessment steps, the nurse must use special equipment.

Basic assessment equipment
Usually, the physical assessment requires an oral or rectal thermometer, stethoscope with a diaphragm for detecting normal and high-pitched sounds and a bell for detecting low-pitched sounds, sphygmomanometer, visual acuity charts, penlight or flashlight, measuring tape and pocket ruler, marking pencil, and a scale.

A complete collection of basic physical assessment equipment includes these additional items:
- a wooden tongue depressor to help assess the pharyngeal cavity
- safety pins to test how well the patient differentiates dull and sharp sensations
- cotton balls to assess fine-touch perception
- test tubes filled with hot and cold water to assess temperature sensitivity
- common, easily identified substances, such as ground coffee and vanilla extract, to evaluate smell and taste sensations
- a water-soluble lubricant and disposable latex gloves. (*Note:* The nurse must be familiar with universal precautions and apply these principles when performing the physical assessment).

Specialized equipment
Certain steps in the physical assessment may require specialized equipment—ophthalmoscope (to assess internal eye structures), nasoscope (to assess the nasal interior), otoscope (to assess the external auditory canal and tympanic membrane), and tuning fork (to test sound conduction during auditory assessment and vibratory sensation during neurologic assessment). Although these devices usually are reserved for nurses with special training and expanded roles, all nurses should be familiar with them and their applications. Other equipment may include the reflex hammer, skin calipers, and vaginal speculum.

Physical assessment techniques

To perform the physical assessment, the nurse uses four basic techniques: inspection, palpation, percussion, and auscultation.

Inspection
Critical observation, or inspection, is the most frequently used assessment technique. When performed correctly, it reveals more than the other techniques. However, an incomplete or hasty inspection may neglect important details or even yield false or misleading findings.

Inspection should be approached in a logical, intelligent manner. While inspecting the patient, the nurse should always maintain objectivity and not be misled by preconceived ideas and expectations.

Unlike palpation, percussion, and auscultation, inspection is not a single, self-contained assessment step. Instead, it occurs continuously throughout the entire examination. Inspection findings enhance and refine the knowledge base.

To inspect a specific body area, first make sure the area is sufficiently exposed and adequately lit. Then survey the entire area, noting key landmarks and checking the overall condition. Next, focus on specifics—color, shape, texture, size, and movement.

Palpation
During palpation, the nurse touches the body to feel pulsations and vibrations; to locate body structures (particularly in the abdomen); and to

CONTINUOUS

assess such characteristics as size, texture, warmth, mobility, and tenderness. Palpation allows detection of a pulse, enlarged lymph nodes, skin or hair dryness, organ tenderness, masses, and measurement of the chest rising and falling with each respiration. Usually, palpation follows inspection as the second technique in physical assessment. Often, it confirms inspection findings.

Correct palpation requires highly developed skills. The nurse should take advantage of the tactile sensitivity specific to each hand region. For instance, the tips and pads of the fingers best distinguish texture and shape, while the flattened finger pads can best palpate tender tissues and detect crepitus. The dorsal surface of the hand best feels warmth; the ulnar surface is best at feeling fine vibrations. Use the thumb and forefinger to grasp tissues for palpation.

Palpation requires patient cooperation. To promote cooperation, explain to the patient what will occur and why, and mention that some forms of palpation or palpation of certain areas may be uncomfortable. If discomfort occurs, ask the patient to describe the discomfort, then document the response in the findings; this information helps in formulating correct nursing diagnoses.

Percussion

During percussion, the nurse uses quick, sharp tapping of the fingers or hands against body surfaces (usually the chest and abdomen) to produce sounds, elicit tenderness, or assess reflexes. Percussing for sound—the most common percussion goal—helps locate organ borders, identify organ shape and position, and determine if an organ is solid or filled with fluid or gas.

Three basic percussion methods include indirect, direct, and blunt percussion. In indirect percussion, the most common method, the examiner taps one finger against an object—usually the middle finger of the other hand—held against the skin surface. Indirect percussion is usually done to elicit sounds, which helps to determine the location and density of underlying organs. Because different organs produce different percussion sounds, sounds are assessed for loudness, duration, and pitch.

When percussing for sound, the nurse creates vibration that penetrates roughly $1\frac{1}{2}''$ to $2''$ (4 to 5 cm) below the skin's surface. Percussion reveals a variety of sounds, including:
• resonance—the long, low, hollow sound heard over an intercostal space above healthy lung tissue
• tympany—the loud, high-pitched, drumlike sound normally heard over a gastric air bubble or gas-filled bowel
• dullness—the soft, high-pitched, thudding sound normally heard over more solid organs, such as the liver and heart.

Abnormal percussion sounds may be heard over body organs. Consider hyperresonance—longer, louder, and lower-pitched than resonance—a classic sign of lung hyperinflation, as in emphysema or acute asthma. Flatness—similar to dullness but shorter in duration and softer in intensity—may be heard over pleural fluid accumulation or pleural thickening.

To enhance percussion technique and improve the results, follow these guidelines:

• As with any other assessment technique, explain to the patient what will occur and why.
• Have the patient void so that a full bladder does not produce dullness.
• Keep fingernails short, and warm hands before starting.
• Make sure the examination area is quiet. Remove any jewelry that may clatter. Keep the area to be percussed free of clothing or examination gowns—especially paper gowns that may make distracting noises.

Auscultation

During auscultation, the nurse listens to body sounds—particularly those produced by the heart, lungs, vessels, stomach, and intestines. Most auscultated sounds result from air or fluid movement—for example, the rush of air through respiratory pathways, the turbulent flow of blood through vessels, and the movement of gas (agitated by peristalsis) through the bowels.

Usually, the nurse performs auscultation after the other assessment techniques. When examining the abdomen, however, always auscultate second—after inspection but before percussion and palpation. That way, bowel sounds are heard before palpation disrupts them.

When auscultating, use a high-quality, properly fitting stethoscope. Maintain a quiet environment, and make sure to sufficiently expose the body area to be auscultated. Instruct the patient to remain quiet and still. Before starting, warm the stethoscope head (diaphragm and bell) in your hand so the cold metal does not startle the patient. Then place the diaphragm or bell over the appropriate area and focus attention on individual sounds, identifying their characteristics. Determine the intensity, pitch, and duration of each sound and check the frequency of recurring sounds.

Approach to physical assessment

The physical assessment may take various forms. A complete physical assessment—appropriate for periodic health checks—includes a general survey, vital sign measurement, height and weight measurement, and assessment of all organs and body systems.

However, in the hospital and many other settings, the nurse rarely has the chance to perform a complete assessment. In such cases, the nurse may conduct a *modified* assessment, using knowledge of the patient's history and complaints. For example, if the patient has a peripheral vascular disease, include skin and peripheral pulse examination in the assessment; if the patient has a herniated lumbar disk, test motor function and sensation in the legs and feet.

The physical assessment requires the same general nursing approach as any other procedure. The nurse gathers and assembles the necessary equipment, explains the reason for the examination, ensures patient comfort, and uses a professional manner to help allay patient anxiety.

Special considerations for pediatric patients

The nurse tailors the assessment to the child's age and developmental level, observing whether certain developmental landmarks have been reached. Whenever possible, smile and look into the child's face while talking in a comforting voice.

When assessing an infant, allow the parent to hold the infant during the examination, as appropriate. Children ages 1 to 2 may be more fearful and harder to examine than infants. If necessary, calm or distract an upset child with a toy or another diversion. Keep in mind that young children typically find eye, ear, and mouth assessment more distressing than assessment of other body areas. For this reason, examine the head last instead of following the standard head-to-toe format. Hip abduction evaluation also can cause distress, so postpone this until late in the examination. Delay assessment of a crying child, if possible. Crying tenses the muscles and produces noise that may prevent accurate assessment.

Children ages 2 to 3 may be the most difficult to assess. These children may dislike being undressed and touched and may cling to their parents. To improve the assessment, develop a supportive relationship with the parent and take the time to gain the trust of both the parent and child. Encourage the parent to participate and let the child sit on the parent's lap. Explain each examination instrument and demonstrate its use on the parent. If appropriate, let the child touch the equipment and help with the assessment, such as by holding the stethoscope in place on the chest. When possible, integrate play into the assessment; for example, let the child pretend to listen to the nurse's heart or to a doll's heart. These creative touches improve cooperation by developing trust and by teaching the child about the body.

By age 4 or 5, a child typically becomes more cooperative and less fearful of the assessment. This child responds especially well when play is incorporated into the assessment.

The older child or adolescent has a better understanding of the goal of assessment. This patient may ask not to have a parent present during the assessment; if so, respect the request. Be sensitive to the patient's increased sense of modesty by providing adequate privacy and letting the patient keep undergarments on until the last minute. Allow the adolescent to ask questions about sexuality and assure the patient that all questions will be kept confidential.

Special considerations for pregnant patients

Assessment of a pregnant patient has a dual focus—the patient and her developing fetus. While assessing the maternal and fetal parameters that mark the normal course of pregnancy—fundal height, nutritional status, weight gain, pelvic size, fetal growth, and the changing appearance of the breasts and vagina—the nurse also checks for evidence of pregnancy-related complications.

Special considerations for elderly patients

When assessing an elderly patient, be aware that aging normally causes physiologic changes and impairs the body's response to stress, illness, and injury. Specific aging-related changes may include reduced muscle strength and range of motion, vital sign changes, slowed reflexes, impaired sensory perception, and slowed or impaired thought processes. To complicate matters, an elderly patient may take many medications, possibly leading to adverse reactions or unexpected drug interactions that can interfere with interpretation of assessment findings.

During the assessment, phrase instructions simply and slowly, addressing one point at a time, and give the patient plenty of time to respond. Because an elderly patient may tire easily and have trouble changing positions, allow extra time for each assessment step. However, do not assume that all elderly patients are frail, move slowly, or are hard of hearing; such preconceptions can interfere with accurate assessment.

Special considerations for patients with disabilities

The nurse may assess a disabled patient during a routine health screening or for a special reason, such as determining eligibility for rehabilitation or setting vocational goals. Whatever the purpose, focus on the patient's functional ability and mental capacity and tailor the assessment to the patient's specific needs, assets, and limitations. Before starting the assessment, take the time to learn as much as possible about the patient's abilities and impairments.

The general survey As the first step in the physical assessment, the general survey provides vital information about the patient's behavior and health status. During this step, the nurse documents initial impressions of the patient in a short statement—a summary that provides an overall picture guiding subsequent assessment.

The general survey requires skilled, focused observation and a professional approach to detect subtle clues from behavior and appearance and to derive an accurate patient profile. During the first contact with the patient, be prepared to receive a large amount of information. The patient's sex, race, and approximate age will be obvious and should be noted. Also note other factors, including signs of distress; facial characteristics; body type, posture, and movements; speech; dress, grooming, and personal hygiene; and psychological state.

Signs of distress

Check for obvious signs of physical or emotional distress. Dyspnea (shortness of breath) suggests a cardiac or respiratory problem, although it sometimes reflects severe emotional distress. Labored respirations or wheezing may indicate asthma or pneumonia. Determine if the patient's dyspnea improves or worsens with position changes.

Pain, another clue to distress, typically shows in a patient's facial expression, body movements, and posture. Check for halting, limited movements and an overly rigid or otherwise odd posture.

Be aware that patients express emotional distress in varying ways. One patient may show distress through jerking hand movements or rapid speech; another may withdraw or sit with head bowed and arms crossed over the chest.

If the patient exhibits any signs of distress during the physical assessment, make sure to explore this thoroughly by asking appropriate questions and conducting a complete symptom analysis. Severe headache, abdominal pain, or chest pain may signal a potentially life-threatening condition and necessitate immediate referral to a nurse practitioner or physician, thus terminating the physical assessment. In any case, patient safety and appropriate intervention are the most important considerations.

Facial characteristics

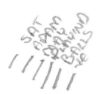

A patient's face provides valuable clues to physical, emotional, and psychological well-being. Observe the face for expression, contour, and symmetry. Obvious tension, staring, trembling, a downcast or shifting gaze, or constant blinking suggests a neurologic or psychological problem. A flat expression with no affect (outward manifestation of feelings) commonly accompanies Parkinson's disease (a progressive, degenerative neurologic disorder) and myasthenia gravis (a neuromuscular disorder causing muscle weakness). In some cases, facial trembling may indicate a psychological disturbance. Be sure to note and further evaluate any abnormalities.

Body type, posture, and movements

Assess the patient's general body type, classifying the build as stocky, average, or slender. Check for cachexia (extreme thinness) or obesity. With an obese patient, assess for abnormal fat distribution, as in Cushing's syndrome (characterized by truncal obesity and thin limbs). Note any unusual physical features; a rounded barrel chest, for example, may signal chronic lung disease.

Observe the patient's gait and other movements for symmetry, coordination, and smoothness. Note any obvious involuntary movements or deformities. Gait problems, such as shuffling, may accompany Parkinson's disease. Limping may stem from a previous injury; spasticity, from cerebral palsy. Note any use of assistive devices, such as a cane, walker, brace, or prosthesis. (Noting this also helps determine whether the patient needs assistance with walking.) Observe the bedridden patient's ability to sit up, turn, and reposition.

Note the patient's posture. Slumping may indicate fatigue or depression; hunching over may reflect guarding (a reaction to abdominal pain). In the classic posture of chronic obstructive pulmonary disease, the patient hunches over a table in an attempt to ease breathing.

Speech

Assess the patient's speech for tone, clarity, vocal strength, vocabulary, sentence structure, and pace. Hoarseness or softness may indicate laryngitis or cranial nerve paralysis. A monotone may reflect depression. Fast, garbled speech may accompany a mental disorder; slow, garbled speech, a cerebrovascular accident (stroke). Note the patient's vocabulary and word usage pattern—possible clues to educational level. (This information may help later when planning the patient's care and teaching sessions.)

Listen carefully to the patient's speech pattern. A patient with expressive aphasia (a neurologic condition impairing the ability to form words) may speak hesitantly and deliberately. Note whether the patient constantly searches for words, repeats the nurse's words, or uses rhyming words (possible clues to a psychological disorder). Also identify other obvious speech characteristics, such as stuttering or lisping.

Dress, grooming, and personal hygiene

A patient's dress, grooming, and personal hygiene may reflect physical and psychological health status. Look for signs of apparent indifference to appearance or inability to perform self-care. Also note whether the patient's hair looks clean and neat, and evaluate facial and oral hygiene.

Closely observe the patient's clothing and note its appropriateness for the season and situation, cleanliness, and general condition. Seasonally inappropriate dress may indicate difficulty making correct decisions. If you detect poor hygiene or clothing repair, assess this in the context of the entire examination rather than assuming it reflects a psychological problem, mental dysfunction, or a vision deficit.

Note any frank odors, such as alcohol, which may indicate alcoholism; urine, suggesting incontinence or poor hygiene; or excessive perfume or cologne, which may reflect an attempt to mask body odor. However, always consider these findings in context.

Psychological state

Behavioral components can supply important clues to the patient's psychological status. Assess the patient's orientation to time, place, and person. Evaluate attention span and attentiveness, noting lethargy, drowsiness, or other signs of a decreased level of consciousness. (For details on assessing mental status and level of consciousness, see Chapter 16, Nervous system.)

Also observe for any bizarre or repeated mannerisms or motions, such as involuntary, spasmodic movements. Check hand position and movement and use of gestures. A patient who clasps the hands tightly, uses wildly flailing gestures, or exhibits hand trembling may be psychologically disturbed.

Special considerations for pediatric patients

When conducting a general survey of an infant or child, expect certain behaviors to vary according to the child's age. A newborn usually lies quietly in the parent's arms or cries when uncomfortable or disturbed. Children ages 6 months to 2 years usually cling to the parent and may be scared and uncooperative. A preschooler may show more confidence and curiosity and, after initial shyness, may cooperate with the assessment. A school-age child typically has a longer attention span and follows instructions better.

Evaluate the same details as for an adult, focusing on signs of distress, facial characteristics, posture, activity level, motor coordination, language function, maturity level, and ability to understand and cooperate with the assessment. Look for signs of anxiety, including thumb sucking, nail biting, and rocking. If a parent is present, observe how the parent and child interact. Note the amount and quality of physical contact and verbal communication and assess how well the parent responds to the child's needs and copes with any crying or uncooperative behavior.

Special considerations for elderly patients

The general survey of an elderly patient resembles that of any adult, but focuses more intensely on certain areas. For example, when observing the patient's skin, gait, and posture, expect the normal physiologic changes of aging. Also stay alert for clues to reduced self-care capacity, such as missing buttons or a misbuttoned shirt, and learn to identify key signs of aging-related disorders.

Although many elderly patients remain alert, independent, and active, some are at risk for special problems, including chronic disease, depression, and confusion. Most have endured numerous losses and have grieved for these losses in a healthy manner. However, some react with prolonged depression, anxiety, or other maladaptive responses. Early signs of depression include a short attention span, emotional lability (instability), and inattention to personal dress or hygiene.

Confusion, another finding in some elderly patients, can result from adverse drug reactions or drug interactions, dehydration, infection, nutritional problems, organic brain changes, and other factors. Unfamiliar surroundings and routines, such as hospitalization or a stay in an extended-care facility, can contribute to confusion.

Special considerations for patients with disabilities

When assessing the patient with a disability, deficit, or deformity that impairs functioning, address any special areas of patient concern (for example, use of a wheelchair or seeing-eye dog). Also assess the patient's functional ability, independence level, and attitude toward the disability and the assessment. As always, avoid stereotyping the patient and be sure to use a caring, sensitive approach.

Cultural and ethnic considerations

Caring for patients of diverse cultural and ethnic backgrounds is commonplace for the nurse. A patient's lifestyle, values, beliefs, and cultural and ethnic customs can influence appearance, behavior, and attitude toward health and illness. Be aware that the nurse's personal values and beliefs may distort the assessment of a patient from a different background. To obtain the most accurate and useful general survey findings, remain as objective as possible and avoid imposing personal values on the patient.

During the general survey, attempt to assess the patient's values and health beliefs accurately. Take care not to mistake cultural preferences in dress, manner, and physical appearance for abnormal behavior or signs of a physical or psychological disorder. For example, behavior that may strike the nurse as apathetic or hostile might be a standard response to stress in patients from a particular family background.

Documenting the general survey

The nurse documents general survey findings in a short, concise paragraph. Include only the information that is essential to communicating an overall impression. Do not comment on everything observed—only the most important points. For example, mention that the patient has a facial rash, but do not describe the rash in detail until later, when documenting the complete physical assessment findings.

Vital signs
Assessment of vital signs—temperature, pulse, respirations, and blood pressure—is a basic nursing responsibility and an important method for measuring and monitoring vital body functions. Vital signs give insight into the function of specific organs—especially the heart and lungs—as well as entire body systems. The nurse obtains vital signs to establish baseline measurements, observe for trends, identify physiologic problems, and monitor a patient's response to therapy.

Taking all vital signs at the beginning of the complete physical assessment can alert the nurse to problems associated with abnormal readings. An acutely ill patient requires frequent vital sign assessment as often as every 1 to 4 hours (postoperatively, as often as every 15 minutes). Be sure to check for trends by comparing new findings to previous measurements; any change warrants further investigation. If the patient's condition calls for more frequent monitoring, do not hesitate to obtain vital signs more often.

General guidelines

To obtain accurate vital sign measurements, the nurse should follow these guidelines:
- To allay patient anxiety, approach the patient calmly and explain what will occur.
- Physical and mental stress may alter vital sign measurements, especially blood pressure, pulse, and respiratory rate. If the patient has an abnormal vital sign reading, maintain a calm demeanor and ask a colleague to confirm the measurement. If the patient expresses concern over the need for repeated measurements, calmly explain that the measurement was slightly high or low and just needs to be rechecked.
- When assessing vital signs in an ill patient, become familiar with the patient's medical diagnosis, treatment, and medication regimen and consider how these factors can affect vital signs. Certain medications, such as beta blockers and digoxin, may lower the pulse rate. Fever may increase the pulse rate and the respiratory rate.

Temperature

The nurse may measure and record temperature in degrees Fahrenheit (° F) or degrees centigrade, or Celsius (° C). Temperature may be measured by the oral, rectal, or axillary route. Unless the physician orders a specific route, choose the one that is best suited to the patient's age and physical condition.

The oral route is appropriate for an alert adult who can close the mouth well and who has not undergone recent oral surgery or is not presently receiving oxygen. Make sure the patient does not breathe through the mouth and has not eaten, drunk a hot or cold beverage, or smoked a cigarette in the past 15 minutes. Smoking, eating, or drinking a hot beverage could raise the temperature; drinking a cold beverage could lower it.

To obtain an oral temperature with a glass-mercury thermometer, place the thermometer tip under the front of the tongue. For the most accurate reading, leave the thermometer in place for about 7 minutes. Because it may break, a glass-mercury thermometer is contraindicated for oral temperature measurement in a young child, a confused patient, or a patient with a frequent cough or a seizure disorder.

Temperature may be measured rectally when the oral route is inappropriate—for example, in an infant or a young child or in a weak, confused, or comatose patient. To obtain the rectal temperature, place the patient in a side-lying or prone position. Lubricate the thermometer bulb with a water-soluble lubricant, and gently insert it into the anus about 1″ to 1½″ (2.5 to 3 cm) in an adult, or about ½″ (1 cm) in a child or an infant. Hold the thermometer in place for about 3 minutes, and stay with the patient during this time.

Avoid the rectal route in a patient with an anal lesion, bleeding hemorrhoids, or a history of rectal surgery. This route also may be contraindicated in a patient with a cardiac disorder because it may stimulate the vagus nerve, possibly leading to vasodilation and a decreased heart rate.

Axillary temperature measurement may be appropriate in the patient who has had oral surgery, who cannot close the lips around a thermometer because of a deformity, or who is using oxygen. Many health care professionals prefer the axillary route for an infant or a small child because it eliminates the risks of thermometer breakage and rectal perforation.

To take an axillary reading, place the thermometer bulb in the patient's axilla (armpit) and position the patient's arm across the chest to keep the thermometer in place. (Hold the thermometer in place if the patient cannot.) Axillary temperature takes the longest to obtain— about 11 minutes.

When used by any route, an electronic thermometer provides the fastest temperature measurement, yielding highly accurate readings in about 30 seconds. The nurse places this thermometer as any other, but changes the disposable cover on the probe for every patient.

Normal and abnormal body temperatures

Normal body temperature ranges from about 96.8° to 99.5° F (36° to 37.5° C). Body temperature varies throughout the day, dropping lowest in the early morning and peaking in late afternoon. Other factors, such as age, sex, physical activity, and environmental conditions, can influence normal temperature ranges. (For details, see *The effect of age on vital signs.*)

In any person, temperature may vary from normal levels during stress, such as from exercise, hard work, or exposure to extreme cold or heat. Temperature also depends on organic body processes. Metabolic diseases, such as hyperthyroidism, and neurologic disorders, such as cerebral hemorrhage (which involves impairment of the hypothalamic regulatory center), can cause body temperature changes. Fever can develop as an inflammatory response to tissue destruction, such as after extensive surgery, during recovery from myocardial infarction, or when the body fights infection.

After obtaining the patient's temperature, interpret the findings. Consider hyperthermia or hypothermia cause for concern. If persistent, a temperature extreme (below 93° F [33.9° C] or above 105° F [40.5° C]) can cause death.

The effect of age on vital signs

Normal vital sign ranges vary with age, as this chart shows.

AGE	TEMPERATURE (° F)	TEMPERATURE (° C)	PULSE RATE (beats per minute)	RESPIRATORY RATE (breaths per minute)	BLOOD PRESSURE (mm Hg)
Newborn	98.6 to 99.8	37 to 37.6	100 to 190	30 to 50	systolic: 50 to 52 diastolic: 25 to 30 mean: 35 to 40
3 years	98.5 to 99.5	36.9 to 37.5	80 to 125	20 to 30	systolic: 78 to 114 diastolic: 46 to 78
10 years	97.5 to 98.6	36.4 to 37	70 to 110	16 to 22	systolic: 90 to 120 diastolic: 56 to 84
16 years	97.6 to 98.8	36.4 to 37.1	55 to 100	15 to 20	systolic: 104 to 120 diastolic: 60 to 84
Adult	96.8 to 99.5	36 to 37.5	60 to 90	12 to 20	systolic: 95 to 140 diastolic: 60 to 90
Older adult	96.5 to 97.5	35.9 to 36.3	60 to 90	15 to 22	systolic: 140 to 160 diastolic: 70 to 90

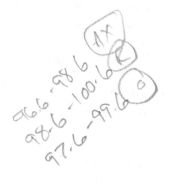

Pulse

By assessing pulses, the nurse can determine how well the heart works as well as the degree of organ perfusion. To assess a patient's pulse, auscultate at the apex of the heart with a stethoscope or palpate a peripheral pulse with the fingers. Although either method can determine heart rate (beats per minute), auscultation proves superior for assessing heart rhythm (regularity).

The pulse can be palpated or auscultated in various locations. Usually, the radial pulse is measured because of its easy accessibility. To do this, palpate the radial artery with the pads of the index and middle fingers for 60 seconds while compressing the artery gently against the radial bone. Do not use the thumb because it has a pulse of its own that could be confused with the patient's pulse.

If the patient has a cast or splint, has a condition that impairs peripheral circulation (such as diabetes or vascular disease), or has undergone a recent invasive vascular procedure (such as angiography or surgery), check all peripheral pulses to ensure adequate circulation to an extremity. If finding a peripheral pulse is difficult, mark the pulse site with a wax marker for future reference. (When marking a pulse site this way, be sure to document it.)

In an emergency, the femoral and carotid pulses may be palpated in a patient with severe cardiovascular compromise. However, take care not to exert too much pressure against the carotid artery because this can stimulate the vagus nerve and cause reflex bradycardia. Also, pressing against both carotid pulses at once is contraindicated because it can interfere with cerebral circulation.

If the patient has a cardiac arrhythmia or is receiving certain cardiac drugs (such as digoxin), auscultate the apical pulse for 60 seconds. To do this, place the diaphragm of the stethoscope over the apex of the heart (located at the fifth intercostal space, approximately at the midclavicular line). Expect to hear a pattern of "lub dub, lub dub," representing heart valve closure. Each pair of sounds represents one beat.

To assess an infant's or a toddler's pulse, auscultate the apical pulse or palpate the femoral pulse. The normal pulse rate varies with age, physical condition, and other factors. (For details, see *The effect of age on vital signs,* page 39.)

In the adult, a pulse rate below 60 (bradycardia) or above 100 (tachycardia) is considered abnormal. However, even in a healthy person, various factors may cause the pulse rate to increase (fear, anger, pain, or exercise) or decrease (sleep, relaxation, or vagus nerve stimulation).

While obtaining the pulse rate, also assess pulse amplitude and rhythm. Document pulse amplitude (which reflects the strength of left ventricular contraction) by using a numerical scale or a descriptive term. A commonly used numerical scale is the 0-to-3 scale. In this scale, 0 indicates an absent pulse; +1, a weak or thready pulse; +2, a normal, easily palpable pulse; and +3, a bounding, forceful, readily palpable pulse.

Normally, the heart rhythm is regular, with approximately the same interval between pulsations. If the patient has an irregular rhythm, describe its pattern. Note whether the rhythm is predictably irregular (indicating that the heart periodically adds or drops a beat) or totally irregular (chaotic). Either pattern may signify cardiac disease. Arrhythmias are best identified by obtaining an electrocardiogram. (For more information, see Chapter 10, Cardiovascular system.)

Occasionally, a patient's pulse may fade on inspiration and strengthen on expiration. Known as a paradoxical pulse, this abnormality can occur with deep breathing or such cardiac problems as tamponade. A paradoxical pulse may indicate an emergency and always warrants further investigation.

Respiration

During respiration, the lungs take in oxygen with each inspiration and expel carbon dioxide with each expiration. When assessing respiration, the nurse focuses on the rate, depth, and rhythm of each breath while staying alert for other evidence of respiratory problems, such as cyanosis (bluish skin), chest pain, anxiety, restlessness, and confusion. A complaint of insufficient air intake or difficulty breathing always warrants further evaluation.

To determine the respiratory rate, count the number of respirations for 60 seconds. (One respiration consists of an inspiration and an expiration.) Do this as unobtrusively as possible—a patient who knows the nurse is counting respirations may inadvertently alter the rate. One unobtrusive method involves holding the patient's wrist against the chest or abdomen as if checking the pulse rate.

As with other vital signs, the respiratory rate varies with age. In adults, it normally ranges from about 12 to 20 breaths per minute. In children, it tends to be faster. (For details, see *The effect of age on vital signs,* page 39.)

The respiratory rate may increase with emotional stress or with various physical problems, including fever. It may decrease with central nervous system depression, as from excessive sedation or anesthesia. Note the depth of each respiration, which reflects tidal volume. The chest should visibly expand and contract with each respiration. Also note the symmetry of chest wall expansion during inspiration. Skeletal deformity, broken ribs, and collapsed lung tissue can cause asymmetrical (unequal) expansion.

Observe thoracic and abdominal muscle use. Women typically use thoracic muscles to breathe, whereas men and children use abdominal muscles. Note any use of accessory respiratory muscles (scalenes, sternocleidomastoid, and abdominal muscles). Accessory muscle use occurs in labored breathing to increase intrathoracic volume and ease the burden of breathing. In children, labored breathing also may cause intercostal muscles to bulge or retract abnormally and may be accompanied by nasal flaring and lip pursing on expiration.

While assessing respiratory rate and depth, note the respiratory rhythm, or pattern. Children and adults normally breathe with a regular rhythm, interspersing respirations with sighs (occasional deep, prolonged breaths that allow full lung expansion). Irregular rhythms in children or adults, such as Biot's or Cheyne-Stokes respirations, commonly result from neurologic disorders. (For more information, see *Respiratory patterns,* page 42.)

Blood pressure

Blood pressure measurement reflects two stages in the cardiac cycle. *Systolic pressure* refers to the maximum pressure exerted on the arterial wall at the peak of systole (left ventricular contraction). *Diastolic pressure* reflects minimum systemic arterial pressure, which occurs during diastole (left ventricular relaxation). The difference between systolic and diastolic readings is called *pulse pressure.*

Many factors affect arterial blood pressure. Physical activity, emotional stress, and body position can cause wide fluctuations. Blood pressure also fluctuates in a 24-hour (circadian) pattern, dropping lowest in the late hours of sleep and peaking in the afternoon and evening. Age

Respiratory patterns

When assessing a client's respirations, the nurse should determine their rate, rhythm, and depth. These schematic diagrams show different respiratory patterns.

Eupnea
Normal respiratory rate and rhythm

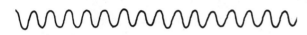

Tachypnea
Increased respiratory rate

Bradypnea
Slow but regular respirations

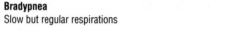

Apnea
Absence of breathing (may be periodic)

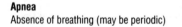

Hyperventilation
Deeper respirations; normal rate

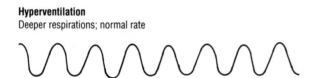

Cheyne-Stokes
Respirations that gradually become faster and deeper than normal, then slower; alternates with periods of apnea

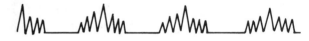

Biot's
Faster and deeper respirations than normal, with abrupt pauses between them; breaths have equal depth

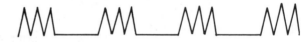

Kussmaul's
Faster and deeper respirations without pauses

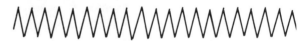

also affects blood pressure. From infancy throughout childhood and adolescence, blood pressure increases gradually, then stabilizes as adulthood begins. In elderly persons, reduced vessel elasticity typically causes increased systolic pressure. (For details, see *The effect of age on vital signs,* page 39.)

Assessing blood pressure

The nurse determines arterial blood pressure (measured in millimeters of mercury [mm Hg]) by using a sphygmomanometer and a stethoscope. To assess blood pressure in an arm or a leg, listen to brachial or popliteal artery pulsations. However, keep in mind that measurements taken over the popliteal artery in the leg produce higher systolic and lower diastolic readings than those obtained from the arm. The nurse who cannot hear a pulse or has reason to doubt a blood pressure finding should always recheck the pressure. To avoid venous engorgement from cuff pressure, wait 30 seconds between attempts.

When assessing a patient's blood pressure for the first time, take measurements in both arms. Consider a slight pressure difference (5 to 10 mm Hg) between arms normal; a difference of 15 mm Hg or more may indicate cardiac disease, especially aortic coarctation (narrowing) or arterial obstruction.

In some cases, the nurse may want to assess orthostatic (postural) blood pressure by taking readings with the patient lying down, sitting, and standing, then checking for differences with each position change. Normally, blood pressure rises or falls slightly with a position change. A drop of 20 mm Hg or more accompanied by an increase in the pulse indicates orthostatic hypotension. Such a decrease, which usually causes dizziness, can result from hypovolemia, medication effects, or prolonged bed rest.

If the pulse cannot be auscultated because the pressure is inaudible, measure blood pressure by palpation. After applying the cuff and palpating the brachial pulse, inflate the cuff until the manometer reads 30 mm Hg above the point at which the pulse can no longer be palpated. Then release the cuff pressure slowly, at a rate of approximately 2 to 3 mm Hg per heartbeat. While doing this, closely observe the manometer. The number that appears when the first palpable pulsation is felt is the systolic reading. Because pulsations continue until the manometer reading falls to zero, determining the diastolic reading may be more difficult. Document a palpated blood pressure by writing, for example, "120/palpated."

Normal and abnormal blood pressure readings

Normal blood pressure varies greatly among individuals. In adults, normal systolic pressure ranges from 100 to 140 mm Hg; normal diastolic pressure, from 60 to 90 mm Hg. However, a series of blood pressure readings establishing a trend is more important than an individual reading. A change of more than 20 mm Hg between readings with no apparent reason for fluctuation (such as a position change or recent physical exertion) warrants further investigation.

Some patients normally have low blood pressure. For most patients, however, consistent readings below 90 mm Hg systolic or 50 mm Hg diastolic indicate hypotension (low blood pressure). Hypotension may result from a condition that reduces total blood volume, such as severe hemorrhage, burns, or diarrhea, or from a condition that decreases cardiac output, such as congestive heart failure.

Consistently elevated readings—above 140 mm Hg systolic and 90 mm Hg diastolic—indicate hypertension (high blood pressure). Hypertension may be primary or essential (of unknown cause) or secondary to an underlying disorder, such as renal disease. (For more information on hypertension, see Chapter 10, Cardiovascular system.)

Consider a pulse pressure difference greater than 40 mm Hg as abnormal. Such a difference can stem from increased systolic pressure caused by rigid, inflexible arteries, or it may be a classic sign of aortic insufficiency (backflow into the heart and consequent low diastolic readings caused by aortic valve incompetence).

Documenting vital signs

The nurse records vital signs in an obvious place on the physical assessment documentation, noting any pertinent information as concisely as possible. In the following example, the patient has a temperature of 98.8° F (37.1° C), measured orally; a pulse rate of 80 bpm, with a regular rhythm and strong amplitude; a respiratory rate of 12 breaths per minute, with a regular rhythm and unlabored quality; and blood pressure readings of 122/90/80 mm Hg measured with the patient lying down, 122/88/80 mm Hg with the patient sitting, and 120/90/82 mm Hg with the patient standing:

T 98.8° F (37.1° C) orally
P 80/minute, regular, +2
R 12/minute, unlabored, regular, and deep
BP 122/80 lying down; 122/80 sitting; 120/82 standing.

Height and weight measurements

With every patient—in any setting—the nurse should record height and weight (anthropometric measurements) as part of the basic assessment profile. In routine physical assessment, these measurements should be taken periodically throughout the patient's life to help evaluate normal growth and development and to identify abnormal patterns of weight gain or loss.

Accurate height and weight measurements also serve other important purposes. In children, they guide dosage calculations for various drugs; in adults, they help guide cancer chemotherapy and anesthesia administration and help evaluate the response to intravenous fluids, drugs, or nutritional therapy.

To weigh an adult or a child who can stand unassisted, the use a standard platform scale with a balance beam. Before taking the measurement, balance the scale by moving the sliding weights to the 0 position and adjusting the movable knob on the back of the scale. The patient removes shoes and wears only a gown or undergarments. Slide the weights down the bar until the indicator balances, and record weight to the nearest 0.5 lb (0.2 kg).

Weighing a patient who cannot stand requires use of a bed scale—either a manual counterbalance scale or an electronic scale with a digital display. Make sure the scale has been calibrated and balanced before each use. To weigh an infant, place the child in a small platform scale with a balance beam and curved sides to hold the infant in place. If possible, weigh the infant naked.

To measure height, use the sliding headpiece on the platform scale; this allows measurement of weight and height at the same time. To ensure accurate measurements, have the patient remove shoes and stand straight, facing away from the scale with feet together and arms hanging relaxed at the sides. Lower the headpiece until it rests lightly on the crown of the head, and record the measurement to the nearest 0.25″ (0.6 cm). Instruct the patient to remain standing straight, then measure again; the two readings should be within 0.25″ of each other. Alternatively, the nurse can measure an adult's height with a measuring tape attached to the wall.

To measure the height of a patient who cannot stand, position the patient supine on a bed. On the sheet, make a mark at the top of the patient's head and another at the bottom of the foot. Then extend these marks to the side of the bed and measure the distance between the marks with a measuring tape.

To measure an infant's height, use a board with a sliding headpiece. Alternatively, the nurse can place the infant on a large sheet of paper on the examining table, make a mark at the top of the head and at the heel of the extended leg, and measure the distance between the two marks with a measuring tape.

STUDY ACTIVITIES

Fill in the blank

1. The stethoscope should contain a _____ for detecting low-pitched sounds and a _____ for detecting normal or high-pitched sounds.

2. In a healthy adult, _____, _____, _____, or _____ can increase the pulse rate; _____, or _____ can decrease it.

True or false

3. Body temperature tends to be highest in the late afternoon and lowest early in the morning.
☑ True   ☐ False

4. When listening to the apical pulse, the nurse hears "lub dub, lub dub." Each "lub" and each "dub" count as single beat.
☐ True   ☑ False

5. One respiration consists of an inhalation and an exhalation.
☑ True   ☐ False

6. Usually, blood pressure in the left and right arms differs by more than 15 mm Hg.
☐ True   ☑ False

7. Accurate weight and height measurements are important in calculating medication doses.
☑ True   ☐ False

Multiple choice

8. The nurse must assess vital signs of Mark Taylor, age 64, who has a cardiac disorder. Which route for temperature measurement may be contraindicated for this patient?

A. Oral, manual
B. Rectal
C. Axillary
D. Oral, electronic

Matching related elements

Match the assessment technique on the left with the description on the right.

9. ___ Inspection

A. Touching the body to feel pulsations and vibrations and to locate structures

10. ___ Palpation

B. Observing critically

11. ___ Percussion

C. Listening to body sounds

12. ___ Auscultation

D. Tapping against a body surface to produce sounds and elicit tenderness

Short answer

13. When percussing, where does the nurse normally expect to hear dullness, tympany, and resonance?

_____

14. Which components should the nurse include when conducting the general survey?

_____

_____

ANSWERS

Fill in the blank

1. bell, diaphragm
2. fear, anger, pain, exercise; sleep, relaxation, vagus nerve stimulation

True or false

3. True.
4. False. Each pair of sounds, "lub dub," constitutes a single heartbeat.
5. True.
6. False. Blood pressure in the left and right arms should differ by 5 to 10 mm Hg. If the difference is greater, suspect a vascular problem, such as aortic coarctation.
7. True.

Multiple choice

8. B. The rectal route may be contraindicated in a patient with a cardiac disorder because it may stimulate the vagus nerve, possibly leading to vasodilation and decreased heart rate.

Matching related elements

9. B
10. A
11. D
12. C

Short answer

13. Normally, dullness is heard over solid organs, such as the liver and heart; tympany is audible over a gastric air bubble or gas-filled bowel, and resonance is heard over healthy lung tissue.

14. During the general survey, the nurse should note any signs of distress, such as pain or dyspnea; observe facial characteristics, such as excessive blinking and absent or inappropriate facial expressions; identify the patient's body type, posture, and movements; evaluate speech, including vocal pitch and strength as well as any slurring or other altered sounds; observe the patient's dress, grooming, and personal hygiene, noting any unusual odors and observing whether dress is seasonally appropriate; explore the patient's psychological state, including evaluating orientation to time, place, and person, and evaluating attention span and level of consciousness.

CHAPTER 4

Activities of daily living and sleep patterns

OBJECTIVES

After studying this chapter, the reader should be able to:
1. Discuss the importance of balance between activity and sleep.
2. Identify the factors affecting activities of daily living.
3. Develop questions used to assess personal care, family responsibilities, work, school, recreation, and socialization activities.
4. Describe normal sleep stages and patterns.
5. Describe the factors affecting sleep.
6. Phrase interview questions that assess a patient's sleep patterns.

OVERVIEW OF CONCEPTS

Maintaining a constant balance between daily activities and sleep is vital to the promotion and maintenance of physiologic and psychosocial health. The nurse must carefully assess the patient's ability to perform activities of daily living (ADLs), the patient's ability to achieve and maintain restful sleep patterns, and the balance between the two. Alterations in ADLs or disturbances in sleep patterns can signal actual or potential health problems.

Activities of daily living

ADLs are the activities necessary to develop and maintain physiologic and psychosocial well-being. These include five components: personal care, family responsibility, work or school, recreation, and socialization. Participating in daily activities promotes physiologic health for children and adults. In children, recreation promotes normal growth and development of the neuromuscular and musculoskeletal systems. In adults, physical activity encourages optimal functioning of each body system and frequently reduces risk factors associated with certain diseases.

Performing ADLs also promotes psychosocial health. Recreation allows children to express emotions—such as joy, fear, and hostility—that encourage emotional growth and build self-concept. In adults, successfully completing ADLs provides a sense of accomplishment. Other activities, such as hobbies, help alleviate stress and tension or serve as a means of self-expression.

A person's interest in and ability to perform necessary ADLs depend on several factors: age and developmental status, culture, physical health, cognitive function, psychosocial function, stress level, and biological rhythms. The nurse must be aware of these factors when performing the assessment.

Assessing ADLs

A thorough assessment ascertains the patient's functional status and identifies actual and potential health problems related to ADLs. It also suggests interventions to help promote the patient's independent function at home and in the community and provides a method for measuring progress. Although ADLs can be assessed in any setting, the nurse ideally performs the assessment in the patient's home. This allows a view of the patient's ability to perform ADLs and reveals environmental resources and physical barriers.

Use the interview and other observation methods to gather information on ADLs. During the interview, gather data from the patient and family, focus on their perceptions of the patient's ability to perform ADLs, and identify the patient's and family's goals for functioning. Also determine whether the patient and family have realistic views, have developed attainable goals, and have similar perspectives. Whenever possible, try to observe the patient performing ADLs. For the hospitalized patient, the nurse can do this subtly, while the patient eats, bathes, or dresses, or, in certain instances, by directly asking the patient to perform specific activities.

Use the assessment to gauge the patient's functional status in performing ADLs. This can help determine whether the patient can function independently, requires the assistance of a person or a device, or depends totally on others. If the patient needs assistance, determine the amount and type required. If the patient depends on devices, inquire about the type of device and its adequacy in resolving the problem. Also evaluate the possible need for other devices.

Personal care activities

When determining a patient's self-care status, assess mobility, ability to prepare and eat meals, and ability to perform elimination, personal hygiene, and dressing and grooming activities. The following questions and rationales offer a guide to assessing personal care activities:

Do you have any difficulty standing, walking, or climbing stairs? Can you get in and out of a chair? Can you get in and out of bed? What assistive devices do you use to aid in mobility? If the patient uses a wheelchair, ask, *Can you propel the chair yourself?*
(RATIONALE: An alteration in mobility may hinder a patient's ability to engage in other ADLs.)

Can you open packages and containers? Can you use utensils for eating? Can you cut your food? Do you have any other problems feeding your-

self? What times do you usually eat? Who prepares your meals? Where do you eat your meals? With whom do you eat?
(RATIONALE: These questions investigate the patient's ability to prepare meals and to eat independently. The ability to feed oneself is an important personal care activity. Besides providing nourishment, meals may provide a time for socialization.)

Can you use the toilet alone or do you need assistance? Do you have any problems with bowel or bladder control? If so, how do you manage these problems? Do you use any assistive devices for elimination, such as catheters or colostomy bags? If so, can you care for these devices? How have elimination problems affected your other activities?
(RATIONALE: An elimination problem can interfere with work, school, recreation, and socialization. These questions give the patient an opportunity to discuss problems, fears, and anxieties regarding elimination and give the nurse a chance to teach the patient how to manage these problems. Keep in mind that elimination is a private matter to adults; the patient or family may hesitate to discuss it because of embarrassment. Ask questions in a matter-of-fact way and try to put the patient at ease.)

What are your usual bathing habits? Do you have any problems with personal hygiene and bathing? Can you get in and out of a tub or shower? Can you shave? Can you care for your teeth, hair, fingernails, and toenails? Can you care for your dentures, hearing aids, or any other prostheses?
(RATIONALE: For many patients, inability to manage personal hygiene activities can reduce self-esteem and self-concept. These questions help explore the patient's ability to perform these activities. Remember that most patients consider personal hygiene activities to be private; they may hesitate to discuss problems. Also, some patients may have experienced a gradual, unnoticed decline in their ability to perform personal hygiene.)

Do you have any problems dressing and grooming? If so, are these problems more pronounced on the left side, the right side, the upper part, or the lower part of your body? Can you fasten buttons, snaps, and zippers? Is dressing easier with certain types of clothing? If so, which ones?
(RATIONALE: Musculoskeletal or neuromuscular abnormalities can disrupt fine or gross motor coordination, making dressing and grooming—activities that most adults perform independently—difficult for the patient. To help prevent frustration with this normal ADL, suggest different types of clothing or assistive devices.)

Family responsibility activities

In any type of family, a patient's family responsibilities reflect his or her developmental status and evolving roles. The following questions offer a guide to assessing family responsibilities associated with ADLs:

What are your living arrangements? Does your home need structural changes so you can take care of yourself and your family? Do you have any problems with shopping or food preparation? Can you do your own laundry? What types of cleaning can you do? If you have a yard, can you care for it? Are you having trouble managing your money, such as getting to a bank? What arrangements have you made for child care? Do your family responsibilities include caring for a sick or disabled person in the home? If so, do you have any problems with this role? Do you care for a pet in your home?

(RATIONALE: These questions help investigate the structure and composition of the patient's family, the patient's developmental status, and the responsibilities the patient has assumed in the family. A patient who cannot perform usual family responsibility activities may develop role and relationship problems. Such a patient may benefit from a referral to a social agency for help with such responsibilities as food management or child care.)

Work and school activities

Work is any formal activity that involves earning a living or preparing to earn a living. A person's work can provide individual identity, sense of worth, and fulfillment. However, work also can be a source of frustration, disappointment, and negative stress. For many people, school is their work. School may offer intellectual stimulation, personal satisfaction, and interpersonal relationships. However, school also may create feelings of frustration and stress and contribute to feelings of low self-esteem. The following offer a guide to assessing the patient's work or school activities associated with ADLs:

What does your typical day involve? Do you work outside the home? Where and what type of work do you do? How many hours per week do you work? What is your work schedule like? Do you have any conflicts between your work schedule and other responsibilities? What is your job like? Is work mainly a source of satisfaction or frustration? Do you engage in any volunteer work?

(RATIONALE: These questions help investigate the type of work the patient participates in and the role of work in the patient's life. A heavy, stressful work schedule may make a person feel he or she is neglecting family and self, thus causing guilt feelings that add to the stress.)

What do you see yourself doing in the future? How do you feel about retirement? What retirement plans have you made?

(RATIONALE: These questions help investigate the patient's view of retirement, including alterations in ADLs caused by retirement.)

Are you going to school? If so, where and for what purpose? What do you like most about school? What do you like least about school? Do you have any problems balancing school activities with other activities and responsibilities?

(RATIONALE: These questions help investigate the nature and demands of any schoolwork and help assess the effects of school on other activities. A patient whose school activities interfere with personal care activities, family responsibilities, or work activities may benefit from counseling.)

Recreational activities

People participate in play, recreation, and exercise for amusement, entertainment, self-fulfillment, or self-improvement. These activities contribute to personal growth, offer an outlet for emotions, provide opportunities for friendships, and help forge bonds among community members. The following questions help investigate recreational activities:

What do you do when you're not working or in school? How do your days off differ from your work or school days? How much recreational time do you have in a day and in a week? Are you satisfied with the amount of your recreational time and what you can do during that time? With whom do you share your recreational time? How would you describe any physical exercise you perform? How often do you get physical exercise? Do you participate in any special exercise program? If so, what kind and for how long? How do you feel after you exercise? Has your physician or nurse practitioner ever restricted your activity or exercise? If so, why? What benefits have you gained from exercise?

(RATIONALE: These questions help investigate the type, amount, timing, purpose, and benefits of the patient's recreational and physical exercise activities. A decrease in usual activity levels may result from a physical disorder and may lead to an emotional problem, such as depression.)

Are you retired? If so, how would you describe your day? What recreational and exercise activities do you participate in now that you are retired?

(RATIONALE: These questions help uncover the types of activities enjoyed by a retired patient, who may have more time for recreation than a younger adult. For a retired patient, recreation and exercise activities may take the place of work activities, providing stimulation, satisfaction, and interpersonal relationships.)

Socialization activities

Relationships significantly influence emotional, intellectual, and personality development. Each individual develops a social network depending on personal choice, occupation, place of residence, gender, age, developmental status, and family size. The following questions offer a guide to assessing socialization activities:

What kinds of things do you do when you are alone? Can you use a phone, write clearly, and see well enough to enjoy reading or watching television? Do you have many close friends? Who would you confide in if you had a problem? Do you depend on your family for help? How often do you get together with family members? Can you travel outside the

home? Which activities are you involved in outside your home? Do you belong to any social groups, such as clubs or church groups? If so, which ones? Do you drive your own car or use public transportation?
(RATIONALE: These questions help investigate the patient's role in society, the structure of the patient's social network, and any barriers to socialization the patient may have. Illness, relocation, or the loss or change of a job can disrupt the patient's usual social network, leading to social isolation, loneliness, and depression.)

Developmental considerations

Devise special questions when assessing a child's ADLs. When possible, try to include the child in the assessment; otherwise, direct questions to the child's parent or guardian. Ask the following questions:

Can your child eat independently? Does your child use utensils or fingers to eat? Does your child eat with other members of the family?
(RATIONALE: The ability to feed oneself is an important personal care activity and, for a child, an important developmental step. A child who eats with other family members not only receives nourishment but also develops social skills.)

Is your child toilet-trained? If so, when did this occur? Does your child have problems with incontinence during the day or bed-wetting at night? How does your child communicate the need to eliminate? Does your child need any type of assistance when going to the bathroom?
(RATIONALE: These questions assess elimination activities, which are important milestones for children. They uncover any special needs the child may have so that these needs can be met during hospitalization, if necessary.)

Can your child get dressed alone? Does your child have any difficulties when dressing?
(RATIONALE: Children gradually assume responsibility for dressing and grooming—two important components of personal care activities. Slowness in assuming these responsibilities may indicate a developmental lag.)

Where does your child go to school? In which grade is your child? What does your child enjoy most and least in school? Has your child's school performance changed recently? If so, in what way?
(RATIONALE: For most older children, school activities are their work activities. Questions such as these evaluate a child's involvement in and feelings about school.)

What is your child's daily schedule? Does your child prefer to play alone, with peers, or with adults? What are your child's favorite activities and toys? Which toys does your child use to feel more secure? Does your child participate in sports? If so, what types? How much time each day does your child have for play? What types of physical exercise does your child perform as a part of normal play?

(RATIONALE: These questions evaluate the type of play the child enjoys and the factors affecting it. Play provides the child with a sense of control, a means of self-expression, and a way to learn about the world. Play also encourages sensorimotor and intellectual development. Culture, gender, age, developmental level, and health status may affect the type of play in which a child engages.)

Observations and documentation

During the assessment, observe the patient for signs of an inability to perform ADLs. For example, when the patient enters the room and sits down, note the degree of mobility. If the patient moves stiffly or unsteadily or requires an assistive device, suspect a mobility problem that affects other ADLs. Also evaluate gross and fine motor coordination. Alterations in gross motor coordination impair ambulation and the ability to move from one position to another; alterations in fine motor coordination hinder the performance of such tasks as buttoning clothes and writing. Document all pertinent observations with other physical assessment findings in the objective portion of the nurse's notes.

Sleep patterns

To assess a patient's sleep patterns, the nurse must know when to refer a patient to a sleep disorder center for specialized diagnostic procedures and treatment.

Sleep stages and patterns

Most adults fall asleep in about 15 minutes, experience two to three brief arousals during the night, and wake up 6 to 10 hours later. During sleep, a person moves about every 15 to 30 minutes, remains immobile for 10 to 30 minutes, and then moves again. Movement and short arousals often take place with changes in sleep stages. Two types of sleep occur: rapid eye movement (REM) sleep and non–rapid eye movement (NREM) sleep. NREM sleep is divided further into Stages 1, 2, 3, and 4.

Sleep stages occur in a repetitive cycle throughout the night. Most adults experience four to six complete sleep cycles per night, with the majority of Stages 3 and 4 sleep occurring early in the night and longer REM-sleep periods occurring in the early morning hours.

Normal sleep patterns (the amount of sleep and the routine time to go to sleep and to awaken) vary among individuals and across groups of people. Many factors, including work or school schedules, can affect the timing and duration of sleep.

The sleep requirement, which varies from person to person, ranges from 4 to 10 hours. On the average, healthy adults between ages 20 and 50 sleep approximately 7.5 hours each night and do not require regular daytime naps. Loss of sleep for one or two nights is not harmful. However, chronic sleep deprivation, such as that experienced by patients suffering from prolonged sleep apnea (absence of spontaneous respirations during sleep), can cause memory problems and mood changes.

Factors affecting sleep patterns

A person's age, exercise level, personal habits, diet, environment, and mood affect the quality and duration of sleep. (For details, see *Factors affecting sleep,* page 56.) Altering one or more of these factors, with the exception of age, often can improve sleep.

Assessing sleep patterns

Asking questions about sleep during the health assessment gives the nurse an opportunity to teach and correct misconceptions as well as collect subjective data about the patient's sleep patterns. Use the following guidelines to assess sleep patterns.

Sleep-wake patterns

Ask the following questions to assess sleep-wake patterns for all patients:

How old are you?
(RATIONALE: Age and developmental status affect the amount, timing, and quality of sleep.)

What do you do for a living? What are your normal working hours?
(RATIONALE: Certain occupations require shift work, which can disrupt sleep.)

What time do you usually go to bed? What time do you usually wake up in the morning?
(RATIONALE: The usual times for retiring and arising provide accurate information about the duration of sleep.)

Do you fall asleep easily? Do you usually sleep all night without waking up? If awakened, do you fall asleep again quickly?
(RATIONALE: Difficulty falling asleep or staying asleep at night may indicate a sleep disorder. If so, a more detailed sleep assessment is necessary.)

Does anything help you to sleep? Does anything make it more difficult to sleep?
(RATIONALE: The answers to these questions provide information about the use of sleeping aids, such as sedatives and hypnotics, and the patient's bedtime rituals.)

Do you feel rested when you awaken in the morning?
(RATIONALE: A complaint of feeling tired on awakening suggests insufficient sleep or lack of restful sleep because of mood changes, medical problems, or a sleep disorder. In this instance, perform a symptom analysis of this complaint.)

Factors affecting sleep

The factors detailed below may affect the quality and duration of sleep.

Age

Sleep patterns change over a person's life span. For example, few children have trouble falling asleep at night or remaining awake during the day. In contrast, many older adults complain of difficulties obtaining enough sleep and frequently develop a dependence on hypnotic drugs to combat age-related changes in their sleep patterns. Individuals spend less time asleep as they grow older, with the most dramatic changes occurring during infancy and childhood. The type (stages) of sleep and the quality of sleep also change with maturation.

Exercise

Although many people advocate regular exercise as a way to improve sleep, little evidence suggests that exercise affects subsequent sleep in any way. Sporadic exercise probably has little effect on sleep unless it is overly vigorous. Then it may cause pain or aching muscles, which can interfere with sleep. Vigorous exercise just before retiring at night may inhibit sleep.

Personal habits

Tobacco smoking alters normal sleep patterns. On the average, cigarette smokers take twice as long to fall asleep as nonsmokers and have lighter sleep with more frequent arousals. Although smokers often complain of feeling tired and irritable when they try to quit smoking, their sleep improves immediately after successful nicotine withdrawal.

Caffeine ingestion often affects sleep. A single cup of coffee before bedtime is unlikely to disrupt sleep, but two or more cups significantly increase sleep latency and reduce total sleep time. Elderly patients are especially sensitive to the arousal effects of caffeine. For instance, after consuming beverages containing caffeine, elderly patients experience an average reduction of 2 hours in total sleep time and a marked increase in sleep latency.

Although alcohol ingestion reduces arousals during the first half of the night, it increases the frequency of arousals during the second half. It also reduces the amount of REM sleep and makes it more fragmented. REM rebound (compensation for REM sleep deprivation by increasing total REM sleep by up to 60%) occurs with chronic alcoholism. Sleep patterns remain disturbed for several months after alcohol withdrawal. Alcohol also exacerbates sleep apnea and age-related sleep disturbances. For example, healthy male snorers over age 40 suffered sleep apneas and other hypoxic events after ingesting alcohol during the evening.

Diet

Food intake also can affect sleep. For instance, a person who is gaining weight may sleep longer and deeper than normal; a person who is losing weight may sleep for shorter periods and may have more fragmented sleep. Although many persons believe that tryptophan (an essential amino acid found in dairy products and other foods) promotes sleep, research shows it has no effect on sleep onset or quality.

Environment

Of all the environmental conditions that can affect sleep, noise—especially occasional loud noise—is particularly disruptive. Such noise interrupts sleep and increases the amount of Stage 1 sleep. Moreover, arousals continue even after a person becomes accustomed to sleeping in a noisy environment.

Sleep also varies with environmental temperature. When the room temperature rises above 75° F (23.9° C), individuals have reduced REM and Stages 3 and 4 sleep, awaken more often, move more frequently, and sometimes have greater dream recall. Cool temperatures below 54° F (12.2° C) can produce unpleasant and emotional dreams as well as difficulty in sleeping.

Sleeping with a partner in the same bed also can disrupt sleep. Sleep improves in quiet surroundings, in a comfortable bed, and without light and noise. Familiar surroundings also promote sleep.

Mood

Mood and expectations strongly influence sleep patterns. Acute and chronic stress can increase arousal and inhibit sleep. In addition, stress may lead to maladaptive behaviors, such as conditioned wakefulness. This occurs when a person learns to associate wakefulness rather than sleep with being in bed, leading to the expectation of not being able to fall asleep. The fear of insomnia becomes a self-fulfilling prophecy, thus triggering a vicious cycle: the harder a person tries to fall asleep, the more aroused the person becomes. In contrast, "good sleepers" expect to have no difficulty sleeping and rarely have trouble falling asleep.

Do you take naps during the day? Can you stay awake when driving, at work, and around the house?
(RATIONALE: Although daytime naps are common for children and elderly patients, most adults can remain awake and alert during the day. If the patient has difficulty staying awake when carrying out ADLs, perform a symptom analysis on this complaint.)

How is your health? Do you have any acute or chronic illnesses? What prescription and nonprescription medications do you take? Do you use alcohol or recreational drugs?
(RATIONALE: Certain medications [such as diet pills], and some ill nesses [such as emphysema] can interfere with sleep.)

Are you satisfied with your sleep? If not, what bothers you about it?
(RATIONALE: The answer to this question uncovers the patient's perception of sleep. If the patient has concerns, perform a further assessment or, if indicated, teach the patient about normal sleep patterns.)

Excessive daytime sleepiness
Ask the following questions to assess a patient with excessive daytime sleepiness:

When did you first notice you had trouble staying awake during the day? When did this begin?
(RATIONALE: The answers to these questions help pinpoint the onset of symptoms. Also question the patient's spouse, friends, or family members about the patient's ability to stay awake during the day.)

Does your sleepiness cause any problems? Can you stay awake while driving? Have you had any accidents because of sleepiness? Do you fall asleep at work, when talking, or while watching TV or reading? Do you fall asleep at unusual times and places?
(RATIONALE: Brief attacks of sleep during activity and rest may indicate narcolepsy or sleep apnea.)

Do you take naps? How long are the naps? Do you feel refreshed after a nap?
(RATIONALE: The responses to these questions provide information about whether the patient can resist naps and about the duration of naps. Naps usually refresh patients with disorders of excessive daytime sleepiness, but only briefly.)

Does anything improve your alertness or make you especially sleepy?
(RATIONALE: The response to this question provides information about methods the patient has used to increase alertness and about conditions that provoke sleepiness.)

Does anything unusual happen—such as a feeling of weakness or a feeling that you will fall down—when you laugh, become angry, or feel startled or surprised?
(RATIONALE: A positive answer to this question indicates cataplexy [attacks of muscle weakness triggered by emotions]. Ask when the symp-

toms first began and what circumstances trigger them. Refer a patient with these symptoms to a sleep disorder center for definitive diagnosis and treatment.)

Have you ever been told you snore? If so, how loudly? Can people in the next room hear you? How about several rooms away? When did you start snoring? Has your snoring recently become louder or more frequent?
(RATIONALE: Snoring often accompanies sleep apnea. The loudness of the snoring provides a rough index of the problem's severity. The patient's bed partner is an excellent source for this information.)

Have you ever been told that you stop breathing at night, that you make grunting or snorting noises, or that you are a restless sleeper? If so, when were you first told this? Have these symptoms recently increased in frequency?
(RATIONALE: Breathing difficulties and restless sleep are common in a patient with obstructive sleep apnea. The patient's bed partner, not the patient, usually notices these signs and symptoms.)

Have you recently gained weight? Do you weigh more now than you did 5 years ago, 10 years ago, or 15 years ago? Has your clothing size increased in recent years?
(RATIONALE: Weight gain often triggers the onset of obstructive sleep apnea.)

Do you drink alcohol? If so, how much?
(RATIONALE: Alcohol exacerbates sleep apnea and may disturb normal sleep.)

Do you have headaches in the morning? How is your memory? Is it worse than it used to be? Have you been told you are more irritable than you used to be?
(RATIONALE: Patients with sleep apnea frequently experience morning headaches, memory loss, and irritability. The spouse or family members are often the first to notice memory and personality changes.)

Does anyone else in your family have similar problems with sleep?
(RATIONALE: Approximately 50% of patients with narcolepsy have family members who suffer from excessive sleepiness.)

Insomnia

Ask the following questions to assess a patient with insomnia:

When did you first notice you had trouble sleeping at night? What was going on in your life at that time? Were you ill, stressed, or having family problems?
(RATIONALE: These questions establish the approximate date of symptom onset and help identify the precipitating circumstances.)

Has the problem worsened, improved, or remained the same? Do you have problems every night or only once in a while?
(RATIONALE: Besides describing the severity of the complaint, the answers to these questions help assess for factors affecting the patient's ability to sleep.)

What do you do when you can't sleep? Do you worry about not being able to sleep? Do you stare at the clock, get up and do something else, or take a sleeping pill?
(RATIONALE: Besides uncovering the use of sleeping pills, these questions can identify behaviors that might increase sleeplessness.)

After a sleepless night, how do you feel the next day? Do you have trouble staying awake? Do you take a nap?
(RATIONALE: Napping, particularly in the evening, may disrupt nocturnal sleep.)

Do you exercise regularly? If so, during what time of day?
(RATIONALE: Regular exercise, especially in the late afternoon, may promote sleep for some individuals. Sporadic exercise or exercise just before retiring may inhibit sleep.)

Do you smoke cigarettes?
(RATIONALE: A smoker may have more trouble falling asleep than a nonsmoker.)

Is your bedroom noisy or uncomfortably hot or cold? Does your bed partner snore or disrupt your sleep?
(RATIONALE: Noise [including snoring], a restless bed partner, or an uncomfortable room temperature can disrupt sleep.)

How would you describe your recent moods? Are you depressed or under stress?
(RATIONALE: Most insomnia results from anxiety or psychological problems.)

Do you have any other concerns about your sleep that you would like to discuss?
(RATIONALE: This open-ended question provides an opportunity for the patient to discuss concerns and for the nurse to reassure the patient that the body obtains all the sleep it needs and that sleep loss rarely leads to illness or other problems.)

Developmental considerations

To assess a child's sleep patterns, ask the parents the following questions:

When does your child go to bed? How long does your child sleep at night? When does your child take naps?
(RATIONALE: Evaluate the child's sleep patterns according to age. Teach the parents about the normal changes that occur with age. For example, many children stop taking naps between ages $2\frac{1}{2}$ to 5 years.)

What is your child's usual bedtime routine? Does it include such activities as eating a snack, listening to a story, or brushing the teeth?
(RATIONALE: Toddlers commonly have elaborate bedtime routines. Use this information to continue the child's usual bedtime routine during hospitalization. Also, if the child has trouble falling asleep at night, assess the child's activities just before bedtime.)

Does your child have any particular security objects, such as a toy or a night-light? Does your child have any security behaviors, such as thumb sucking?
(RATIONALE: Use this information to continue the child's usual routine during hospitalization. Also, reassure parents that many children need security objects and behaviors and will relinquish these with maturity.)

Does your child have any sleep difficulties? Does your child have trouble falling asleep? Does your child awaken during the night (if not appropriate for the child's developmental age)? Does your child have nightmares or night terrors? If so, please describe. Does your child wet the bed, snore, or breathe loudly when sleeping?
(RATIONALE: Many problems associated with going to bed and awakening at night are caused by inconsistent routines, lack of parental limit-setting, and the parent's response to the child awakening at night. For example, feeding and holding the child whenever the child awakens at night positively reinforce nighttime awakenings. Reassure the parents that children commonly have night terrors and nightmares between ages 2 and 4. Provide information about enuresis, if appropriate. Also, loud, noisy breathing or snoring suggests sleep apnea, which requires referral to a sleep disorder center for evaluation and treatment.)

Do you have any other concerns about your child's sleep patterns that you would like to discuss?
(RATIONALE: This open-ended question gives the parents the chance to discuss any additional concerns.)

Observation and documentation
While assessing the patient's sleep-wake patterns, observe for clues to a sleep disorder. If the patient is hospitalized, note excessive daytime sleepiness or insomnia and document this information along with vital signs and other objective (physical) assessment findings.

STUDY ACTIVITIES

Short answer
1. Gerald Franklin, age 68 and single, is hospitalized after surgery to treat an arterial ulcer caused by peripheral vascular disease. After discharge, he will have to limit his mobility while the surgical site heals; he will not be able to leave home or to stand for more than a few minutes at a time. To assess Mr. Franklin's ability to perform ADLs and to

prepare him for discharge, the nurse should obtain which additional information about the patient?

_____

_____

2. Thomas Birdsey, age 48, weighs 300 lb. He tells the nurse that, for years, he has been feeling very sleepy during the day. He states he has not experienced any new emotional upset or other stress. His partner, who has accompanied him on this medical visit, reports that Mr. Birdsey snores loudly. Which sleep disturbance should the nurse suspect? What further information should the nurse obtain to assess this sleep disturbance?

_____

_____

3. To assess a child's ADLs, the nurse should investigate which major abilities and activities of the child?

_____

4. When assessing a patient's sleep patterns, the nurse should ask the patient about the use of tobacco, alcohol, and caffeine. Briefly explain how each factor affects sleep.

_____

Fill in the blank

5. The patient's _____ is the ideal setting for assessing ADLs.

6. Meals supply nourishment and offer a time for _____.

7. The two main types of sleep are called _____ sleep and _____ sleep.

8. The sleep requirement ranges from _____ hours to _____ hours.

9. _____ disrupts sleep more than any other environmental condition.

10. Consumption of _____ may exacerbate sleep apnea.

11. Stress and _____ are common causes of insomnia.

ANSWERS **Short answer**

1. Because Mr. Franklin will have limited mobility, his ability to perform normal ADLs will be significantly impaired. To develop his discharge plan, the nurse should determine the following: How well can

Mr. Franklin bathe and dress and undress himself? What is the physical layout of Mr. Franklin's home? Will he be able to get to and from the bathroom by himself, given his limits on activity? Will someone be available to purchase groceries for him and assist with meal preparation? (Good nutrition is especially important after surgery to promote wound healing. If no friend or family member is available to assist the patient, homemaker services may be needed.) Given the complexity of Mr. Franklin's needs, the nurse should arrange for a visiting nurse consultation.

2. The nurse should suspect sleep apnea. The nurse should find out more about Mr. Birdsey's snoring by asking his partner the following questions: Has the snoring become louder or more frequent? Does Mr. Birdsey ever stop breathing or make grunting noises while sleeping? If so, when did these problems first arise? Have they have gotten worse over time? The nurse also should ask Mr. Birdsey how long he has weighed 300 lb and how much he weighed 5, 10, and 15 years ago. If he weighed less in previous years, the nurse should ask whether his snoring was less pronounced then.

3. Depending on the child's age, the nurse should investigate the child's ability to eat independently, perform elimination activities independently, and dress independently. The nurse also should explore the child's involvement in and feelings about school and play.

4. Smokers take twice as long to fall asleep and have lighter sleep with more arousals. Drinking alcohol reduces arousals during the first half of sleep, but increases the number of arousals during the second half of sleep; it also decreases REM sleep. Caffeine ingestion may increase sleep latency and reduce total sleep time.

Fill in the blank

5. home

6. socialization

7. rapid eye movement (REM), non–rapid eye movement (NREM)

8. 4, 10

9. noise

10. alcohol

11. anxiety

CHAPTER 5

Nutritional status

OBJECTIVES

After studying this chapter, the reader should be able to:

1. Discuss the relationship between nutrient intake and health.
2. Describe how pregnancy can place the patient at nutritional risk.
3. Give examples of appropriate health history questions to ask the patient when assessing nutritional status.
4. Assess a patient's dietary patterns using a dietary recall method.
5. Differentiate normal from abnormal nutritional findings obtained by inspection, palpation, and anthropometric measurements.
6. Describe how to adapt assessment techniques for children and elderly patients.
7. Document nutritional assessment findings.

OVERVIEW OF CONCEPTS

From birth, the quality of a person's life is affected by the quality and quantity of nutrients consumed and used. The body's nutritional status—the balance between nutrient intake and energy expenditure or need—reflects the degree to which the physiologic need for nutrients is being met. Proper nutrition promotes growth, maintains health, and helps the body resist infection and recover from disease or surgery. Malnutrition impedes these natural processes.

Three basic types of nutrients—carbohydrates, proteins, and fats—supply the body with energy. Vitamins and minerals also are necessary for normal functioning.

Basic nutrients

Carbohydrates, the primary source of energy, are composed of carbon, hydrogen, and oxygen; one gram of carbohydrate yields 4 kcal. Carbohydrates are ingested as starches (complex carbohydrates) and sugars (simple carbohydrates).

Proteins are complex, nitrogenous, organic compounds composed of carbon, hydrogen, oxygen, and nitrogen atoms arranged as amino acids (organic compounds containing nitrogen). One gram of protein yields 4 kcal. An adequate daily intake of protein is essential to health because proteins are necessary for growth, maintenance, and repair of all body tissues and for efficient performance of regulatory mechanisms.

Like carbohydrates, fats are composed of carbon, hydrogen, and oxygen. The major fats are the glycerides (primarily triglycerides), phospholipids, and cholesterol. One gram of fat yields 9 kcal. Fats are a major source of energy and give taste and flavor to food. Because fats reduce gastric motility and remain in the stomach longer than other foods, they delay the onset of hunger sensations; thus they have high satiety value.

Vitamins and minerals

Vitamins are biologically active organic compounds that are essential for normal metabolism; they contribute to enzyme reactions and are essential to normal growth and development. Although relatively small amounts of vitamins are needed, inadequate vitamin intake leads to deficiency states or disorders. Vitamins are classified either as water-soluble (C and B-complex) or fat-soluble (A, D, E, and K).

Minerals also are essential to good nutrition. They participate in the metabolism of many enzymes, in the membrane transfer of essential compounds, in the maintenance of acid-base balance and osmotic pressure, in nerve impulse transmission, and in muscle contractility. Minerals also contribute to growth. Calcium, phosphorus, magnesium, sodium, chloride, potassium, and sulphur—are considered macronutrient or major minerals (greater than 0.005% of body weight). Zinc, iron, copper, iodine, cobalt, chromium, manganese, selenium, molybdenum, and fluorine are considered micronutrient or trace minerals (less than 0.005% of body weight).

Health history

The nutritional health history includes a dietary history, intake record, and psychosocial assessment. Besides confirming good nutrition or detecting an altered nutritional status, the health history identifies potential nutrition-related health problems, detects the need for education, and permits realistic planning for short- and long-term goals.

Health and illness patterns

Use this part of the health history to help identify actual or potential nutrition-related health problems.

Current health status

Begin the assessment by inquiring about the patient's current health status. Then explore factors related to nutritional status by asking these questions:

Have you made any recent changes in your diet? If so, please describe the changes.
(RATIONALE: A decreased intake may stem from an acute illness or loss of income; it contributes to weight loss and may lead to nutritional deficiency. An increased intake may lead to weight gain but does not rule out a nutritional deficiency.)

Have you experienced any unusual stress or trauma, such as surgery, a change in employment, or family illness?

(RATIONALE: Stress and trauma increase the nutritional requirements for essential nutrients, including protein, vitamins, and calories.)

Have you experienced any significant weight gain or loss or a change in appetite?
(RATIONALE: Significant changes may indicate an underlying disease. For example, weight gain may signal an endocrine imbalance, such as Cushing's syndrome or hypothyroidism; weight loss may be related to cancer, a gastrointestinal disorder, diabetes mellitus, or hyperthyroidism. In uncontrolled diabetes mellitus, weight loss usually is accompanied by an increased appetite.)

Do you take any vitamin or mineral supplements or diet pills? If so, what is the purpose, starting date, dose, and frequency of each? When did you last take them?
(RATIONALE: The patient's response may indicate a nutritional deficiency requiring supplementation or reveal that the patient perceives a nutritional deficiency and self-prescribes supplements or is taking potentially dangerous appetite suppressants.)

Do you take any prescription or over-the-counter drugs?
(RATIONALE: The patient's response may reveal routine drug use that can cause nutritional deficiencies or related problems. For example, diuretics deplete the body's potassium and magnesium stores; cholestyramine impairs the absorption of folic acid and fat-soluble vitamins.)

Do you drink alcoholic beverages? If so, what kind, how often, and in what amount?
(RATIONALE: Alcohol intake provides calories but no essential nutrients. It depletes the body of vitamin B_{12}, thiamine, magnesium, and folic acid. The chronic alcohol abuser may eat little and derives virtually all calories from alcohol.)

Do you smoke or use tobacco? If so, how much? How long ago did you start?
(RATIONALE: Tobacco use may decrease the appetite. It also depletes vitamins, particularly vitamin C.)

How much per day do you consume of the following: coffee, tea, cola, and cocoa?
(RATIONALE: These beverages contain caffeine. In moderate amounts of 50 to 200 mg daily, caffeine is relatively harmless. However, intake of greater amounts can cause nervousness and intestinal discomfort and may interfere with appetite. The caffeine content of beverages ranges from 3 mg per cup of decaffeinated coffee and 50 mg per cup of brewed black tea to 85 mg per cup of brewed coffee; a 12-oz serving of cola contains 32 to 65 mg of caffeine.)

Past health status

Ask the following questions to explore the patient's history for information related to nutritional health or disorders:

Have you had any major or chronic illnesses? Have you had recent surgery?
(RATIONALE: Any of these may affect the patient's daily living patterns by interfering with the ability to walk, open food containers, shop for groceries, prepare food, or chew or swallow food, thereby altering nutritional intake.)

Do you have any food allergies? If so, can you describe what happens when you eat the offending food?
(RATIONALE: Food allergies may cause the patient to eliminate certain foods, increasing the risk for nutritional deficiencies. Also, some foods—especially nuts—can cause dangerous allergic reactions.)

Have you ever had, or been told you have, an eating disorder, such as anorexia nervosa or bulimia, or a problem with substance abuse? If so, have you ever had treatment for this problem? What was the result of the treatment?
(RATIONALE: Eating disorders and substance abuse compromise nutritional status and should be considered potentially life-threatening. The patient requires ongoing evaluation and appropriate referral.)

Have you tried to lose or gain weight within the past 6 months? If so, please describe the diet or program you followed.
(RATIONALE: Certain diets can alter a patient's nutritional status. The nurse should explore the patient's diet to make sure it is well-balanced.)

Family health status

Next, explore possible genetic or familial disorders that may affect the patient's nutritional status:

Do you have a family history of Crohn's disease, ulcers, allergies, or food intolerance (such as lactose intolerance)?
(RATIONALE: These genetic or familial disorders may affect food digestion or metabolism and can alter the patient's nutritional status.)

Developmental considerations for pediatric patients

Nutritional needs vary greatly as a child ages. The following questions help determine if those needs are being met.

Infant (neonate to age 1): For a bottle-fed infant, omit questions that relate specifically to breast-feeding. Ask the following questions:

If the infant is breast-fed, how often and how long does he or she nurse at each breast? How much water does the infant drink, and how often? What type of formula do you use? How much and how often do you give formula? Do you give the infant supplementary food or cereal?
(RATIONALE: During the first few months of life, energy needs are high in relation to body size. The normal full-term neonate needs 110 to 120 calories per kg of body weight every 24 hours. For an infant under

4 months, human milk and properly prepared formula supply adequate fluid intake under normal circumstances. Early solid feeding is a risk factor for obesity and anemia; solid food usually is not introduced until the fourth to sixth month for formula-fed infants and the sixth month for breast-fed infants. Cereal is usually the first solid food added to the infant's diet. Strained fruits and vegetables may be introduced gradually. Formula or breast milk should be the major source of nutrition during the infant's first year.

Do you give your child vitamin or iron supplements? If so, what type and why?
(RATIONALE: If the child's diet is adequate, vitamins are not needed. Excessive iron supplementation may cause iron overload.)

Toddler (age 1 to 3): Ask the following questions to evaluate a toddler's nutritional status:

How much fluid does your child drink in a typical day? How much of it is milk or juice? Does the child drink any soda or sweetened beverages? Does the child use a bottle? How often and what kinds of snacks does the child eat? Is the child allergic to any foods? Does the child particularly like or dislike any food(s)?
(RATIONALE: Growth rate slows during this time, but muscle mass development and bone mineralization increase. At age 1, a child needs approximately 1,000 kcal daily; by age 3, the daily requirement increases to 1,300 to 1,500 kcal. Excessive amounts of juices and other fluids may increase the child's appetite for solid foods. Using a bottle may cause dental caries.)

Preschooler (age 3 to 6): Ask the same questions as for a toddler as well as the following question:

Does the child attend a day-care center, nursery school, kindergarten, or other group?
(RATIONALE: A child who spends time in a group should be receiving a nutritionally balanced diet.)

School-age child (age 6 to 12): Ask the same questions as for the toddler, and this additional question:

What does the child eat for breakfast?
(RATIONALE: Breakfast is the most important meal for a school-age child. Eating breakfast has been correlated with improved school performance. Nutrition information usually is included in the curriculum.)

Adolescent (age 12 to 18): To determine the nutritional intake of an adolescent, ask the following questions about the types, amounts, and frequency of foods and other substances consumed and investigate the possibility of eating disorders:

What do you eat in a typical day? What snacks and fluids do you eat and drink? Do you follow any special diet? Have you gained or lost weight recently?

(RATIONALE: Adolescence is a time of rapid growth, with the onset of puberty increasing nutritional requirements. The growth rate varies widely among individuals and includes gender-related differences. Eating disorders commonly begin during adolescence. Ask the adolescent about alcohol, tobacco, caffeine, and drug use as you would an adult.)

Developmental considerations for pregnant patients

Ask a pregnant patient the following questions:

Has your diet changed since you became pregnant? If so, in what way?
(RATIONALE: The mother's nutritional status during pregnancy affects the child's future health. A pregnant woman needs an increased intake of protein and other nutrients, particularly calcium, iron, and folic acid. A pregnant adolescent has even greater nutrient needs—those of the developing fetus as well as her own. The daily requirement for folic acid doubles from 0.4 mg to 0.8 mg during pregnancy because of increased fetal needs. Some pregnant women have pica [a craving for nonfood substances, such as starch or clay].)

Are you taking any vitamins or other supplements?
(RATIONALE: Physicians, nurse practitioners, and nurse midwives usually prescribe vitamin supplements for pregnant patients. Proper iron and folic acid intake is especially important.)

How has your weight changed since you have become pregnant?
(RATIONALE: The pregnant woman should increase her caloric intake by about 300 kcal daily–but should not overeat in the mistaken belief that she must eat for two. She should gain 1 lb (.45 kg) per week during the last 2 months of pregnancy; by delivery, her weight gain should total 25 to 30 lb (11.4 to 13 kg). If her weight gain is below normal, obtain a complete 24-hour diet history, focusing on the reasons for the poor weight gain.)

Developmental considerations for breast-feeding patients

The following questions help evaluate the nutritional status of a breast-feeding mother:

How are you and your baby doing? Have you noticed any problems? Is anything going particularly well?
(RATIONALE: Asking such general, open-ended questions encourages the patient to elaborate on the breast-feeding experience. Often, further questions will arise during the discussion. The breast-feeding woman should have a diet similar to the pregnant woman, including vitamin supplementation.)

Developmental considerations for elderly patients

Ask an elderly patient the following questions:

Do you wear dentures? If so, do you have any problems with them? Do you have any other problems with chewing?
(RATIONALE: Poorly fitted dentures may decrease nutritional intake and limit variety in diet.)

Do you have any bowel problems? Do you use laxatives or enemas?
(RATIONALE: Constipation is a common problem in the elderly because intestinal motility typically decreases with age. Factors that may contribute to constipation include poor dietary fiber intake, physical inactivity, and adverse drug reactions. Elderly patients may rely on laxatives and enemas for bowel control—a habit that ultimately may cause severe constipation.)

Has your diet changed as you have grown older?
(RATIONALE: Protein, vitamin, and mineral requirements usually remain the same during aging, while caloric needs decrease. Reduced activity may lower energy requirements by about 200 calories/day for men and women ages 51 to 75, 400 calories/day for women over age 75, and 500 calories/day for men over age 75.)

Do you get any help with meals, such as from family members or "Meals on Wheels"?
(RATIONALE: Participation in community-based food programs and help from family members can improve the nutritional status of many elderly patients.)

Health promotion and protection patterns
The following questions help determine what the patient is doing to maintain an adequate nutritional intake and prevent deficiencies.

Exercise and activity patterns
A patient's activity level may affect nutritional status. The following questions help assess this possibility:

How active are you? Give an example of a typical day's activities. Do you follow a special exercise program? If so, describe it.
(RATIONALE: The response will reveal whether the patient is active or sedentary and will help determine the patient's caloric requirements.)

Nutritional patterns
To assess the nutritional adequacy of the patient's dietary intake and related factors, obtain a dietary history. Use any of the following methods: 24-hour dietary recall, 3-, 7- or 14-day dietary inventory or diary, or agency dietary history questionnaires. When compared with recommended dietary allowances, dietary intake data obtained from the patient show where diet counseling is needed.

For the 24-hour dietary recall, ask the patient to recall everything consumed as food or drink within the past 24 hours. When recording the responses, include the amount, type of food or drink, and how it was prepared. Note whether any sauces or other substances were added. Ask if this is a typical day; if not, ask why. If the patient was ill on the day of the 24-hour recall, consider repeating the process when the patient is well.

The U.S. Department of Agriculture recently revised its dietary guidelines to reflect the use of a nutritional "pyramid" whose layers consist of the basic food groups. The bread, cereal, rice, and pasta group is at the base of the pyramid; six to eleven daily servings of this group are recommended. One level higher includes the fruit group (two to four daily servings) and the vegetable group (three to five daily servings); these foods are high in fiber and rich in water-soluble vitamins. The milk, yogurt, and cheese group (two to three daily servings) and the meat, poultry, fish, eggs, and nuts group (two to three daily servings) comprise the next higher level. Fats, sweets, and oils are at the top of the pyramid; these foods should be used sparingly.

Stress and coping patterns

Understanding the degree of stress in the patient's life and the usual way of coping with stress aids the nutritional assessment. Explore stress by asking this question:

Does the stress of your job, daily schedule, or other factors influence your appetite or ability to eat regular meals?
(RATIONALE: Stress at work and long work hours can interfere with mealtimes, setting the stage for nutritional deficiencies. Also, many people overeat in response to stress, whereas others eat less.)

Socioeconomic patterns

Economic, cultural, and sociologic factors can markedly affect the patient's nutritional patterns and health status. To uncover such factors, ask the following questions:

Do you have access to a stove, refrigerator, and food storage space?
(RATIONALE: Inadequate cooking facilities, refrigeration, or food storage can lead to nutritional problems.)

Do you receive food stamps, Social Security payments, supplemental Social Security payments, or assistance from welfare or the Women, Infant, Child (WIC) program?
(RATIONALE: Even with help, most public assistance recipients live at, near, or below the poverty line. These patients may be unable to purchase adequate food, increasing their risk for nutritional deficiencies.)

Role and relationship patterns

This portion of the history is important because body image and relationships with others are frequently interrelated with food intake.

Self-concept

Self-concept and dietary intake are closely related. To explore the patient's self-concept, ask the following questions:

Do you like yourself physically? Are you content with your present weight?
(RATIONALE: The patient's answers may reveal beliefs about weight that can lead to serious eating disorders, such as obesity, anorexia nervosa, or bulimia.)

Social support patterns

Nutrition and eating are affected by social support patterns. The following question helps evaluate the patient's social support pattern:

Do you eat alone or with others?
(RATIONALE: Mealtimes should be relaxing, not a time for the family or social group to air grievances. Stressful mealtimes can lead to eating disorders and poor nutrition. On the other hand, eating alone all or most of the time may cause the patient to neglect nutrition.)

Physical assessment

Overt clinical signs of altered nutritional status occur late in the course of the problem. Whenever possible, the nurse should anticipate nutritional problems early to avoid serious consequences. However, keep in mind that many patients have marginal nutritional problems that are hard to detect. The following paragraphs describe the steps to follow during the physical assessment.

The physical assessment includes inspection, palpation, and collection of anthropometric data (height and weight; body frame size; skinfold evaluation; and, in infants and children, head and chest size). In some cases, assessment also includes measurement of midarm and midarm muscle circumference. To prepare for the physical assessment, obtain a standing platform scale with height attachment; use an infant scale when appropriate and a stature measuring device if the patient is a child. Also obtain skinfold calipers, a measuring tape, and a recumbent measuring board.

Many patients are uncomfortable being weighed and measured. Before beginning this part of the assessment, try to provide privacy and take a few minutes to establish rapport with the patient.

Inspection

Begin by inspecting the patient's overall appearance. The skin should be smooth, free of lesions, and appropriate for the patient's age. The hair should be shiny. The mouth, mucous membranes, lips, tongue, and gingivae should be pink and free of lesions; the teeth, intact, firmly attached, and in good repair. The eyes should be clear with pink conjunctivae. The nails should be smooth, without cracks or fissures. The thyroid should not appear enlarged. (For more information about these structures and their normal assessment findings, see their respective chapters). Abnormalities in these and other areas may indicate a nutritional deficiency. (See *Detecting nutritional deficiencies,* page 72.)

Some nutritional deficiencies can impair the musculoskeletal system. For example, marasmus (severe protein–calorie malnutrition caused by inadequate caloric intake or, more rarely, a metabolic defect) can cause growth retardation and muscle wasting. Kwashiorkor, caused primarily by protein deficiency, leads to marked edema of the extremities.

Detecting nutritional deficiencies

Information obtained from the patient's health history and physical assessment may indicate a nutritional deficiency. This chart links abnormal assessment findings with their possible implications.

SITE	ASSESSMENT FINDINGS	POSSIBLE DEFICIENCY
Conjunctivae	Roughness, dryness	Vitamin A
	Mild irritation	Vitamin B$_2$ (riboflavin)
	Hemorrhage	Vitamin C (ascorbic acid)
Cornea	Clouding	Vitamin A
Lips	Cheilosis (scales and fissures)	Vitamin B$_2$, vitamin B$_6$, or iron
Gingivae	Swelling, bleeding	Vitamin C
Tongue	Irritation (glossitis)	Vitamin B$_{12}$
Skin	Dryness and flaking	Protein
	Pellagra (dryness and flaking in sun-exposed areas)	Niacin
Nails	Thin, spoon-shaped	Iron
	Dull, transverse ridging	Protein
Hair	Thinning, pigment changes	Copper, zinc, or protein
	Easily plucked	Protein
Muscles	Wasted, tender upon palpation	Protein, calories (if patient's weight is 60% to 80% of predicted weight: marasmus)
Extremities	Edema	Protein, calories (kwashiorkor)

Palpation

Palpation helps detect enlarged glands, including the thyroid, parotid, liver, spleen, and others that may indicate a nutrition-compromising disorder. Enlargement of a specific gland can indicate a particular nutritional deficiency. For example, thyroid enlargement is characteristic of iodine deficiency; liver or spleen enlargement may occur with an iron deficiency. (For information on palpating the glands and their normal assessment findings, see Chapter 12, Gastrointestinal system, and Chapter 19, Endocrine system.) When performed on the teeth and tongue, palpation may reveal signs of deficiency.

Anthropometric measurements

Considering the patient's height in relation to weight may provide clues to undernutrition or overnutrition. Always take a baseline measurement. Comparison with standard measurements shows whether the patient's weight, height, and body frame are above or below that standard, revealing whether the patient is undernourished or overnourished. Measured daily, the patient's weight reflects changes in hydration, which helps assess fluid retention and the effectiveness of diuretic therapy or dialysis.

To determine the ideal weight for an adult patient (age 18 and over), first determine body frame size. Then, based on body frame size, compare the patient's height and weight with the values on a standard height-weight chart. After locating the patient's ideal weight-for-height, use that value to calculate the percentage of ideal weight the patient's present weight represents. The patient who has had an unmonitored weight loss of 10% over 6 months or who is either 20% above or 20% below the standard is at risk for nutritional disorders and should be referred for further evaluation and appropriate follow-up.

Development considerations for pediatric patients

In a child under age 2, measure length with the child supine. Weigh an infant nude, because diapers vary greatly in weight. Use growth charts to compare the height and weight measurements; these charts reflect measurements of the population of American children taken as a whole. Plot the data on a growth chart; measurements that fall between the 5th and 95th percentiles represent normal growth for most patients. The most important factor in tracking percentiles on a growth grid is a consistent position. The child should remain at about the same position during the early childhood years; from late childhood to early puberty, many children show a rapid gain in position. A fall in position warrants close monitoring and possibly further evaluation because it may indicate a serious nutritional or developmental problem.

In infants and children, measure head and chest circumference. (See *Measuring head and chest circumference,* page 74.) Because the brain grows rapidly during the first 2 years, head circumference can reflect an abnormal development rate, giving some indication of nutritional status. Chest circumference is routinely measured only in the newborn; it should be roughly 10% smaller than the head circumference. If chest circumference exceeds head circumference, the child should be referred to a physician or a nurse practitioner.

Developmental considerations for elderly patients

Personally measure an elderly patient's height. The patient's self-report may be inaccurate because the patient may be unaware of a height loss. Height decreases with age as a result of changes in intervertebral disks, vertebrae, and posture.

Other assessment skills

Midarm circumference, triceps skinfold thickness, and midarm muscle circumference help gauge the amount of skeletal muscle and adipose tissue, which indicate protein and fat reserves. (For information about these procedures, see *Anthropometric arm measurements,* page 75.)

If any of the above measurements fall between the 5th and 25th percentiles, the patient may have moderate nutritional depletion; report this finding and conduct serial measurements. If the measurements fall

Measuring head and chest circumference

Head and chest circumference are anthropometric measurements taken as part of the physical assessment of infants and children. To obtain accurate results, the nurse should follow these procedures.

Head circumference

To measure an infant's head circumference, wrap a nonstretching measuring tape around the head, just above the supraorbital ridges and over the most prominent part of the occiput.

Chest circumference

To measure an infant's chest circumference, wrap the tape around the chest at the nipples. Take the measurement between inspiration and expiration.

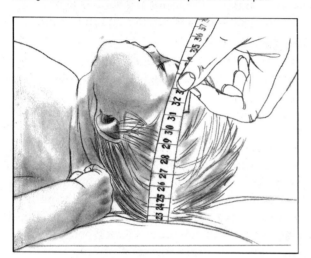

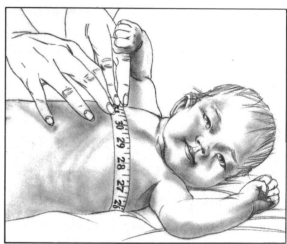

at or below the 5th percentile or at or above the 95th percentile, refer the patient for further evaluation.

Documentation Evaluation of history, physical, and laboratory data places the patient in one of these categories that describe nutritional status:
- Adequate nutrition. The patient exhibits no deficits in body fat stores, lean body mass, visceral proteins, or immunologic competence.
- Marasmus. Body fat and lean body mass are depleted. Body weight is 60% to 80% of the standard range, reflecting loss of muscle and fat. Decreased triceps skinfold thickness and reduced arm muscle circumference indicate loss of body fat and skeletal tissue.
- Kwashiorkor. This deficiency state indicates protein loss, often from the stress of trauma or infection. It also can occur in an acutely ill, hospitalized patient receiving intravenous glucose (which contains some calories) with no protein supplementation.

The following example illustrates the documentation of some normal findings in a nutritional assessment:

Weight: 150 lb
Height: 5′10″

Anthropometric arm measurements

Measurements of the midarm circumference, triceps skinfold thickness, and midarm muscle circumference provide information about skeletal muscle and adipose tissue, which helps determine the patient's protein and calorie reserves. To obtain these measurements, the nurse follows this procedure.

1. Locate the midpoint on the patient's upper arm, using a nonstretching tape measure, and mark the midpoint with a felt-tip pen.

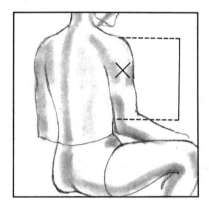

2. Determine the triceps skinfold thickness by grasping the patient's skin between the thumb and forefinger approximately 1 cm above the midpoint. Place the calipers at the midpoint and squeeze them for about 3 seconds. Record the measurement registered on the handle gauge to the nearest 0.5 mm. Take two more readings, then average all three to compensate for possible error.

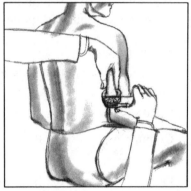

3. From the midpoint, measure the midarm circumference. Calculate midarm muscle circumference by multiplying the triceps skinfold thickness (in centimeters) by 3.143 and subtracting the result from the midarm circumference.

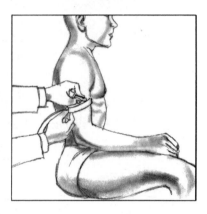

4. Record all three measurements as percentages of the standard measurements by using the following formula:

$$\frac{\text{actual measurement}}{\text{standard measurement}} \times 100$$

Compare the patient's percentage measurement to the standard shown at right. A measurement less than 90% of the standard indicates caloric deprivation; a measurement over 90% indicates adequate or more than adequate energy reserves.

MEASUREMENT	STANDARD	90%
Triceps skinfold	Men: 12.5 mm Women: 16.5 mm	Men: 11.3 mm Women: 14.9 mm
Midarm circumference	Men: 29.3 cm Women: 28.5 cm	Men: 26.4 cm Women: 25.7 cm
Midarm muscle circumference	Men: 25.3 cm Women: 23.2 cm	Men: 22.8 cm Women: 20.9 cm

Adapted with permission from Blackburn, G., Bistrian, B., Maini, B., Schlamm, H., and Smith, M., "Nutritional and Metabolic Assessment of the Hospital Patient." *The Journal of Parenteral and Enteral Nutrition* 1(1):11-22, 1977.

Vital signs: within normal limits (BP 126/82, T 98.4° F, P 82/minute, and R 18/minute).

Additional notes: Body frame size, small. Triceps skinfold thickness, 12.4 mm; midarm circumference, 28.2 cm; midarm muscle circumference, 22.8 cm. No abnormalities noted upon inspection. Skin without blemishes; nails short; hair shiny; mouth, tongue, and gingivae free of lesions. Extremities equal in size with normal range of motion. No glandular enlargement present.

The following example illustrates the documentation of some abnormal findings in a nutritional assessment:

Weight: 138 lb

Height: 5'11"

Vital signs: within normal limits except for pulse (104/minute) and respiration (28/minute).

Additional notes: Body frame size, large. Triceps skinfold thickness, 10 mm; midarm circumference, 22.8 cm; midarm muscle circumference, 20 cm. Eyes sunken and dry. Skin dry and scaly. Cheilosis present; glossitis present; nails split and spoon-shaped. Extremities thin.

STUDY ACTIVITIES

Matching related elements

Match the clinical finding in the left column with its most likely cause in the right column.

1. ___ Cheilosis	**A.** Vitamin C deficiency
2. ___ Conjunctival hemorrhage	**B.** Protein deficiency
3. ___ Pellagra	**C.** Iron, vitamin B_2, or vitamin B_6 deficiency
4. ___ Easily plucked hair	**D.** Protein-calorie deficiency
5. ___ Muscle wasting	**E.** Niacin deficiency

Fill in the blank

6. Proteins contain _____ kcal/g, carbohydrates contain _____ kcal/g, and fats contain _____ kcal/g.

7. Tobacco use is especially likely to deplete vitamin _____; alcohol use commonly depletes vitamin _____.

8. A pregnant women needs an increased intake of _____, _____, _____, and _____.

9. Reduced activity may lower energy requirements by _____ calories/day for patients between ages 51 and 74; by _____ calories/day for patients over age 75.

Short answer

10. Clifford Samuelson, age 47, complains of nervousness. While obtaining his health history, the nurse discovers that he drinks 5 cups of brewed coffee with milk, 2 cups of brewed black tea, and one 12-ounce can of cola each day. What is his total daily caffeine intake in milligrams? What impact could this have on his complaint?

_____

11. Marjorie Love, age 16, is the first-time mother of a 3-month-old infant. During a clinic visit, the nurse asks Ms. Love what she is feeding her infant. What response from Ms. Love would indicate she is feeding her infant appropriately? What response would indicate inappropriate feeding?

_____

12. Maria Rodriguez, age 80, has severe arthritis. She lives alone and has few family members in the area. The nurse obtains a 24-hour diet history, which reveals a low-calorie, nutritionally deficient diet. Which additional subjective data does the nurse need to fully assess this patient's nutritional status?

_____

_____

13. Tom Stormcloud, age 8, is brought to the nursing clinic for a well-child visit by his father, a single working parent. They both admit that Tom does not eat breakfast on school mornings because "time is very tight". Why is breakfast of particular importance to a child of Tom's age? How should the nurse incorporate information about Tom's eating habits in the care plan?

_____

ANSWERS

Matching related elements

  1. C
  2. A
  3. E
  4. B
  5. D

Fill in the blank

  6. 4, 4, 9
  7. C, B_{12}

8. protein calcium, iron, folic acid

9. 200, 400

Short answer

10. Mr. Samuelson's caffeine intake is 557 to 590 mg/day—well above the 50 to 200 mg/day that is considered a moderate intake. This excessive intake may be causing or contributing to his nervousness.

11. Ms. Love should report that she is providing breast milk or formula only. Giving whole milk, juice, or solid foods to a 3-month-old infant would be inappropriate.

12. The nurse should find out if arthritis has limited the patient's ability to obtain or prepare foods. The nurse also should ask Ms. Rodriguez if she is getting assistance from any community-based feeding programs, such as "Meals on Wheels," as well as help from family or friends. In addition, the nurse should find out if she eats alone (which could cause her to neglect nutrition), if she has any problems chewing food, and if she wears dentures. Poor-fitting dentures and other dental problems can limit the food selection.

13. Eating breakfast improves school performance in the school-age child. The nurse should help Tom and his father devise a morning schedule that gives Tom the opportunity to eat breakfast.

CHAPTER 6

Skin, hair, and nails

OBJECTIVES After studying this chapter, the reader should be able to:

1. Identify the structures and appendages of the skin.

2. Give examples of appropriate health history questions for assessment of the skin, hair, and nails.

3. Identify behavior patterns harmful to the skin.

4. Describe how to assess the patient's skin using inspection and palpation.

5. Differentiate between normal and abnormal skin conditions.

6. Describe the characteristics of common skin lesions, using appropriate terminology.

OVERVIEW OF CONCEPTS The skin and its appendages protect underlying structures, help regulate body temperature, and serve as a sensory organ. Because changes in the skin can indicate health changes, assessment of this system is an essential part of the physical assessment.

The skin (integument) is the largest body organ, comprising 15% of total body weight and covering a surface area of 2 square meters. Its two distinct layers, the epidermis and dermis, lie above a third layer of subcutaneous fat. Numerous epidermal appendages exist throughout the skin: hair, nails, sebaceous glands, and two types of sweat glands, apocrine glands, which are found in the axilla and groin near hair follicles, and eccrine glands, which are located over most of the body (except the lips). (For illustrations, see *Anatomy of the skin and its appendages,* page 80.)

Health history Skin assessment begins with a complete health history. When assessing the skin, remember that skin disorders may involve or stem from other organ system problems, and that minor symptoms or systemic complaints should not be discounted. To lessen the patient's anxiety about the assessment, explain that questions about other parts of the body and general health are necessary to understanding the skin problem.

Begin with questions about present problems, followed by a full investigation of the patient's health and illness patterns, health promotion and protection patterns, and role and relationship patterns. Obtain as

Anatomy of the skin and its appendages

As this illustration shows, the skin is a complex structure containing cells, blood vessels, hair follicles, glands, and other networks. The skin appendages—hair, nails, and sebaceous, eccrine, and apocrine glands—derive from the epidermis and may extend into the dermal layers.

Skin

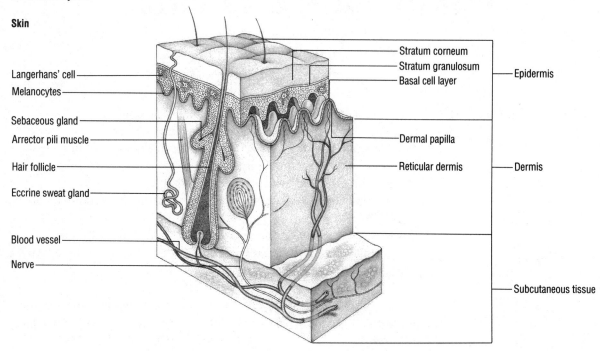

Langerhans' cell
Melanocytes
Sebaceous gland
Arrector pili muscle
Hair follicle
Eccrine sweat gland
Blood vessel
Nerve

Stratum corneum
Stratum granulosum
Basal cell layer — Epidermis
Dermal papilla
Reticular dermis — Dermis
Subcutaneous tissue

Hair   **Nails**

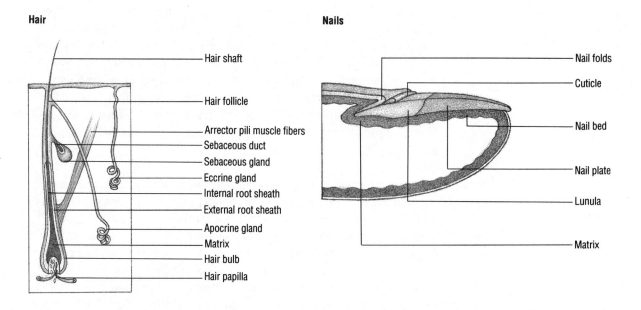

Hair shaft
Hair follicle
Arrector pili muscle fibers
Sebaceous duct
Sebaceous gland
Eccrine gland
Internal root sheath
External root sheath
Apocrine gland
Matrix
Hair bulb
Hair papilla

Nail folds
Cuticle
Nail bed
Nail plate
Lunula
Matrix

much information as possible about the patient's general health, using terms familiar to the patient, and make pertinent observations. These observations may provide additional insight into the problem and serve as a guide for further data collection. (*Note: Skin change* refers to variation from normal; *skin disorder* refers to a problem affecting function.)

Health and illness patterns

To assess important health and illness patterns, explore the patient's current, past, and family health status as well as developmental status.

Current health status

Carefully document presenting signs and symptoms in the patient's words. Then use the PQRST method to obtain a complete description of these complaints. (For information on this method, see *Symptom analysis,* page 15.) Ask questions to determine the onset and course of the problem, symptoms, and any treatments used. To assess the patient's current health status further, ask the following questions:

What aspect of your skin problem bothers you the most?
(RATIONALE: This question allows the patient to identify the most important personal aspect of the problem.)

Where on your body did the skin problem begin?
(RATIONALE: Certain skin problems have a characteristic pattern of progression (for example, pityriasis rosea [viral rash] begins on the trunk and spreads to proximal extremities.)

When did you first notice these changes?
(RATIONALE: Knowing the progression of the skin changes can provide important information.)

Please describe the initial problem in as much detail as possible, even if that problem has already disappeared. Can you also describe how the problem spread and in what order other areas were affected?
(RATIONALE: The shape, size, color, location, and distribution of the problem give clues to the cause of the disorder. So do the sensations associated with it and any pattern of migration. For example, chicken pox [varicella] spreads from the trunk to the limbs; shingles [herpes zoster] spreads in a distinct pattern along cutaneous nerve endings.)

Do you have other symptoms?
(RATIONALE: Symptoms in other body systems may be associated with certain skin disorders. For example, systemic prodromal symptoms, such as malaise, fever, and cold symptoms, are associated with chicken pox.)

How does your skin feel?
(RATIONALE: Try to obtain the patient's description before asking about specific sensations, such as itching, burning, stinging, tingling, numbness, pain, tenderness, malaise, or achiness.)

Can you relate the skin problem to a cause or event, such as stress, contact with a particular substance, or a change in activities?
(RATIONALE: Relating the skin problem to a clearly defined cause or event may help establish its etiology.)

Does anything make the problem worse?
(RATIONALE: Aggravating factors are part of the diagnostic pattern for many skin disorders. Ask specifically about changes related to food, heat, cold, exercise, sunlight, stress, pregnancy, and menstruation. Herpes simplex, for example, is frequently aggravated by sunlight, menstruation, or stress.)

Does anything make the problem better?
(RATIONALE: A positive answer, with specific drug or treatment description, may help the nurse plan appropriate interventions.)

Does the problem seem to be getting better or worse?
(RATIONALE: Determining the course of the skin problem aids differential diagnosis.)

Are you taking any prescription or over-the-counter drugs? Have you taken any in the recent past? Have you ever experienced a skin problem after taking a medication?
(RATIONALE: Both prescription and nonprescription drugs may cause certain skin problems or aggravate others. Many common medications, such as penicillins, can cause hivelike and macular or papular eruptions. Tetracyclines commonly produce photosensitivity; corticosteroids may cause skin atrophy, ecchymosis, and acne. Do not overlook vaccines, especially when assessing pediatric patients.)

Have you used any topical compresses, lotions, or creams to resolve your skin problem?
(RATIONALE: If a home remedy is not harmful and the patient believes it helps, try to incorporate it into the care plan.)

Do you have any other illness, such as arthritis, inflammatory bowel disease, or infections?
(RATIONALE: A review of body systems effectively elicits information on conditions that may produce associated skin findings.)

Have you noticed any unusual overall or patchy hair loss?
(RATIONALE: Overall hair loss may result from systemic illness, such as anemia or thyroid disease, or from any treatment that affects the hair growth cycle, such as chemotherapy. Patchy hair loss may stem from hair styles, secondary syphilis, scalp infections, or infestations, such as lice.)

Have you noticed any changes in your nails?
(RATIONALE: Nail changes from aging and systemic illness are common. Fungal infections and psoriasis can cause characteristic nail changes.)

Past health status

During this part of the health history, explore the patient's medical history for additional related information. Ask the following questions:

Have you recently experienced fever, malaise, or upper respiratory or gastrointestinal problems?
(RATIONALE: Many common skin eruptions are related to viral infections. Recent infections and illness as well as treatment regimens may contribute to skin disorders.)

Have you ever experienced anything similar to what you have now?
(RATIONALE: Some skin disorders, such as psoriasis, can recur.)

Have you had any allergic reactions to medications, foods, or other substances, such as cosmetics?
(RATIONALE: Past and present allergies, including those caused by cutaneous, ingested, or inhaled allergens, may predispose the patient to other skin disorders.)

Have you had any sexually transmitted diseases? What safe sex measures do you practice?
(RATIONALE: To ensure prompt diagnosis and appropriate patient teaching, the nurse must determine the patient's risk factors for acquiring sexually transmitted diseases that affect the skin, such as genital warts, herpes simplex, and syphilis. Viral and fungal infections of the skin may herald human immunodeficiency virus infection.)

Family health status

When inquiring about family health status, try to elicit information suggesting a familial tendency to skin disease and allergies. Ask the following questions:

Has anyone in your family had a skin problem? If so, what was it and when did it occur?
(RATIONALE: Some skin disorders, such as skin cancer, atopic [allergic] dermatitis, acne, or psoriasis, have familial tendencies; contagious skin problems, such as chicken pox and scabies, may be transmitted to the patient from a family member.)

Does anyone in your family have allergy-related disorders, such as asthma, allergic rhinitis, or eczema?
(RATIONALE: The patient's problem may stem from an atopic [allergic] response that may be identified through knowledge of allergies in other family members.)

Developmental considerations for pediatric patients

Encourage the child to participate in the interview as fully as age permits, relying on the parent or guardian for information the child cannot provide. Include the following questions:

Is the infant breast-fed or formula-fed?
(RATIONALE: Breast-fed infants have fewer allergies because they are not exposed to foreign proteins as early as formula-fed infants.)

Has the child had any skin problems related to a particular formula or a food added to the diet?
(RATIONALE: Food allergies often manifest as skin problems in infants and young children.)

Has your infant had any diaper rashes that did not clear up readily with over-the-counter skin preparations?
(RATIONALE: Severe, unremitting diaper rash may be caused by fungal or bacterial infection.)

How often do you bathe your infant?
(RATIONALE: Too-frequent bathing can lead to dry skin. Conversely, infrequent bathing can lead to intertrigo [superficial dermatitis in the skin folds].)

What products do you use on the infant's skin?
(RATIONALE: The infant may be allergic to soaps or other skin preparations.)

Is your child attending nursery or elementary school?
(RATIONALE: Contact with other children increases early exposure to communicable diseases with exanthems [skin eruptions accompanied by inflammation], such as measles or scarlet fever.)

Has the child been scratching the scalp? Does the scalp flake in circular patterns? Has the child lost an unusual amount of hair? Has the child been pulling the hair?
(RATIONALE: The child may have pediculosis or ringworm [tinea capitis]. Both conditions injure the hair roots, weaken hair follicles, and may damage hair. A hair-pulling habit [trichotillomania] may cause patchy hair loss.)

For a school-age child or an adolescent, ask the following questions to assess additional developmental considerations:

Do you play where you might come in contact with bugs, weeds, or bushes?
(RATIONALE: A child may develop transient or permanent hypersensitivity to insect bites or contact dermatitis from plant oils. The resulting itching can lead to scratching, excoriation, and possibly infection.)

Does your face, upper back, or chest ever break out? If so, how do you feel about your skin appearance?
(RATIONALE: The adolescent may be self-conscious about acne and reluctant to talk about it until rapport is established. Knowing what exacerbates the problem, how the patient feels about it, and what skin preparations are used helps establish an effective therapeutic regimen.)

Developmental consideration for pregnant patients
Itching (pruritus) and dry skin (xerosis) may occur in this patient. Symptomatic treatment with mild soaps and emollients frequently improves the comfort level. However, any rash has the potential for infec-

tion and warrants serious attention. To assess a pregnant patient, ask the following question:

Have you noticed any changes in your skin during your pregnancy?
(RATIONALE: The answer provides an opportunity to discuss normal changes with the patient and to explore abnormal changes more fully.)

Developmental considerations for elderly patients
When assessing an elderly patient, ask the following questions:

How has your skin changed as you have gotten older?
(RATIONALE: The answer allows the nurse to assess the patient's perception of changes and provides an opportunity to discuss and clarify normal changes and to explore abnormal ones.)

Have you noticed any difference in the way your wounds or sores heal?
(RATIONALE: Healing capacity decreases with age. Diseases, such as diabetes mellitus and peripheral vascular disease, also affect healing.)

Have you developed more moles recently? If so, where? Have any of your moles changed in appearance, become painful, developed a discharge, or bled? Have you seen any shiny papules or crusted lesions on skin areas exposed to the sun?
(RATIONALE: Development of pigmented lesions, such as nevi, later in life may represent a cancer [melanoma] risk. Sun-induced [basal cell and squamous cell] skin cancers may occur on skin surfaces chronically exposed to ultraviolet light.)

Health promotion and protection patterns
The following questions help identify factors in the patient's environment that may cause or aggravate skin disorders, and help determine how the patient's lifestyle relates to the skin problem.

What type of soap, skin creams, or lotions do you use? Do you use ointment, oil, or styling spray on your hair? How often do you shampoo, and what products do you use? Do you use makeup or scents? If so, what type? Do you shave with a blade or an electric razor? Do you use a depilatory? Do you color your hair?
(RATIONALE: Skin changes, such as acne and contact dermatitis, may result from cosmetic and grooming practices. Information on such personal habits are pertinent for some skin disturbances, particularly localized ones. For example, dying the hair may have preceded scalp or hair changes.)

How would you describe your usual skin exposure to the sun? Did you have blistering sunburns as a child?
(RATIONALE: This question investigates the patient's sun-protection practices and the potential for exacerbating age-related and familial skin cancers.)

What type of work do you do or have you done?
(RATIONALE: Skin disorders may be caused by exposure to occupational substances, such as paint, aerosol sprays, petroleum products, weed killers, and cleaning solvents.)

What are your recreational activities? Do these activities expose you to sun or other light, chemicals or other toxins, animals, the outdoors, or foreign travel?
(RATIONALE: Recreational activities, such as craft work, gardening, camping, outdoor sports, and tanning, may expose the patient to sources of skin problems. Foreign travel may expose the patient to skin diseases that are uncommon in North America.)

Have you recently experienced any life stressors?
(RATIONALE: Stress may contribute to some skin diseases, and some skin diseases may cause stress by inducing changes in the patient's self-image.)

What concerns do you have about your skin problem and its treatment?
(RATIONALE: Many treatments for skin disorders are expensive and time-consuming, limiting the patient's ability to carry out the regimen. The patient may express concern about the cost of medications.)

Role and relationship patterns
Once patient trust has been established, explore sensitive areas of physical appearance and social or sexual practices related to the skin disorder. Such questions might include:

How has your skin problem affected your daily activities?
(RATIONALE: This question may provide information on limitations related to physical or emotional discomfort or distress. For example, gloves may be required when washing dishes because pain occurs when water contacts the affected area.)

How does the affected area look to you?
(RATIONALE: Skin appearance is important to the patient because it provides an initial impression to others. The patient's perception of this appearance can affect self-image, self-esteem, and participation in activities.)

Has your skin problem interfered with your role as a spouse (or student, parent, or other) or with your sexuality?
(RATIONALE: The patient's self-esteem and sexual feelings and expression may be severely diminished. Do not underestimate the psychological ramifications of skin disease or the need to provide an opportunity to discuss such feelings.)

Physical assessment
To assess the patient's skin, hair, and nails thoroughly, evaluate the features that reflect skin composition and function, such as body weight, fluid balance, and appearance.

Physical assessment of the skin, hair, and nails requires inspection and palpation. Implementation of these techniques demands good observation skills but requires only simple equipment. Before beginning, wash the hands. Then gather the following items:
• a bright, even light source
• a penlight
• a metric rule that marks centimeters (preferably clear lucite)
• a magnifying glass
• gloves
• a Wood's lamp (optional).

The nurse should examine the entire skin surface, maintaining the patient's modesty with appropriate draping. A systematic approach to assessment includes inspection and palpation of all skin, hair, nails, and mucous membranes, even if the patient reports only a local lesion. The patient may not recognize subtle skin changes or asymptomatic skin disturbances. Also, the patient may be too embarrassed to mention a lesion in the genital area.

Body weight, fluid balance, and appearance

To assess fluid status, weigh the patient daily at the same time on the same scale every day with the same amount of clothing. Recent weight changes (over the previous 48 hours) reflect changes in fluid status rather than body mass, and may affect skin turgor (resiliency).

Compare the patient's stated age with the general appearance. Long-term excessive sun exposure, acute or chronic illness, and long-term smoking can cause a patient to look older than his or her actual age.

Skin diseases associated with systemic disorders also may affect the mucous membranes, which normally appear smooth and moist with a consistent pink color and an intact surface. Blood vessels usually do not predominate. The most readily examined mucous membranes include the conjunctivae and the oral mucosa. (For a description of assessing the conjunctivae, see Chapter 8, Eyes and ears; for a description of assessing the oral mucosa, see Chapter 7, Head and neck.) Pale mucous membranes may indicate anemia; a blue tinge (cyanosis) may indicate carbon dioxide excess associated with cardiopulmonary disorders.

Dry mucous membranes suggest dehydration. Other mucous membrane conditions and lesions may be caused by pressure; burns; actinic (sun) damage; contact with tobacco, chemicals, or allergens; adverse drug reactions; infections with viruses, bacteria, fungi, or animal parasites; or systemic causes, including leukemia, thrombocytopenia, pernicious anemia, metabolic disorders, collagen vascular disease, autoimmune disease, and underlying cancers. Because skin disorders may result from metabolic, endocrine, gastrointestinal, hepatic, cardiovascular, blood, respiratory, renal, or psychological disorders, always correlate skin findings with body system assessments.

Inspection

During this part of the assessment, inspect the skin, hair, and nails.

Skin

Begin by observing the patient's overall appearance from a distance of 3′ to 6′, noting complexion, general color, color variations, and general appearance. Also note any body odor. Particular odors are associated with certain skin problems; for example, a distinct, sickly sweet odor is a sign of *Pseudomonas* infection.

Because abnormal skin variations require identification and description, be sure to note disturbances in pigmentation (areas that are lighter or darker than the rest of the skin), freckles, moles (nevi), and tanning (usually considered normal variations). Usually benign, nevi that occur in large numbers (up to 40) or change in size, color, border or symmetry may indicate dysplastic changes. Freckles and nevi are examples of focal or localized hyperpigmentation (increased pigmentation).

Color. Skin color varies from person to person, depending on race and ethnic origin. These variations usually range from whitish pink to ruddy with olive or yellow tones, or to warm yellow, brown, or black. Oxyhemoglobin (oxygen combined with hemoglobin) in red blood cells imparts a warm, lively color to healthy skin. Skin color also varies normally in different parts of the body, although overall coloring should remain fairly even—especially within a body region. For example, the face, neck, hands, and arms frequently darken from sun exposure; the areola is darker than the surrounding breast; and the genitalia may have a darker color. Some alterations in the normal pigmentation pattern may result from changes in melanocyte distribution or function, which may cause increased pigmentation (hyperpigmentation)—such as in birthmarks and freckles—or decreased pigmentation (hypopigmentation) as seen in vitiligo (a complete lack of pigment).

Vascular changes. Inspection detects vascular changes; palpation differentiates these from nonvascular changes. Because the epidermis has no vasculature, all vascular lesions (even those visible in the epidermis) originate in the dermis. Some skin areas readily reflect vascular changes. For example, the flush areas across the cheeks, nose, neck, upper chest, and genitalia often exhibit an increased pinkness in response to vasodilation from blushing, excitement, sexual stimulation, or fever.

Alterations in skin vasculature usually appear as red pigmented lesions. Some vascular lesions occur in persons in good health. For example, blood vessel hypertrophy (enlargement) may result in hemangiomas, which vary from bright red to purple. Usually soft and easily compressed, hemangiomas range from 1 to 3 mm in diameter. These lesions blanch (lose color or fade) slightly when palpated and compressed. To demonstrate blanching, press on the lesion with a lucite ruler, diascope, or glass slide and note the color change. Permanently dilated superficial blood vessels (telangiectasia or spider veins) may indicate disease, but frequently are normal.

Skin lesions. Throughout the assessment, carefully observe and document any lesion according to the following considerations:

Morphology (clinical description) of the lesion. Note the size (measure and record its dimensions), shape or configuration, color, elevation or depression, existence of peduncles (that is, connection of lesion to the skin by a stem or stalk), and texture. Note the odor, color, consistency, and amount of exudate. Use a flashlight or penlight to assess the color of the lesion and elevation of its borders. Side-lighting permits differentiation of solid and fluid content of a lesion. Use a Wood's lamp to assess fungal lesions and a magnifying glass to inspect tiny lesions.

Identifying lesion morphology is the most crucial part of the physical assessment because morphology often is closely related to histology (microscopic anatomy). Describe lesions accurately, keeping in mind that two or more types can coexist. In some cases, lesions change during the natural course of a disease. For example, the rash of chicken pox begins with macules that progress rapidly to papules, then to vesicles, and finally to pustules and crusts. Scratching, rubbing, and applying medication also may alter the original, or primary, lesion. These modified lesions are described as secondary lesions.

Distribution. Lesion distribution may vary with the disease progression or external factors. Note the pattern upon first inspection; many skin disorders involve specific skin areas. Assessment of distribution includes the extent of involvement; the pattern of involvement (such as symmetry or distribution in areas that are exposed to sunlight); and characteristic locations, such as dermatomes (along cutaneous nerve endings), flexor or extensor surfaces, intertriginous areas, or palms or soles.

Location (related to total skin area). Note whether the pattern of lesions is localized (in one small area), regionalized (in one large area), or generalized (over the entire body). Also note which areas they affect, such as flexor or extensor surfaces, along clothing or jewelry lines, or if they appear randomly.

Configuration or pattern (arrangement of lesions in relation to each other). Configuration may help determine the cause. Note whether lesions are discrete (separate and distinct), coalesced or confluent (fused or blended), grouped (positioned close together), diffuse (scattered), linear (arranged in a line), annular (distributed in a ring), or arciform (arranged in a curve or arc). Also note gyrate or polycyclic (concentric), herpetiform (along the course of cutaneous nerves), and iris configurations. (For illustrations of lesion patterns, see *Assessing lesion distribution and configuration,* pages 90 and 91.)

Document lesion configurations carefully because some diseases have definite, readily identifiable configurations. Herpes zoster vesi-

Assessing lesion distribution and configuration

When a patient has skin lesions, the nurse must assess their distribution and configuration to help pinpoint their cause.

Distribution

To assess distribution, note the location of all lesions. Then characterize the distribution pattern as localized (over a small area), regionalized (over a larger area), or generalized (over the whole body). Further characterize the distribution, if possible, by one of the distribution patterns shown below.

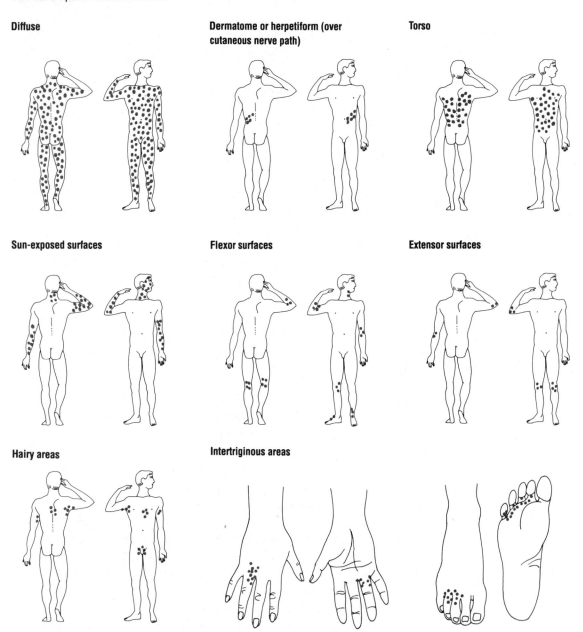

Diffuse

Dermatome or herpetiform (over cutaneous nerve path)

Torso

Sun-exposed surfaces

Flexor surfaces

Extensor surfaces

Hairy areas

Intertriginous areas

Assessing lesion distribution and configuration *(continued)*

Configuration
To assess configuration, observe the relationship of the lesions to each other. Then characterize the configuration by one of the patterns illustrated below.

Discrete
Individual lesions are separate and distinct.

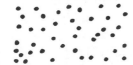

Annular (circular)
Lesions are arranged in a single ring or circle.

Grouped
Lesions are clustered together.

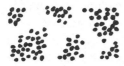

Polycyclic
Lesions are arranged in concentric circles.

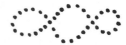

Confluent
Lesions merge so that discrete lesions are not visible or palpable.

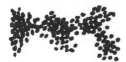

Arciform
Lesions form arcs or curves.

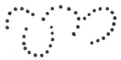

Linear
Lesions form a line.

Reticular
Lesions form a meshlike network.

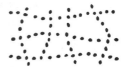

cles, for example, characteristically appear in a linear pattern; those of herpes simplex usually appear in groups.

Individual characteristics. Assessment involves descriptive terms, such as annular, iris, linear, round, oval, and arciform, as well as a description of the color and consistency or "feel" of the lesion. For example, a lesion may be pink or red, or red in the center and pink at the edges, and soft or firm in consistency. Besides lesions, document the characteristics of any breaks or other skin changes, including abrasions, scratches, cuts, bruises, or scars from previous injuries.

Hair and scalp
When assessing the hair, note its quantity, texture, color, and distribution. Hair distribution varies greatly among individuals and is affected by race and ethnic origin. Cultural differences in grooming and hair ar-

rangement may affect the appearance of scalp hair. For example, traction from repeated braiding may cause scalp hair loss.

Assessment of the scalp should reveal a surface, free of debris, with equal distribution of hair follicles. Variations in hair growth and distribution, including hereditary baldness and excessive facial hair, occur naturally and are not preventable.

Nails

Careful nail assessment provides information that reflects not only health status but also lifestyle and level of self-care. Inspect the nails for color, consistency, smoothness, symmetry, and freedom from ridges and cracks as well as for length, jagged or bitten edges, and cleanliness.

Assess the angle between the fingernail and the nail base (usually about 160 degrees) by placing the lucite ruler across the dorsal surface of the finger and the nail, then observing the angle formed where the proximal nail fold meets the nail plate. In clubbing (abnormal enlargement of the distal phalanges caused by decreased oxygen supply to peripheral tissues), this angle reaches 180 degrees or more. Caucasians normally have pink nail beds (easily visible through the translucent nail), whereas those of dark-skinned persons may appear brown, with occasional longitudinal lines.

Abnormal findings

Some of the most common disorders of the skin, hair, and nails are discussed below.

Skin

Generalized or diffuse hyperpigmentation usually accompanies a systemic disorder, such as Addison's disease, a nutritional deficiency, or adverse drug reactions. Focal, macular, hypopigmented lesions occur in vitiligo (characterized by the complete absence of melanocytes) and postinflammatory hypopigmentation.

Other abnormal skin variations include hypertrophic changes from increased numbers of cells. Such changes usually involve the epidermis and include scales, papules, plaques, and lichenification (skin thickening and hardening from continuous irritation, such as rubbing). Dermal layer changes frequently involve the connective tissue and may cause nodules. Skin thickening or induration may follow collagen buildup, a change associated with epidermal hypertrophy. Hypertrophy of subcutaneous fat is visible only if tissue mass significantly increases, as in obesity. Small, local accumulations of fat are called lipomas.

Thinning or atrophy of the skin, which makes the skin appear smooth or finely wrinkled, accompanies aging and may follow long-term use of topical steroids. Atrophy of the dermis usually follows destruction of dermal tissue by an inflammatory condition. Such atrophy appears as a skin depression.

Erosions (ulcerations) may accompany atrophy. They result from superficial damage, such as maceration and excoriation. Dried exudate from erosions forms crusts. Erosions may involve the entire thickness of the epidermis and subcutaneous layers. (For illustrations of common abnormal skin lesions, see *Primary and secondary skin lesions,* pages 94 and 95.)

Inspection may reveal a wide variety of vascular lesions. It may detect flushing, hemangiomas (small, usually benign tumors consisting of blood vessels) and telangiectasia (permanent dilation of groups of superficial capillaries, common in pregnancy and hepatic cirrhosis). Erythema (redness that can be blanched caused by vasodilation) may be localized or generalized and may accompany wheals (a condition in which intravascular fluid leaves the capillaries, causing local edema). Purpura occurs when blood seeps into the dermis after blood vessel disruption. With palpable (papular) purpura, raised purple lesions may represent an inflammatory process disrupting the blood vessel walls, such as sepsis or collagen vascular disease; an adverse reaction to some drugs; or edematous disseminated intravascular coagulation. Such lesions herald the progress of a potentially fatal condition. Nonpalpable (macular) purpura produces macular purple lesions and occurs secondary to clotting disorders or capillary fragility. Immediately report either type of purpura to the physician for further evaluation.

Additional vascular lesions may occur, such as a cherry angioma (a round, raised, bright red, 1- to 3-mm lesion that usually appears on the trunk, partially blanches, and occurs with aging), a spider angioma (a round, central lesion of up to 2 mm, surrounded by fine vascular "legs," that appears on the upper half of the body, blanches with pressure, and may accompany liver disease, vitamin B deficiency, or pregnancy), ecchymosis or bruise (a large, irregularly shaped, hemorrhagic area, ranging from purple or purplish blue to green, yellow, or brown in color), or petechiae (small, 1- to 3-mm, red or purple hemorrhagic spots, possibly from vascular leaks or a decreased platelet count).

Changes in the sebaceous glands also may cause skin changes. Increased sebum production, for example, causes the skin to look and feel oily but does not necessarily cause skin lesions. Blockage or impaction of a sebaceous gland outlet produces a comedo (blackhead), the classic lesion of acne. Inflammation around the follicles may cause formation of pustules, papules, nodules, and cysts, resulting in acne.

Sweat gland changes also may cause observable differences. Anhidrosis (absence of sweat) results from atrophic changes in sweat glands; hyperhidrosis (increased sweating) occurs in response to such stimuli as highly seasoned or excessively hot foods or emotional stress. Blockage of eccrine sweat glands may cause miliaria (commonly called prickly heat or heat rash), which is characterized by pruritus, erythema, small papules, and vesicles.

Hair

Hair loss (alopecia), whether normal or pathologic, may be diffuse or patchy. Diffuse hair loss may be caused by hormonal and genetic

Primary and secondary skin lesions

Primary skin lesions appear on previously healthy skin in response to disease or external irritation. Secondary lesions result from changes in the primary lesion, usually related to the disease process. The chart below, arranged alphabetically, illustrates the most common primary and secondary lesions.

PRIMARY LESIONS

Bulla
Fluid-filled lesion greater than 2 cm ($^3/_4$″) in diameter (also called a blister); for example, severe poison oak or ivy dermatitis, bullous pemphigoid, second-degree burn

Comedo
Plugged pilosebaceous duct, exfoliative, formed from sebum and keratin; for example, blackhead (open comedo), whitehead (closed comedo)

Cyst
Semisolid or fluid-filled encapsulated mass extending deep into dermis; for example, acne

Macule
Flat, pigmented, circumscribed area less than 1 cm ($^3/_8$″) in diameter; for example, freckle, rubella

Nodule
Firm, raised lesion; deeper than a papule, extending into dermal layer; 0.5 to 2 cm ($^1/_4$″ to $^3/_4$″) in diameter; for example, intradermal nevus

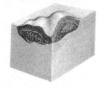

Papule
Firm, inflammatory, raised lesion up to 0.5 cm ($^1/_4$″) in diameter; may be same color as skin or pigmented; for example, acne papule, lichen planus

Patch
Flat, pigmented, circumscribed area greater than 1 cm ($^3/_8$″) in diameter; for example, herald patch (pityriasis rosea)

Plaque
Circumscribed, solid, elevated lesion greater than 1 cm ($^3/_8$″) in diameter. Elevation above skin surface occupies larger surface area in comparison with height; for example, psoriasis

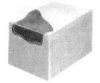

Pustule
Raised, circumscribed lesion usually less than 1 cm ($^3/_8$″) in diameter; contains purulent material, making it a yellow-white color; for example, acne pustule, impetigo, furuncle

Tumor
Elevated, solid lesion larger than 2 cm ($^3/_4$″) in diameter, extending into dermal and subcutaneous layers; for example, dermatofibroma

Vesicle
Raised, circumscribed, fluid-filled lesion less than 0.5 cm ($^1/_4$″) in diameter; for example, chicken pox, herpes simplex

Wheal
Raised, firm lesion with intense localized skin edema, varying in size and shape; color varies from pale pink to red; disappears in hours; for example, hive (urticaria), insect bite

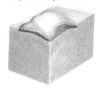

Primary and secondary skin lesions *(continued)*

SECONDARY LESIONS

Atrophy
Thinning of skin surface at site of disorder; for example, striae, aging skin

Crust
Dried sebum, serous, sanguineous, or purulent exudate overlaying an erosion or weeping vesicle, bulla, or pustule; for example, impetigo

Erosion
Circumscribed lesion involving loss of superficial epidermis; for example, rug burn, abrasion

Excoriation
Linear scratched or abraded areas, often self-induced; for example, abraded acne lesions, eczema

Fissure
Linear cracking of the skin extending into dermal layer; for example, hand dermatitis (chapped skin)

Keloid
Thick, red, or dark firm scar formed by hyperplasia of fibrous tissue; more common in Blacks and Asians; for example, surgical incision

Lichenification
Thickened, prominent skin markings caused by constant rubbing; for example, chronic atopic dermatitis

Scale
Thin, dry flakes of shedding skin; for example, psoriasis, dry skin, newborn desquamation

Scar
Fibrous tissue caused by trauma, deep inflammation, or surgical incision; red and raised (recent), pink and flat (6 weeks), or pale and depressed (old); for example, a healed surgical incision

Ulcer
Epidermal and dermal destruction; may extend into subcutaneous tissue; usually heals with scarring; for example, decubitus or stasis ulcer

changes (male or female pattern hair loss), systemic infections, hypothyroidism, or a reaction to chemicals or medications. Anticancer drugs commonly cause hair loss because of their effects on rapidly dividing cells. Patchy hair loss may accompany scalp infections, such as ringworm, which typically produces reddened bald patches with broken-off hair stumps; bacterial infections of the scalp (folliculitis, furuncles, and carbuncles); secondary syphilis; and chicken pox. Traumatic alopecia (hair loss caused by plucking or breaking the hair) may result from permanent waving, using hot combs, wearing pony tails, or trichotillomania.

Nails

Exogenous causes of nail color changes include contact with such agents as silver nitrate or gentian violet, cosmetics, or occupational chemicals and trauma. Endogenous causes include poisons, drugs, lymphatic disease, endocrine disorders, cardiovascular disorders, metabolic and congenital disorders, and infection. White spots or streaks on the nails (leukonychia) may result from trauma, cardiovascular or liver disease, or renal failure. Yellow nails may accompany lymphatic abnormalities or thyrotoxicosis, but also may result from nicotine staining (in heavy cigarette smokers). Green nails usually suggest *Pseudomonas* infection; blue nails may be caused by drugs, such as zidovudine (distal discoloration only), or vascular disease. Gastrointestinal disease or nutritional disorders may cause bright pink nails. Renal disease causes a pigmentary change—a vertical brown line at the free edge of the nail.

Additional nail abnormalities may be present. Beau's lines (transverse depressions in all nails) may signal severe, acute illness; malnutrition; or anemia. Fingernail clubbing, which causes fingertip enlargement and a spongy, swollen nail base, often indicates a cardiopulmonary disorder. Koilonychia (spoon-shaped nails with a concave curve) is associated with chronic eczema, nail bed tumor, systemic diseases, and anemia. Onycholysis (partial separation of the distal nail edge) may occur in heart disease and other chronic disorders. Paronychia (erythema, swelling, and thickening of the skin around the nail edges) usually results from moniliasis but may also occur with diabetes, bacterial infections, third-stage syphilis, or leprosy. Pterygium (nail matrix inflammation accompanied by fusion of the proximal nail fold to the nail bed) may indicate peripheral vascular disease, trauma, or lichen planus.

Palpation

Use the following guidelines when palpating the skin. Wash the hands before and after each patient encounter, and wear gloves when palpating moist skin lesions or mucous membranes.

Skin

Palpation allows assessment of skin texture, consistency, temperature, moisture, and turgor. It also permits evaluation of changes or tenderness of particular lesions. Also, touching the skin reassures the patient that the nurse is not afraid of making physical contact.

Texture and consistency. Skin texture refers to smoothness or coarseness; consistency refers to changes in skin thickness or firmness and relates more to changes associated with lesions. Always note the general texture of the skin and the location of any changes, such as roughness. Skin texture may vary with age and nutrition, as in the thin, fragile skin of an elderly or emaciated patient. Skin thickness also varies with age and body area. For example, thin skin covers the eyelids, whereas thick skin covers the soles, palms, elbows, and other areas subject to local pressure or rubbing.

Temperature. Assess temperature by using the dorsal surfaces of the fingers or hands, which are most sensitive to temperature perception. The skin should feel warm to cool, and areas should feel the same on both sides of the patient's body.

Moisture. To prevent confusing the patient's moisture with that of the nurse, assess for moisture with the relatively dry dorsal surface of the hands and fingers. Moisture normally varies in different parts of the body; the greatest amounts are found on the palms, soles, and skin folds (intertriginous areas).

Turgor. Assess skin turgor (elasticity) by gently grasping and pulling up a fold of skin, releasing it, and observing how quickly it returns to normal shape. Normal skin usually resumes its flat shape immediately. This technique also helps in assessing skin mobility, which may be diminished in connective tissue disorders.

Lesions. Palpating skin lesions provides details about their morphology, distribution, location, and configuration, as described earlier.

Hair
To palpate the patient's hair, rub a few strands between the index finger and thumb, then feel for dryness, brittleness, oiliness, and thickness.

Nails
When palpating the nails, assess the nail base for firmness and the nail for firm adherence to the nail bed; sponginess and swelling accompany clubbing.

Abnormal findings
Skin texture may vary with disease, as in the smooth, soft skin of hyperthyroidism or the coarse, dry skin of hypothyroidism. Dermal flow may affect skin temperature; for example, the entire skin surface may feel warm in a patient with vasodilation caused by fever, whereas it may feel cold in a patient in shock because of local constriction of peripheral vessels. Localized temperature changes also may reflect underlying conditions. For instance, localized warmth may indicate inflammation or infection, whereas coolness of the legs may signal decreased peripheral circulation related to arteriosclerosis. Although skin feels drier during the winter, severe dryness can indicate dehydration. Increased

perspiration may result from abnormally increased sweat gland function.

When assessing skin turgor, describe abnormal findings as *tenting*, because of the shape the pinched skin assumes. Decreased turgor may occur in the elderly patient from decreased elastin content, but it more commonly results from dehydration; increased turgor may occur with edema.

Essential hypertrichosis (hirsutism, or excessive hair growth) occurs in women on the face and legs; the amount ranges from a few hairs to extreme overgrowth. Suspect an underlying endocrine disorder in recent hypertrichosis.

Gentle pressure on the nail causes blanching of the nail bed as blood is forced out of the capillaries; color should return rapidly on release of pressure as blood returns to the capillaries. Known as capillary refill, this maneuver evaluates both central cyanosis (when accompanied by mucosal cyanosis) and peripheral cyanosis (independent of mucosal cyanosis) related to reduced peripheral blood supply.

Cultural considerations

Normal skin variations in a dark-skinned patient require careful assessment. A pigmented line of demarcation (Futcher's line) that extends diagonally from the shoulder to the elbow, and deep pigmentation of ridges in the palm, occur normally in some individuals with dark skin. Yellow-brown pigmentation of the sclera in a Black patient is normal and does not indicate jaundice. The Black patient also may normally have a freckled or patchy appearing oral mucosa, with dark brown or even blue gingivae; do not confuse such coloring with cyanosis.

Common skin disorders also appear differently on dark skin. Lesions that are deep red in Caucasians may be deep purple in Blacks. Many inflammatory conditions lead to chronic pigment changes.

Developmental considerations for pediatric patients

The thin, delicate skin of an infant may appear mottled from the development of the cutaneous capillary network. An infant with less subcutaneous tissue may appear redder than one with thicker subcutaneous tissue. A dark-skinned infant may appear lighter at birth than at age 2 to 3 months, when melanocytes are fully functional. A normal physiologic jaundice (related to the destruction of excess red blood cells) may occur 2 to 3 days after birth but should resolve in about a week.

Although the full-term infant has all necessary skin structures at birth, most of these structures are functionally immature. For example, nails remain quite thin for the first 18 months. The premature infant has soft nails and light-appearing skin because of incomplete melanization and less prominent accumulation of sebum (vernix caseosa). The immature sweat glands of the premature infant may also interfere with thermoregulation. Desquamation (shedding of the epidermis) normally begins a few days after birth, especially on the infant's wrist and ankle creases. Neonates may have profuse hair or no hair at all; hair present at birth is usually shed within the first 3 months. Most abundant on the scalp, face, and genitals, sebaceous glands secrete sebum, which may contribute to cradle cap (sebum accumulation manifested as a yellow, greasy crusting with matted hair). The skin of a dehydrated or malnourished infant or young child readily demonstrates tenting in response to skin turgor tests.

Other normal skin variations in an infant, such as milia (small white papules on the face) and nevus flammeus (port-wine stain), may distress the parents. Provide information and reassure the parents that the changes are normal.

Diaper dermatitis (rash), also common in infants, may result from numerous causes, such as infrequent diaper changes, poor hygiene, psoriasis, seborrhea, and candidiasis. The condition, which first appears as a smooth erythematous eruption, with or without scales and vesicles, tends to spare the skin creases. Establish the underlying cause before initiating therapy. For example, candidiasis, a superficial fungal infection, commonly occurs in the diaper area as a scaly, red, papular rash, and on the oral mucosa as a widespread, creamy or bluish white film. Both manifestations require antifungal treatment. Viral and bacterial infections that commonly occur in children also cause many skin lesions.

Between infancy and puberty, the skin changes very little, although the texture may coarsen. Changes in hair texture and distribution and sebaceous and sweat gland activity increase at puberty.

The adolescent patient may be particularly modest, so take special care to preserve privacy while assessing the skin, hair, and nails. During inspection, look for increased skin and scalp oiliness. Assess for characteristic adult body odor from functional maturation of apocrine glands, as well as pubic and axillary hair and male or female body hair patterns. Acne, common in the prepubertal and adolescent patient, also causes much concern. Lesions typically occur as comedones, papules, pustules, nodules, and cysts on the face, back, and upper chest. Establishing a trusting, caring relationship while assessing the adolescent patient increases cooperation during planning and implementation of skin care and treatment regimens.

Developmental considerations for pregnant patients

Pregnancy may affect the skin, hair, and nails. Melanocyte activity increases during pregnancy and may cause generalized hyperpigmentation. Scars, moles, and the areola tend to darken, and a brownish black streak (linea nigra) may appear on the midline of the abdomen. Facial skin may darken, a condition called chloasma or the mask of pregnancy. Other common manifestations of pregnancy include striae (stretch marks), spider angiomas, varicose veins, brittle nails, and increased sweating. A pregnant patient also may experience hair changes, such as straightening, increased oiliness, or partial hair loss.

Developmental considerations for elderly patients

In the elderly patient, the epidermis may thin and flatten so that it looks like parchment, and blood vessels may become more visible. Skin permeability makes the skin more susceptible to absorption. The dermis becomes less elastic from loss of collagen and elastin fibers, and wrinkles develop. The subcutaneous tissue layer may diminish, resulting in increased bony prominence and less protection from pressure. Decreased numbers of functioning sebaceous and sweat glands cause skin dryness and impair thermoregulation. Although usually age-related, the same changes may occur at a younger age because of photo-aging (actinic damage from sun exposure).

Elderly patients commonly have gray or white hair, from decreased numbers of functioning melanocytes. Changes in hair-growth stages within the hair follicles, decreased androgen production in the elderly male patient, and a decreased ratio of estrogen to androgen in the elderly female patient may cause changes in hair distribution, including baldness; growth of coarse hair in men's ears and on women's faces; and loss of axillary and pubic hair. Decreased peripheral circulation, particularly in the toes, typically increases the thickness and fragility of toenails and turns them yellow.

Documentation The following example shows correct documentation of normal physical assessment findings:

Weight: 134 lb

Vital signs: T 98.6° F, P 72/minute and regular, R 18/minute and regular, BP 130/70.

Additional notes: Black female patient, age 60. Skin warm to touch; color medium brown; smooth and pliable; minimal wrinkling and good turgor. Skin somewhat thickened and rough on extensor surfaces of knees. Two hypopigmented patches on left anterior calf, approximately 1½″ and 2″ in diameter. About 15 to 20 dark brown to black, rough, dry, flat nevi 0.5 to 1 cm in diameter, scattered on thorax.

Mucous membranes moist, slight bluish brown cast throughout oral mucosa. Palpebral conjunctiva also brownish, and bulbar conjunctiva yellowish.

Scalp hair is coarse, tightly curled terminal hair with even distribution, showing some graying on crown, worn short (1½″) all over head. Skin is moist in intertriginous areas of breasts.

Nails well-groomed, with good capillary refill and normal 160-degree angle; some thickening and longitudinal ridges on toenails.

The following example shows correct documentation of abnormal physical assessment findings:

Weight: 100 lb

Vital signs: T 99° F, P 100/minute and irregular, R 20/minute and regular, BP 90/60.

Additional notes: Female patient, Caucasian, age 27. Takes Motrin (400 mg) prescribed by gynecologist t.i.d. 3 days before menses, sometimes q.i.d. during days 1 and 2. Skin color golden tan from recent beach vacation, pale white in areas covered by bikini. No scars; skin has good turgor. Several lichenified, hyperpigmented patches at flexural folds of arms.

Lesion on upper lip at border: small group of ruptured vesicles coated with yellow crust. Center of largest vesicle ulcerated and tender to palpation. (Patient says constant annoyance #3 on 1 to 10 scale, increases to #5 or #6 when touched; tried coating lesions with camphor ice.)

Mucous membranes moist, oral mucosa pink, with thick, rough, reddened area inside lower lip on right side. Palpebral conjunctiva pale.

Terminal scalp hair bleached pale blond, worn long and permed; many broken hair ends noted, dark roots in some areas, some scalp irritation with scaling at nape of neck and above ears.

Nails clean and well-groomed, toenails short and polished; fingernails long, tapered, and polished.

STUDY ACTIVITIES

Multiple choice

1. Which of the following is a secondary skin lesion?
   A. Plaque
   B. Comedo
   C. Erosion
   D. Vesicle

2. Which of the following is a primary skin lesion?
   A. Bulla
   B. Crust
   C. Keloid
   D. Scale

3. Bob Rutter, age 26, seeks care for a skin rash. During the physical assessment, the nurse notes that the rash covers most of the patient's back. What is the distribution of this rash?
   A. Localized
   B. Regionalized
   C. Generalized
   D. Intertriginous

4. When inspecting Mr. Rutter's skin, the nurse notes that the lesions are arranged in single rings. Which configuration does this represent?
   A. Arciform
   B. Reticular
   C. Polycyclic
   D. Annular

5. During a prenatal visit, Rhonda Stone, age 22, displays a brownish black streak on the midline of her abdomen. What is this skin change?

   A. Striae

   B. Chloasma

   C. Linea nigra

   D. Spider angioma

Fill in the blank

6. The two distinct layers of the skin are the _____ and _____.

7. A _____ is a primary, raised, firm lesion with intense, localized edema that may disappear in hours.

8. An encapsulated mass of semisolid or fluid matter, such as seen in acne, is called a _____.

9. _____ is an allergic skin disorder that frequently is familial.

10. _____ lesions spread from the trunk to the limbs; _____ lesions spread along cutaneous nerve endings.

11. A drug history is helpful in skin assessment because, for example, _____ can cause photosensitivity and _____ can cause hivelike and macular or papular eruptions.

12. _____ are skin regions found along cutaneous nerve endings.

ANSWERS

Multiple choice

1. C. An erosion is a secondary skin lesion caused by superficial damage.

2. A. A bulla is a primary skin lesion and also is called a blister.

3. B. A localized rash covers a small area; a regionalized rash covers a larger area; a generalized rash covers the whole body.

4. D. Lesions in an annular configuration are arranged in a single ring or circle. Arciform lesions form arcs or curves; reticular lesions form a meshlike network; and polycyclic lesions form concentric circles.

5. C. During pregnancy, generalized hyperpigmentation can cause linea nigra and darkening of scars, moles, and areolae.

Fill in the blank

6. epidermis, dermis

7. wheal

8. cyst

9. Atopic dermatitis

10. Chicken pox (varicella), shingles (herpes zoster)

11. tetracycline, penicillins

12. Dermatomes

CHAPTER 7

Head and neck

OBJECTIVES   After studying this chapter, the reader should be able to:
1. Discuss the anatomy of the head and neck.
2. Give examples of appropriate health history questions to ask the patient when assessing the head and neck.
3. Describe how to inspect, palpate, percuss, and auscultate the structures of the head and neck.
4. Describe normal findings from a head and neck assessment for patients of all ages.
5. Describe common abnormalities that may be found during head and neck assessment.
6. Document head and neck assessment findings.

OVERVIEW OF CONCEPTS   Head and neck assessment includes evaluation of the head, face, nose, sinuses, mouth, and neck. (For illustrations of these structures, see *Anatomy of the head and neck*, page 104.)

   The health history is vitally important in head and neck assessment because of the wide range of disorders that can affect these structures. Such disorders range from an episodic illness or injury to a life-threatening disease. For example, headache may result from work-related tension—a bothersome but treatable condition—or from a much more serious problem, such as a brain tumor or stroke (cerebrovascular accident [CVA]). To detect a serious underlying condition, the nurse must conduct a symptom analysis.

Health history   Because of the many structures of the head and neck, the nurse should construct health history questions that elicit information on diverse topics, ranging from headaches to oral hygiene. To gather information about the patient's chief complaint and current status, use the PQRST method. (For a detailed explanation of this method, see *Symptom analysis,* page 15.) Because some head and neck problems are emergencies, the nurse may have to delay the complete health history until the patient's condition is stabilized.

Anatomy of the head and neck

Before assessing the head and neck, the nurse should be familiar with their structures.

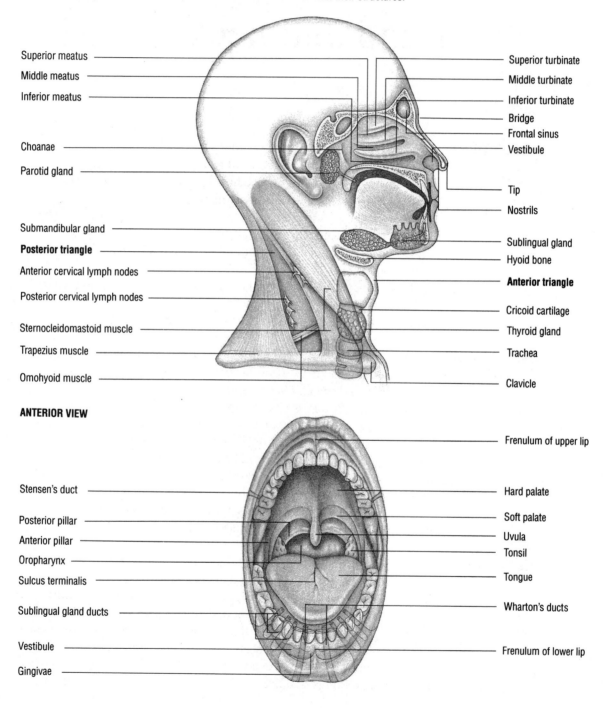

Superior meatus
Middle meatus
Inferior meatus

Choanae
Parotid gland

Submandibular gland
Posterior triangle
Anterior cervical lymph nodes
Posterior cervical lymph nodes

Sternocleidomastoid muscle
Trapezius muscle
Omohyoid muscle

Superior turbinate
Middle turbinate
Inferior turbinate
Bridge
Frontal sinus
Vestibule

Tip
Nostrils

Sublingual gland
Hyoid bone
Anterior triangle

Cricoid cartilage
Thyroid gland
Trachea

Clavicle

ANTERIOR VIEW

Stensen's duct

Posterior pillar
Anterior pillar
Oropharynx
Sulcus terminalis

Sublingual gland ducts

Vestibule
Gingivae

Frenulum of upper lip

Hard palate

Soft palate
Uvula
Tonsil

Tongue

Wharton's ducts

Frenulum of lower lip

Health and illness patterns

Begin compiling the health history by investigating the patient's current, past, and family health status. Use the following questions to help elicit the most valuable information.

Have you ever had head trauma, skull surgery, or a jaw or facial fracture? If so, when? Have you had any problems since the injury?
(RATIONALE: Head trauma, skull surgery, or jaw or facial fractures can change the configuration of the skull or face, producing abnormalities that should be observed in a physical assessment. Be sure to note any sequelae of a serious injury.)

Do you have frequent headaches? If so, where does your head hurt? What is the pain like? How often and during what part of the day do the headaches occur? What brings them on? What makes them better?
(RATIONALE: Answers to these questions can help distinguish one type of headache from another. For example, a muscle contraction [tension] headache usually produces a tight sensation in the occipital or temporal area and is relieved by mild analgesics or rest. Headache from a brain tumor typically causes a dull, deep pain that worsens in the morning and improves as the day progresses; analgesics provide little relief.)

Have you ever had a sinus infection, tenderness, or facial swelling? If so, when?
(RATIONALE: Sinus infections tend to recur in persons susceptible to such infections. Tenderness usually accompanies sinus infections. Facial swelling may be caused by severe sinusitis.)

Do you have any nasal discharge or postnasal drip? If so, describe it. When does it occur?
(RATIONALE: Nasal discharge and postnasal drip typically result from infections, allergies, or environmental irritants. Thick, purulent discharge suggests infection; a watery discharge suggests an allergy or irritant.)

Do you have frequent or prolonged nosebleeds?
(RATIONALE: Epistaxis [nosebleed] can occur with overuse of nasal sprays, elevated blood pressure, hematopoietic disorders [such as leukemia and thrombocytopenia], and other problems.)

What over-the-counter (OTC) drugs, prescription medications, or recreational substances do you currently use?
(RATIONALE: OTC drugs and prescription medications can cause numerous adverse reactions affecting the head and neck. In particular, chronic use of OTC nasal sprays can lead to mucosal irritation. Cocaine, an illegal stimulant, is commonly inhaled through the nose and may erode the nasal septum.)

Have you ever had mouth lesions, ulcers, or cold sores? If so, do they recur?
(RATIONALE: Herpes simplex produces vesicles that rupture and leave painful, crusting ulcers [cold sores] that typically recur. Aphthous stomatitis also produces painful, recurrent ulcers [canker sores].)

Do you have any trouble swallowing or chewing?
(RATIONALE: Painful swallowing accompanied by hoarseness may indicate cancer of the larynx or esophagus. Difficulty chewing or swallowing may result from dental problems, such as malocclusion, or from neuromuscular disorders, such as CVA.)

Do you have any allergies? If so, please describe your symptoms.
(RATIONALE: Some allergic reactions manifest in the head and neck. For example, hay fever [seasonal rhinitis] commonly causes nasal and eye irritation.)

Have you ever had a neck injury or difficulty moving your neck?
(RATIONALE: Neck injuries can cause chronic pain and restrict neck movement. Other causes of restricted neck movement include cervical arthritis and inflamed lymph nodes.)

Developmental considerations for pediatric patients
Ask the child's parent or guardian the following questions:

Is the child's drinking water treated with fluoride?
(RATIONALE: Fluoride helps prevent dental caries, especially in children. If the child's water is not fluoridated, ask what other measures the family takes to prevent caries, such as taking fluoride supplements.)

Does the child use a pacifier or suck the thumb?
(RATIONALE: These habits misalign the upper teeth as they erupt.)

Developmental considerations for elderly patients
Ask an elderly patient the following question:

Do you wear dentures? If so, how well do they fit?
(RATIONALE: Ill-fitting dentures can cause reluctance to speak, difficulty with eating, or gingival lesions.)

Health promotion and protection patterns
The following questions help the nurse assess behavioral patterns that may affect the patient's health status.

Do you smoke cigarettes, cigars, or a pipe? Do you chew tobacco or use snuff?
(RATIONALE: Any tobacco use increases the risk for head and neck cancers.)

Do you grind your teeth?
(RATIONALE: Bruxism [grinding of teeth, especially while sleeping] can be a sign of stress.)

Does a job or recreational activity put you at risk for head injury? If so, do you wear a helmet to protect your head? Do you wear a seat belt when you are in an automobile?
(RATIONALE: Answers to these questions will show how highly the patient regards personal safety. They also may point to a need for safety teaching.)

How often do you brush and floss your teeth? When was your last dental examination?
(RATIONALE: These questions elicit information about the patient's dental health habits.)

Role and relationship patterns
A head or neck problem can affect the way a patient feels about roles and relationships with others. The following question can reveal such difficulties:

Does your head or neck problem affect the way you feel about yourself or the way you relate to your family?
(RATIONALE: Many head and neck problems cause chronic pain, which may interfere with the patient's ability to care for self and others.)

Physical assessment

For a complete head and neck assessment, the nurse uses the four major examination techniques—inspection, palpation, percussion, and auscultation—and the following equipment: stethoscope, tape measure, glass of water, tongue depressor, gloves, 4″ × 4″ gauze pad, small flashlight, and nasal speculum or ophthalmoscope handle with nasal attachment. Universal precautions should be observed.

Examining the head and face
First, observe the patient's spontaneous facial expression, noting any tics, twitching, or other abnormal movements. Inspect the head and face for abnormalities in size, shape, contour, or symmetry. Observe the head; it should be erect and midline, and the patient should be able to hold it still. Inspect the face for symmetry, paying special attention to the palpebral fissures and nasolabial folds. Check that the eyes are equidistant both midline and laterally and that they align horizontally with the helix, the prominent outer rim of the ear.

Look for facial lesions, rash, swelling, or redness. Keep in mind that certain facial features are characteristic of race. Examine the scalp and hair, observing how the hair is distributed on the scalp and face and whether it is appropriate to the sex. (For more information about this part of the assessment, see Chapter 6, Skin, hair, and nails.) Also note facial color. Pallor or cyanosis (bluish skin tone) usually appears first in the oral mucous membranes. Yellow skin and sclerae may indicate jaundice.

Next, palpate the head and face to learn more about their condition, observing universal precautions. Use the fingertips to discriminate skin surface textures and the pads of the fingers to determine the configuration and consistency of bony structures or skin lesions.

Palpate the head for symmetry and contour. The head should feel symmetrical and be free of lumps and other lesions. It should not be tender to the touch. The scalp should be free from dryness, lesions, or scars and should move freely over the skull. The hair should not feel excessively dry, oily, or brittle and should not be easily plucked.

Next, gently palpate the face to assess skin tone and facial contours, using both hands simultaneously and comparing one side to the other. The face should feel smooth, and the patient should not feel any tenderness or pain. Facial contours should feel symmetrical, with no swelling, edema, or masses. Simultaneously palpate the muscles on both sides of the face while the patient smiles, frowns, grits the teeth, and puffs out the cheeks. This maneuver evaluates facial muscle tone. Check for symmetrical muscle movement with each of these maneuvers.

When palpating the face, be sure to check the temporal artery pulses; they should be of equal strength and rhythm. Palpate the temporomandibular joints (located anterior to and slightly below the auricle) to assess how easily they move, whether they are properly aligned (approximation), and whether they cause any discomfort. To palpate this area, place the middle three fingers of each hand bilaterally over each joint, then press gently on the joints as the patient opens and closes the mouth. The temporomandibular joints should move smoothly and without pain.

Finally, auscultate the temporal arteries using the bell of the stethoscope. Auscultation should not reveal any sounds in these arteries. If any bruits are detected, notify the physician promptly for further evaluation.

Abnormal findings

Skull deformities may result from various causes, including head trauma and surgical removal of part of the skull. In an adult, an abnormally large head may indicate acromegaly, a disorder of excessive growth hormone characterized by enlarged and thickened skull bones, increased mandible length, and increased prominence of the nose and forehead.

Abnormalities in facial color, shape, or symmetry may stem from a systemic disorder. For example, cyanosis of the lips and oral mucosa may occur in serious cardiovascular disorders, such as congestive heart failure, or in serious respiratory disorders, such as chronic obstructive pulmonary disease. A blank or masklike facial expression may indicate Parkinson's disease. Facial pallor can result from shock or anemia. Yellow skin and sclerae suggest jaundice, usually resulting from liver disease.

Examining the nose and sinuses

Inspect the nose for symmetry and contour, noting any areas of deformity or swelling. The nose should be intact and symmetrical, with no edema or deformity. Note any nasal flaring, which may indicate respiratory distress. If nasal discharge is present, note its character and amount.

Next, palpate the nose, checking for painful or tender areas, swelling, and deformities. Evaluate nostril patency by gently occluding one nostril with a finger and having the patient inhale and exhale through the other.

To assess the sinuses, inspect, palpate, and percuss the frontal and maxillary sinuses. First, inspect the external skin surfaces above and lateral to the nose for inflammation or edema. Then palpate the sinuses by placing the thumb over each sinus and pressing gently. For the frontal sinuses, place the thumb just above the eye, under the bony ridge of the orbit. For the maxillary sinuses, place the thumbs on each side of the nose in the area just below the zygomatic bone. Note any unusual warmth over the sinuses. To percuss the sinuses, gently tap the index finger over the areas mentioned above. Neither maneuver should elicit tenderness.

Abnormal findings

Inspection of the nose may reveal asymmetrical bones or cartilages, causing a deviation to one side. Marked flaring of the nostrils may indicate respiratory distress, especially in a child. Nonpatent nostrils may indicate simple nasal congestion, a nasal fracture, or a deviated septum.

The type and amount of drainage from the nostrils provides clues to its origin. Bloody drainage may be minor from frequent blowing, or major from spontaneous or traumatic epistaxis. Thick white, yellow, or green drainage usually occurs with infection, such as in sinusitis. Clear, thin drainage may be associated with allergic or viral rhinitis (nasal irritation). Rarely, cerebrospinal fluid leakage from a basilar skull fracture causes copious, clear nasal discharge.

Pain or discomfort elicited by sinus palpation may indicate sinus congestion or infection. Sinusitis often is accompanied by fever or purulent nasal discharge as well as warmth over the sinus region. Swelling over sinus areas also may indicate congestion or infection.

Examining the mouth and oropharynx

Observe universal precautions. Ask the patient to remove any partial or complete dentures to allow better visualization of the inside of the mouth and throat. Note how the dentures fit and how easily the patient can remove them.

Next, note any unusual breath odors. Inspect the oral mucosa by inserting a tongue depressor between the teeth and the cheek to examine the membranous tissue. It should be moist, smooth, and free of lesions. Note the color of the mucosa; it is usually pink, although in dark-skinned patients, it may be bluish-tinted or patchily pigmented. Assess for tenderness at Stensen's duct openings—small, white-rimmed openings located at the level of the second molar in each cheek.

When examining the oral mucosa, observe the gingivae and teeth. Gingival surfaces should appear pink and moist, with no spongy or edematous areas. Check tooth color, which normally varies from bright white to ivory. Tooth edges should be smooth, with no areas of unusual wear. Note any missing, broken, or loose teeth. To assess occlusion of the upper and lower jaw, ask the patient to close the mouth gently. The upper teeth should extend slightly beyond and over the lower teeth.

The tongue should appear moist, pink, and slightly rough, with a midline depression and a V-shaped division (sulcus terminalis linguae) separating the anterior two thirds from the posterior third. The tongue should fit comfortably into the floor of the mouth. Note any lesions or bleeding. Geographic tongue (superficial, irregular areas of the tongue with exposed tips of the papillae) is normal.

The position of the tongue in the mouth helps evaluate the function of cranial nerve XII, which controls tongue movement. To perform this assessment, ask the patient to stick out the tongue, then observe for midline positioning, voluntary movement, and tremors. Next, ask the patient to touch the tip of the tongue to the roof of the mouth; observe the underside for lesions or other abnormalities. The bottom surface of the tongue should be smoother and pinker than the top surface. Also inspect the lingual frenulum (the membrane that anchors the tongue to the floor) and the submandibular (Wharton's) ducts. Saliva should be visibly pooled on the floor of the mouth.

Inspect the superior labial frenulum (the membrane that attaches the upper lip to the gingivae) and the inferior labial frenulum (the membrane that attaches the lower lip to the gingivae) for irritation and signs of inflammation.

Examine the oropharynx, using a tongue depressor and flashlight, if necessary. Observe the position, size, and overall appearance of the uvula and tonsils. Then, place the tongue depressor firmly at the midpoint of the tongue—almost far back enough to elicit the gag reflex—and ask the patient to say "ah." The soft palate and uvula should rise immediately.

Observe the tonsils for unilateral or bilateral enlargement. The tonsils should be the same color as the rest of the pharyngeal mucosa. Grade tonsil size on a scale of 0 to + 4. A grade of 0 (normal) indicates that both tonsils are behind the pillars (the supporting structures of the soft palate); +1, that the tonsils peak from the pillars; +2, that the tonsils are between the pillars and the uvula; +3, that the tonsils touch the uvula; and + 4, that one or both tonsils extend to the midline of the oropharynx.

Evaluating the gag reflex is the last step of the basic mouth and oropharynx assessment. With the tongue depressor, gently touch the posterior aspect of the patient's tongue. (*Note:* Use this technique cautiously in a patient with nausea because it may induce vomiting.) Gagging indicates that cranial nerves IX and X (the glossopharyngeal and vagus nerves) are intact.

Abnormal findings

Any abnormalities warrant further evaluation and appropriate referral to a physician or nurse practitioner. An unusual breath odor may indicate a serious systemic disorder. For example, an ammonia breath odor may be caused by chronic renal failure; fecal breath odor, by a gastrointestinal obstruction or disorder; fetid breath odor, by streptococcal pharyngitis; and fruity breath odor, by diabetic or starvation ketoacidosis.

Abnormalities of the oral mucosa may point to various disorders. Reddened mucosa often results from infection; cyanotic mucosa may indicate hypoxia (oxygen deficiency). Pale mucous membranes suggest anemia. A painless oral lesion may indicate oral cancer or syphilis and warrants prompt evaluation.

Marginal redness, retraction, swelling, or bleeding of the gingivae may be a sign of gingivitis. Absent or broken teeth, cavities, or malocclusion (improper alignment of the upper and lower teeth) can cause chewing difficulties, leading to poor nutrition.

On the tongue, a smooth dorsal surface, beefy red color, white coating, or patches on the anterior surface suggest an infection. An irritated, beefy red tongue may indicate vitamin B_{12} deficiency. Deviation of the tongue to one side may indicate a problem with cranial nerve XII. Nodules or ulcers, especially painless lesions, may be cancerous.

The oropharynx may be reddened from various conditions, such as infection or irritation. In viral pharyngitis, the throat is usually mildly red. In streptococcal pharyngitis, the pharynx is bright red, possibly with patches of white discharge. Cigarette smoking and allergies also may cause pharyngeal redness; a reddened pharynx typically is accompanied by enlarged tonsils.

Note a decreased or absent gag reflex, which suggests possible neurologic dysfunction and increases the patient's risk for aspiration. Deviation of the uvula to one side when the patient says "ah" could indicate pathology of cranial nerve IX or X. Record the direction and extent of any deviation.

Examining the neck

Begin by inspecting the skin for lesions and by palpating for masses along the chains of lymph nodes. (For further information, see Chapter 18, Immune system and blood, and Chapter 19, Endocrine system.) Observe the neck area for jugular vein distention and visible pulsations in the carotid and jugular veins. (For more information, see Chapter

10, Cardiovascular system.) The neck should be free of masses, lymph node enlargement or tenderness, and venous distention.

Next, check the neck muscles for strength and symmetry. Have the patient move the neck through its entire range of motion, including extension, flexion, and lateral bending, The neck should be supple, moving easily and without discomfort. (For more information on major neck muscles, see Chapter 17, Musculoskeletal system.) To evaluate innervation of the neck, shoulder, and upper arm muscles, have the patient slowly and carefully rotate the neck through the entire range of motion, then shrug the shoulders and lift the arms.

Inspect and palpate the trachea for its position; it should be midline in the neck. Place the index finger or thumb along each side of the trachea and assess the space between the trachea and sternocleidomastoid muscle. It should be equal on each side; narrowing on either side indicates tracheal deviation to that side. (For information on evaluating the thyroid, see Chapter 19, Endocrine system.)

To assess the ability to swallow, have the patient sip water with the head tipped back slightly. Normally, the larynx, trachea, and thyroid rise with swallowing. Palpate down the posterior neck over the bony prominences of the cervical vertebrae, checking for tenderness.

Abnormal findings

Neck pain and stiffness can result from many disorders, including trauma, cervical arthritis, and osteoporosis. If tracheal deviation is detected, consider the possibility of a neck or mediastinal tumor. Muscle spasm and tenderness may result from simple tension, but sometimes are caused by a neck injury that does not involve the vertebrae. Nuchal rigidity (severe muscle stiffness at the nape of the neck) is characteristic of meningitis.

Developmental considerations for pediatric patients

To assess the head of a child under age 2, measure head circumference and assess the fontanels. The head circumference, which provides information about nutritional and growth disturbances, should increase on a predictable basis. (For information on this procedure, see Chapter 5, Nutritional status.) Record the result on the child's growth chart, and compare it to the normal range for the child's age group. An abnormal measurement or a change from the former growth pattern requires further evaluation by a physician or nurse practitioner.

Assess the fontanels—particularly the large anterior fontanel–by inspecting and then gently palpating with the pads of the index and middle fingers. The fontanels should feel soft, yet firm, and should appear almost flush with the scalp surface with slight visible pulsations. For the most accurate findings, examine the fontanels when the infant is quiet and seated upright. Pressure from postural changes or intense crying can cause the fontanels to bulge or seem abnormally tense. Also palpate the sutures; they should feel smooth and should not override one another or feel separated.

When examining a neonate's head and face, remember that the shape may be altered by the molding that occurs during vaginal delivery. Absence of molding may indicate premature closure of the sutures (craniosynostosis), a condition that requires immediate evaluation.

Be aware that congenital syndromes can alter a child's facial appearance. For example, a child with congenital hypothyroidism (cretinism) has coarse facial features, a low hairline, and sparse eyebrows. One with Down's syndrome typically has a small, rounded head; prominent epicanthal folds; small, low-set ears; and oblique palpebral fissures.

Assess whether the nares are patent bilaterally. Most infants under age 6 months breathe only through the nose, not through the mouth; nasal congestion may cause considerable respiratory distress.

In an infant, an unusually large or small tongue may indicate a congenital abnormality. Macroglossia (a grossly enlarged tongue) may occur in cretinism, Down's syndrome, and other disorders. A tight frenulum—a congenital abnormality that may cause speech problems—prevents the child from touching the tip of the tongue to the upper lip.

Evaluate the tonsils according to the child's developmental stage. Tonsils are small in the neonate, enlarge progressively until age 5, then start to decrease at age 10 and continue to shrink through adolescence. In a neonate, raised white spots called Epstein's pearls may occur normally along the gum line or on the hard palate. These spots usually disappear a few weeks after birth.

An infant's neck should move easily in all directions. However, the muscles are not sufficiently developed to enable the infant to turn the head from side to side until about age 2 weeks; to lift the head 90 degrees when prone until about age 2 months; or to hold the head upright when seated until about age 3 months. Infants and young children normally have very short necks.

Developmental considerations for pregnant patients

After the 16th week of pregnancy, many women develop a blotchy, brownish hyperpigmentation of the face called melasma ("mask of pregnancy"). Although cosmetically bothersome, this skin disorder is benign and usually fades after delivery. Slight gingival swelling also may be normal during pregnancy.

Developmental considerations for elderly patients

Typically, an elderly patient's face is wrinkled from an overall reduction in subcutaneous fat. This fat loss also may make the nose seem more prominent or the bony ridges over the brow more noticeable. An elderly patient usually exhibits some gingival recession and may have loose teeth and gingival inflammation. With aging, salivary output decreases, causing oral dryness and eating difficulties. Longitudinal and latitudinal fissures in the tongue also can occur with aging. Many elderly patients have a decreased range of motion and may experience neck pain from osteoporosis, arthritis, or other disorders.

Documentation

The following illustrates the documentation of some normal physical findings in a head and neck assessment:

Head held upright, facial features are symmetrical. Facial skin color is appropriate for race. Skin is free of lesions, palpable lumps, or tenderness. Temporal pulses are equal and nontender. Auscultation of the head vessels reveals no bruits. Temporomandibular joint moves freely; no tenderness or discomfort present. Nose is symmetrical, nontender, and free of drainage; no sinus tenderness present. Oral and pharyngeal mucosa are pink and moist; teeth are intact. Lips, gingivae, and tongue are free of lesions. Neck has full range of motion and is not tender.

The following illustrates the documentation of some abnormal physical findings in a head and neck assessment:

Head held at midline, with right facial drooping and flattening of nasolabial fold. Tongue is not held at midline, shifts slightly to right; appears moist and pink. Tender, mobile, 1-cm lump, without change in skin temperature and color, noted under left eye over orbital bone. Temporal pulses are +1 on right side and +2 on left; bruit noted on right. Temporomandibular joint on right side does not approximate. No sinus tenderness or nasal discharge present. Gingivae are erythematous and edematous and bleed slightly when palpated. Range of motion is limited by pain; patient cannot flex and rotate neck.

STUDY ACTIVITIES

Fill in the blank

1. The nurse should suspect jaundice if the patient's _____ and _____ are yellow.

2. Muscle movement should be _____ on both sides of the face when the patient smiles, frowns, grits the teeth, and puffs out the cheeks.

3. A blank or masklike facial expression suggests _____.

4. Marked nostril flaring may indicate _____.

5. An ammonia breath odor suggests _____; fecal breath odor suggests _____.

Matching related elements

Match the developmental assessment finding on the left with the patient group on the right.

6. ___ Epstein's pearls   **A.** Elderly patients

7. ___ Melasma   **B.** Pregnant patients

8. ___ Gingival recession   **C.** Infants

9. ___ Head molding   **D.** Neonates

Multiple choice

10. Rosa Garcia, age 35, complains of recurrent headaches. The health history reveals that the headaches cause tightness in the temporal area and usually are relieved by rest or aspirin. What is the most likely cause of Ms. Garcia's headaches?

    A. Brain tumor
    B. Sinus infection
    C. Head trauma
    D. Muscle contraction

11. Lisa Flynn, age 5, who is complaining of a sore throat, is brought to the clinic by her father. She says her throat started bothering her the previous day. When assessing Lisa, the nurse notes that her tonsils touch the uvula. How should the nurse grade this enlargement?

    A. + 1
    B. + 2
    C. + 3
    D. + 4

ANSWERS

Fill in the blank

    1. skin, sclerae
    2. symmetrical
    3. Parkinson's disease
    4. respiratory distress
    5. chronic renal failure, gastrointestinal obstruction or disorder

Matching related elements

    6. C
    7. B
    8. A
    9. D

Multiple choice

10. D. Muscle contraction (tension) headaches usually produce a tight sensation in the occipital or temporal area and are relieved by mild analgesics or rest. Headache due to a brain tumor typically causes deep, dull pain that worsens in the morning and is not relieved by analgesics.

11. C. A grade of + 1 indicates that the tonsils peak from the pillars; + 2, that the tonsils are between the pillars and the uvula; + 3, that the tonsils touch the uvula; and + 4, that one or both tonsils extend to the midline of the oropharynx.

CHAPTER 8

Eyes and ears

OBJECTIVES

After studying this chapter, the reader should be able to:

1. Identify the major structures of the eye.

2. Demonstrate the five acuity tests performed for vision testing.

3. Explain how vision testing for children differs from that for adults.

4. Compare common eye assessment findings for an elderly patient with those for a young adult.

5. Demonstrate how to assess the external and internal eye of an adult and a child.

6. Identify the major structures of the ear.

7. Demonstrate how to assess the external and internal ear of an adult and a child.

8. Discuss possible adverse effects of drugs on hearing.

9. Document assessment findings for a patient with a common eye or ear ailment.

OVERVIEW OF CONCEPTS

Although the eyes and ears differ in structure and function, they share several important features. For example, they are two of the main sources of perception, responsible for sight and hearing. Also, the eyes and ears may be evaluated with similar techniques: screening tests (for vision or hearing), inspection, palpation, and advanced assessment skills (using an ophthalmoscope or an otoscope).

Some eye or ear disorders can signal a serious neurologic problem, such as a brain tumor or an acoustic nerve (cranial nerve VIII) damaged by an adverse drug reaction. Other disorders may indicate an episodic illness, such as conjunctivitis (inflammation of the conjunctivae) or otitis media (middle ear infection). Regardless of the cause, a patient may be especially anxious about an eye or ear disorder because vision and hearing are vital.

This chapter presents the eye and its assessment followed by the ear and its assessment.

Anatomy and physiology review: The eye

The eye is the sensory organ of sight that transmits visual images to the brain for interpretation. The eyeball is about 1″ (2.5 cm) in diameter and occupies the bony orbit, a skull cavity formed anteriorly by the frontal, maxillary, zygomatic, acromial, sphenoid, ethmoid, and palatine bones. Nerves, adipose tissue, and blood vessels cushion and nourish the eye posteriorly. Extraocular (external) and intraocular (internal) structures form the eye, and extraocular muscles and nerves control it. (For an illustration of intraocular structures and of the retina, see *Intraocular muscles and structures,* page 118.)

Every object reflects light. For an individual to perceive an object clearly, reflected light must pass through the intraocular structures, including the cornea, anterior chamber, pupil, lens, and vitreous humor. The retina focuses light into an upside-down and reversed image. This stimulates nerve impulses to travel from the retina through the optic nerve and optic tract to the visual cortex of the occipital lobe, which then interprets the image.

Health history: The eye

The following questions are designed to help evaluate the patient's eyes. They include rationales that explain the significance of the answers.

Health and illness patterns

To assess important health and illness patterns, use the following guidelines to explore the patient's current, past, and family health status, as well as the patient's developmental status.

Current health status

Ask about the patient's current eye health status, using the PQRST method to gain a complete description of any problems. (For an explanation of this method, see *Symptom analysis,* page 15.) If the patient reports eye pain or a sudden change in the ability to see, arrange for immediate referral to an ophthalmologist.

During the interview, observe the patient's eye movements and focusing ability for clues to visual acuity and eye muscle coordination. To investigate further, ask the following questions about eye function:

Do you have any problems with your eyes?
(RATIONALE: Eye problems can indicate such conditions as diabetes, hypertension, or neurologic disorders as well as ophthalmologic disorders. Decreased visual acuity affects the ability to carry out activities of daily living safely, including medication administration.)

Do you wear eyeglasses or contact lenses? If you wear contact lenses, what type? When was your last eye exam?
(RATIONALE: This establishes the patient's need for assistance with vision and the pattern of seeking eye care. Eyeglasses that fully correct-

Intraocular muscles and structures

The nurse can view some intraocular structures, such as the sclera, cornea, iris, pupil, and anterior chamber through inspection. However, others, such as the retina, must be seen through an ophthalmoscope.

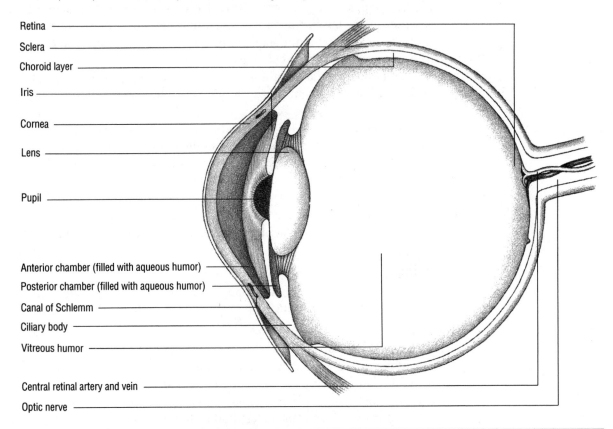

Retina
Sclera
Choroid layer
Iris
Cornea
Lens
Pupil
Anterior chamber (filled with aqueous humor)
Posterior chamber (filled with aqueous humor)
Canal of Schlemm
Ciliary body
Vitreous humor
Central retinal artery and vein
Optic nerve

ed a problem 5 years ago may be of little help now. Improperly fitted or prolonged wearing of contact lenses can cause eye inflammation and corneal abrasions.)

For what eye condition do you wear glasses or contact lenses?
(RATIONALE: Besides providing information about any existing eye condition, the answer allows the nurse to adjust the diopters for nearsightedness or farsightedness in the ophthalmoscopic examination.)

Past health status
During the next part of the health history, ask the following questions to gather additional information about the patient's eyes.

Have you ever had blurred vision?
(RATIONALE: Blurred vision can indicate the need for corrective lenses

or suggest a neurologic disorder, such as a brain tumor, or an endocrine disorder, such as poorly controlled diabetes.)

Have you ever seen spots, floaters, or halos around lights? If yes, is this a sudden change or has it occurred for a while?
(RATIONALE: The sudden appearance of spots, floaters, or halos may indicate retinal detachment or glaucoma. However, be aware that many people have chronic floaters normally.)

Do you suffer from frequent eye infections or inflammation?
(RATIONALE: Frequent infections or inflammation can indicate low resistance to infection, eye strain, allergies, or occupational or environmental exposure to an irritant.)

Have you ever had eye surgery or an eye injury?
(RATIONALE: Changes caused by eye surgery or injury may appear as abnormalities upon ophthalmoscopic examination. Also, a history of eye surgery or injury is significant.)

Do you have a history of high blood pressure or diabetes?
(RATIONALE: Both high blood pressure and diabetes can cause retinopathy, changes in the retina that can lead to blindness.)

Are you currently taking any prescription medications for your eyes? If so, which ones and how often?
(RATIONALE: Use of prescription eye medications should alert the nurse to an eye disorder. For example, a patient who is taking pilocarpine probably has glaucoma.)

What other medications are you taking, including prescription drugs, over-the-counter (OTC) medications, and home remedies?
(RATIONALE: Certain medications and preparations can cause vision disturbances.)

Family health status
Investigate the eye health of the patient's family by asking the following question:

Has anyone in your family ever been treated for cataracts, glaucoma, or macular degeneration?
(RATIONALE: These conditions have a familial tendency.)

Developmental considerations for pediatric patients
When assessing a child who is old enough to participate, include the child in the interview along with the parent or guardian by using age-appropriate words. For an infant, gather information about visual acuity and eye muscle coordination by observing the steadiness of the infant's gaze at the parent's face or nearby objects.

For additional information about the child's developmental status, ask the following questions:

Does your infant gaze at you or other objects and blink at bright lights and quick, nearby movements?
(RATIONALE: Failure to gaze and blink appropriately could indicate impaired vision.)

Does the child squint frequently?
(RATIONALE: Squinting implies a vision disturbance, such as farsightedness or light sensitivity.)

Does the child often bump into or have difficulty picking up objects?
(RATIONALE: A positive response suggests astigmatism—a condition that distorts or blurs vision because of an irregularly shaped lens.)

If the child attends school, does the child have to sit at the front of the room to see the chalkboard? Does the child sit close to the television at home?
(RATIONALE: If so, the child could be nearsighted.)

Developmental considerations for elderly patients
Ask the following questions about eye disorders common to aging:

Do your eyes feel dry?
(RATIONALE: Dry eyes or a feeling of sand or grittiness is common in elderly patients because of decreased lacrimal gland secretion.)

Do you have difficulty seeing in front of you but not to the sides?
(RATIONALE: In macular degeneration, a common form of blindness in older patients, central vision deteriorates but peripheral vision remains intact.)

Do you have problems with glare, discerning colors, or seeing at night?
(RATIONALE: With age, the lens may thicken and turn yellow, leading to glare and poor color discernment. Lens opacity that occurs with cataracts causes night blindness.)

Can you read the labels on medication bottles?
(RATIONALE: Safe medication use depends on the ability to read instructions.)

Health promotion and protection patterns
Questions related to health promotion and protection patterns indicate the patient's involvement in personal health care. Ask the following questions to elicit this information:

When was your last eye examination?
(RATIONALE: This question may reveal changes that led the patient to have an examination. Examinations by an optometrist or ophthalmologist are recommended at least every 2 years.)

Does your health insurance cover eye examinations, glasses, and lenses?
(RATIONALE: If not, the patient may forgo eye examinations or buying glasses or lenses for economic reasons.)

Does your occupation require close use of your eyes, such as long-term reading or prolonged use of a video display terminal?
(RATIONALE: These activities can cause severe eye strain and dryness.)

Does the air where you work or live contain anything that causes you eye problems?
(RATIONALE: Cigarette smoke, formaldehyde, insulation, or occupational materials, such as glues or chemicals, can cause eye irritation.)

Do you wear goggles when working with power tools, chain saws, or table saws or when engaging in sports?
(RATIONALE: Serious eye irritation or injury can occur with these activities.)

Role and relationship patterns
Vision disturbances can influence many roles and relationships. To discover the extent of this influence, ask the following question:

If you are visually impaired, do you have difficulty fulfilling home, work, or social obligations?
(RATIONALE: Visual impairment can seriously affect the patient's ability to carry out roles and activities of daily living. The patient may need the assistance of an occupational therapist.)

Physical assessment: The eye

Assessment of the eye includes testing the patient's vision and extraocular muscles, inspecting and palpating external ocular structures, and inspecting internal structures with an ophthalmoscope.

Test the patient's vision before inspecting and palpating. To test vision, obtain a Snellen eye chart, a piece of newsprint, an eye occluder or 3″ × 5″ card, a penlight, a pencil or other narrow cylindrical article, and an ophthalmoscope.

Vision and extraocular function
The nurse typically tests visual functions by checking near and distant visual acuity, color perception, and peripheral vision. Perform these tests in a well-lit room where the amount of light can be controlled. Record the results of visual acuity testing for each eye separately and for both eyes together, noting whether the patient wears corrective lenses. Also record the results of the color perception test. Refer any patient with abnormal findings for further evaluation.

Distance vision
To test the distance vision of a patient who can read English, use the Snellen alphabet chart containing various-sized letters. If the patient is illiterate or cannot speak English, use the Snellen E chart, which dis-

plays the letter E in varying sizes and positions. The patient indicates the position of the E by duplicating the position with his or her fingers.

The Snellen chart contains lines of letters that decrease in size with each succeeding line. Each line is labeled with a number containing a numerator and a denominator. The numerator, which is always 20, is the distance in feet between the chart and the patient. (Be sure to position the patient 20′ from the chart.) The denominator, which ranges from 10 to 200, indicates from what distance a normal eye can read the chart. For example, if the patient reads a line identified by the numbers 20/20, this means the patient can read from 20′ what a person with normal vision also can read from 20′. If the patient can read only a line identified by the numbers 20/100, this means the patient can read from 20′ what a person with normal vision can read from 100′. On the other hand, if the patient can read a line labeled 20/10, this means the patient can read at 20′ what a person with normal vision can read from 10′.

Test each eye separately by covering first one eye and then the other with an opaque 3″ × 5″ card or an eye occluder. Afterward, test binocular vision by having the patient read the chart with both eyes uncovered. The patient who normally wears corrective lenses for distance vision should wear them for the test. Have the patient start with the line marked 20/20; if the patient reads more than two letters incorrectly, direct the patient up to the next line (20/25). Continue until the patient can read a line correctly with no more than two errors. That line indicates the patient's distance visual acuity. If the patient reads the 20/20 line correctly, move down until the patient makes more than two mistakes. The last line read with fewer than two mistakes indicates the patient's distance visual acuity.

Near vision

To test near vision, hold either a Snellen eye chart or a card with newsprint 12″ to 14″ (30.5 to 35.5 cm) in front of the patient's eyes. The patient who normally wears reading glasses should wear them for the test. As with distance vision, test each eye separately and then together. Any patient who complains of blurring with the card at 12″ to 14″ or who cannot read it accurately requires retesting and referral to an ophthalmologist if necessary.

Abnormal findings. Poor near vision can signal cataracts or presbyopia, in which the lens loses elasticity and the ciliary muscles weaken.

Color perception

A patient with color blindness cannot distinguish among red, green, and blue. Of the many tests used to detect color blindness, the most common involves asking a patient to identify patterns of colored dots on colored plates; the patient who cannot discern colors will miss the patterns. Detecting color blindness early allows a child to learn to compensate for the deficit and alerts teachers to the student's special needs.

Extraocular muscle function

To assess extraocular muscle function, use the following techniques. First, inspect the eyes for position and alignment, making sure they are parallel. Next, perform the six cardinal positions of gaze test and the corneal light reflex test.

The six cardinal positions of gaze test evaluates the function of each of the six extraocular muscles and tests the cranial nerves responsible for their movement (cranial nerves III, IV, and VI). The normal eye muscles work together so that when the right eye moves upward and inward, the left eye moves upward and outward. These movements are commonly called extraocular movements (EOMs).

To test the six cardinal positions of gaze, stand directly in front of the patient, hold an index finger about 18″ (45 cm) away from the patient's nose, and ask the patient to watch the finger. Slowly trace a large *H* in the air by moving the finger to the patient's right, pausing, then moving up about 8″ (12 cm) and pausing again. Next, move the finger down about 16″ (40 cm), then through the midline, repeating the actions on the other side. This will cause the patient's eyes to travel through the six cardinal positions of gaze. Throughout the test, the eyes should remain parallel as they move.

The corneal light reflex test assesses the ability of extraocular muscles to hold the eyes steady (parallel) when fixed on an object. With the patient looking straight ahead, shine a penlight on the cornea from about 12″ to 15″ (30 to 37 cm) away. The light should fall at the same spot on each cornea. If it does not, suspect dysfunction of one of the extraocular muscles.

Abnormal findings. Testing the six cardinal positions of gaze can reveal exophoria, a mild outward deviation of the eye, or esophoria, an inward deviation. Both conditions are caused by muscle weakness. Tropia is a more severe ocular muscle weakness that produces permanent misalignment of the optic axes of the eyes (strabismus), in which the eyes turn outward (exotropia) or inward (esotropia).

Testing the corneal light reflex is an important first step in strabismus screening and should be conducted on a regular basis on children. An asymmetrical corneal light reflex is common in strabismus. If strabismus remains untreated, the affected eye weakens from disuse (amblyopia). This occurs because the optic cortex receives two images instead of one, suppresses one of the images to avoid diplopia, and causes a "lazy," or nonfunctioning, eye. As appropriate, refer the patient for further evaluation.

Peripheral vision

Assessing peripheral vision tests the optic nerve (cranial nerve II) and measures the ability of the retina to receive stimuli from the entire visual field. The nurse can evaluate peripheral vision by comparing the patient's vision field with the nurse's. However, if the nurse does not have normal vision, this test may be subjective and inaccurate.

The normal range of peripheral vision is a circle of 4' at a distance of 20' from the eye. Each eye has its own peripheral visual field, with the two fields overlapping. The eyes should be tested separately and together.

To test peripheral vision, instruct the patient to cover one eye. Hold a finger at the edge of the expected visual field, and ask the patient to identify how many fingers are being held up. Next, move to the lower edge of the expected field, holding up a different number of fingers and asking for a response. Repeat this procedure at the left and right borders. If the patient cannot see within the normal range, slowly move the finger into the expected field, noting where it becomes recognizable. Repeat the process on the opposite side, then with both eyes together. This test allows the nurse to evaluate not only the margins of the visual field but also what the patient sees within the field.

Abnormal findings. Decreased peripheral vision along with a history of seeing rainbows or halos around lights may indicate glaucoma. Peripheral visual field defects can result from lesions on the retina, in the occipital lobe, or at any point along the optic nerve. Because nerves from both eyes cross at the optic chiasm and both optic tracts terminate in the occipital lobe, a lesion in either location affects the visual fields of both eyes. However, damage or lesions on one optic nerve affect the visual field in that eye only. The nurse should promptly refer the patient with these findings to an ophthalmologist.

Inspection

After testing the patient's vision, perform the inspection techniques described below.

Eyelids, eyelashes, eyeball, and lacrimal apparatus

Inspect these structures for general appearance. Normally, the eyes are bright and clear. The eyelids should close completely and, when opened, the margins of the upper lids should fall slightly over the iris. The eyelids should be free of edema, scaling, or lesions, and the eyelashes should be equally distributed along the upper and lower lid margins. Inspect the palpebral folds for symmetry and the eyes for nystagmus (involuntary oscillations) and lid lag (unequal eyelid movement). Check the eyes for excessive tearing or dryness and the puncta for inflammation and swelling.

Conjunctivae and sclerae

Using universal precautions, inspect the bulbar conjunctivae for clarity. Check the palpebral conjunctivae only if a problem is suspected, such as a foreign body. Next, inspect the color of the sclerae, keeping in mind that the color varies with race. Most Caucasians have white sclerae; in patients with dark complexions, the sclerae may have small, dark-pigmented spots or an overall buff color.

Cornea, anterior chamber, and iris

To inspect the cornea and anterior chamber, shine a penlight into the patient's eye from several side angles (tangentially). Normally, the cornea and anterior chamber are clear and transparent. The iris appears flat and the cornea is slightly convex. The surface of the cornea is shiny and bright, with no scars or irregularities.

Pupils

Examine the pupil of each eye for equality of size, shape, reaction to light, and accommodation. To test pupillary reaction to light, darken the room. Have the patient stare straight ahead at a fixed point, then sweep a penlight beam from the side of the left eye to the center of its pupil. Both pupils should respond; the pupil receiving the direct light typically constricts directly, while the other pupil constricts simultaneously and consensually. Repeat the process on the other side. The pupils should react immediately, equally, and briskly (within 1 to 2 seconds). If the results are inconclusive, wait 15 to 30 seconds and try again. The pupils should be round and equal before and after the light flash.

To test for accommodation, ask the patient to stare at an object across the room; normally, the pupils dilate. Then ask the patient to stare at the nurse's index finger or at a pencil held about 2′ (60 cm) away. The pupils should constrict and converge equally on the object. To document a normal pupil assessment, use the abbreviation PERRLA (pupils equal, round, reactive to light, and accommodation) and the terms *direct* and *consensual.*

Abnormal findings. In ptosis, the upper eyelid falls below the middle of the iris. An oculomotor nerve lesion or a congenital condition in children can cause the eyelid to fall at or below the pupil.

Conjunctivitis usually is self-limiting and does not cause permanent damage. Bacterial conjunctivitis (pinkeye) is a contagious disease characterized by yellow or green purulent drainage accompanied by conjunctival vessel engorgement. Usually, antibiotic therapy is required to resolve it. Viral conjunctivitis is contagious and common in upper respiratory infections. It produces a copious, watery eye discharge but does not require antibiotic therapy.

Scleral color change may indicate a potentially severe systemic problem. Jaundice from liver disease manifests first in the sclerae, which becomes yellow. However, scleral thinning, common in elderly patients and neonates, may give the sclerae a bluish tone.

Corneal abrasions cause corneal inflammation, pain, and light sensitivity (photophobia). Such abrasions can occur after prolonged wearing of contact lenses or after injury from a foreign object, such as a fragment of metal or glass; they can be visualized only with special examination with staining. Any patient with an opacity of the cornea needs further evaluation.

A cataract is an opacity in the lens that makes seeing through the pupil difficult. Cataracts can be congenital or, in a young adult or a child, can result from a metabolic disorder, such as diabetes mellitus. However, most cataracts occur result from lens degeneration caused by aging.

Anisocoria, a difference in pupil size, affects up to 25% of the population. However, new onset pupil inequality may result from a central nervous system disorder or trauma. An irregular pupil contour may result from trauma or iritis. Pupillary constriction (miosis) is caused by use of narcotics or pilocarpine, a medication prescribed for glaucoma. Pupillary enlargement (mydriasis) can result from trauma or a systemic reaction to sympathomimetic and parasympathetic drugs.

Palpation

After inspection, palpate the eye and related structures. Using universal precautions, gently palpate the eyelids for swelling and tenderness. Next, palpate the eyeball by placing the tips of both index fingers on the eyelids over the sclerae while the patient looks down. The eyeballs should feel equally firm.

To palpate the lacrimal sac, press the index finger against the patient's lower orbital rim on the side closest to the patient's nose. While pressing, observe the punctum for abnormal regurgitation of purulent material or excessive tears, which could indicate blockage of the nasolacrimal duct.

Abnormal findings. Excessive hardness of the eyeball could indicate increased intraocular pressure, as in glaucoma.

Developmental considerations for pediatric patients

To perform a successful and accurate eye assessment on a preschooler, consider the child's age and behavioral development. Also consider appropriate ways to allay the child's anxiety before the examination and to divert the child's attention during the examination. For example, use a brightly colored toy, a piece of yarn, or a puppet to divert a toddler's or preschooler's attention while inspecting external ocular structures, testing pupillary functions, assessing the corneal light reflex, and checking the six cardinal positions of gaze. The parent can assist with the examination by soothing, distracting, or holding the infant or child.

Few infants or children under school age can cooperate long enough for an ophthalmoscopic examination or an assessment of visual fields. However, the nurse should check for a red reflex (a bright orange glow in the pupil) to verify lens patency.

Brief periods of nystagmus are normal in an infant who is not yet focusing. However, if nystagmus is continuous, the infant requires further examination by a specialist. Children normally may demonstrate a slight nystagmus when gazing to either side.

Developmental considerations for elderly patients

Although assessment procedures for the elderly patient are the same as those for a younger adult, findings vary because of normal aging-related changes. With aging, eyebrows and eyelashes thin as the number of hair follicles decreases; tear production also decreases, leading to the complaint of dry eyes.

Other noticeable changes include clouding of the cornea and small, somewhat fixed pupils; both changes are caused by sclerotic changes in the iris. Lipid deposits may cause a thin, gray-white ring surrounding the cornea. This finding, called arcus senilis, is normal in elderly patients. Most patients over age 85 show almost no pupil reaction to accommodation, and only one third react to light. Also, as the lens thickens and yellows, light perception diminishes and colors become distorted, with blues and purples appearing green. The yellow lens also leads to glare and decreases visual acuity in dim light; thus, elderly patients require more light to read or perform other fine work. Loss of lens elasticity and transparency decreases the ability of the elderly patient to discriminate clear objects, such as windows, and may impair distance perception.

Peripheral vision also may decrease normally with age. Because intraocular fluid reabsorption diminishes, glaucoma may occur. A sudden decrease in peripheral vision accompanied by eye pain signals acute glaucoma, a medical emergency that requires immediate evaluation by an ophthalmologist.

Ethnic considerations

Asians have epicanthic folds—skin folds covering the inner canthus, similar to those seen in individuals with Down's syndrome.

Ophthalmoscopic examination

After becoming proficient at basic eye assessment techniques, the nurse is ready to learn the more advanced techniques of ophthalmoscopic examination and tonometry. The ophthalmoscope allows the nurse to observe the retina and its structures, the lens, and the vitreous body. The ophthalmoscopic examination is a complex psychomotor skill and requires much practice to master.

Documentation: The eye

The following example illustrates how to document some normal physical assessment findings for the eye:

Snellen alphabet chart demonstrates 20/20 vision in both eyes without corrective lenses. Palpebral fissures are symmetrical. Eyelids are free of lesions. Corneal light reflex appropriate. EOMs intact with no abnormal movements bilaterally. PERRLA direct and consensual. Sclerae, conjunctivae, and corneas clear bilaterally.

The following example illustrates how to document some abnormal physical assessment findings for the eye:

Structures of the ear

This illustration shows the anatomic structures of the external, middle, and inner ear.

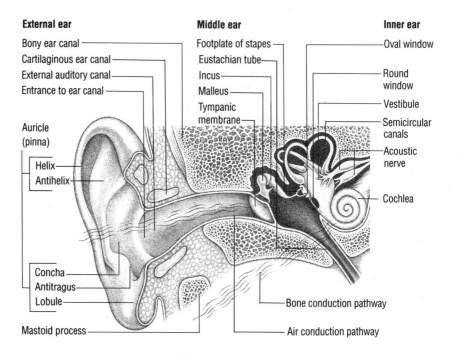

External ear
Bony ear canal
Cartilaginous ear canal
External auditory canal
Entrance to ear canal
Auricle (pinna)
Helix
Antihelix
Concha
Antitragus
Lobule
Mastoid process

Middle ear
Footplate of stapes
Eustachian tube
Incus
Malleus
Tympanic membrane

Inner ear
Oval window
Round window
Vestibule
Semicircular canals
Acoustic nerve
Cochlea

Bone conduction pathway
Air conduction pathway

Visual acuity of 20/50 in right eye; 20/30 in left eye with corrective lenses using Snellen chart. Corneal light reflex at 8 o'clock in right eye, center of pupil in left eye. EOMs not intact, with limited lateral range in right eye. Lens opaque bilaterally.

Anatomy and physiology review: The ear

The ear contains three anatomic parts: external ear, middle ear, and inner ear. The external flap, called the auricle or pinna, and the external auditory canal compose the external ear. The tympanic membrane (eardrum) separates the external ear from the middle ear at the proximal portion of the auditory canal. The middle ear is a small, air-filled cavity in the temporal bone that contains three small bones—malleus, incus, and stapes. It leads to the inner ear, a bony and membranous labyrinth. (For illustrations, see *Structures of the ear.*)

The ear is a sensory organ that has the functions of hearing and maintaining equilibrium. The auricle picks up sound waves and channels them into the auditory canal, where they strike the tympanic membrane. The membrane vibrates and, in turn, vibrates the handle of the malleus. Vibrations travel from the malleus to the incus to the stapes, through the oval window, and through the fluid of the cochlea to the round window. The membrane covering the round window shakes the delicate hair cells in the organ of Corti, which stimulates sensory endings of the cochlear branch of the acoustic nerve (cranial nerve VIII). The nerve sends the impulses to the auditory area of the brain's temporal lobe, which interprets the sound.

The semicircular canal in the inner ear helps maintain balance and equilibrium. Within this canal, fluid circulates in relation to head movement. This fluid bathes the cristae and its hair cells. When hair cells are stimulated, impulses are transmitted to vestibular nerves, allowing the brain to orient the person to the motion.

Health history: The ear

Before beginning the interview, find out if the patient hears well. If a hearing problem exists, look directly at the patient and speak clearly when interviewing. Keep in mind that hearing problems can seriously affect the ability to carry out activities of daily living and can adversely affect every aspect of life.

Health and illness patterns

To assess current health and illness patterns related to the ear, use the following guidelines to explore the patient's current, past, and family health status as well as the patient's developmental status.

Current health status

Using the PQRST method, ask for a complete description of any ear-related problem. Usually, complaints of hearing loss and tinnitus (ringing or other noise in the ears) are long-standing, whereas complaints of ear pain, discharge, and dizziness are more acute. Ask the following questions:

Have you recently noticed any difference in your hearing in one or both ears?
(RATIONALE: The pattern of hearing loss gives clues about its cause. For example, otitis media [middle ear infection] may cause a sudden decrease in hearing in the affected ear, as well as pain. Acoustic neuroma [tumor of the eighth cranial nerve] usually causes a gradual decrease in hearing in one ear, accompanied by dizziness.)

Do you have ear pain?
(RATIONALE: Ear pain can indicate a middle or inner ear infection, an ear canal obstruction by ear wax [cerumen], or a foreign body.)

Do you have any drainage from your ears? If so, can you describe it?
(RATIONALE: Otorrhea [drainage from the ear] can result from buildup of fluid pressure, leading to rupture of the tympanic membrane. In otitis media, otorrhea usually is bloody and purulent. Otitis externa [infection of the ear canal] also can cause otorrhea.)

Do you smoke cigarettes? Does anyone in your household smoke?
(RATIONALE: Cigarette smoking or exposure to passive smoke at least doubles the risk of otitis media in both adults and children.)

Past health status

Ask the following questions to gather additional information about the patient's ears:

Have you had an ear injury? If so, describe the injury and treatment.
(RATIONALE: Some injuries can cause permanent hearing impairment.)

Have you ever experienced ringing or crackling in your ears?
(RATIONALE: Tinnitus can result from hypertension, ossicle dislocation, blockage by cerumen, or idiopathic causes. Crackling results from fluid in the middle ear.)

Have you had many ear infections?
(RATIONALE: A patient with a history of many ear infections may have tympanic membrane scarring or other ear damage, leading to hearing loss.)

Have you had problems with balance or dizziness?
(RATIONALE: Vertigo or poor balance can indicate a neurologic or otologic disorder.)

Have you been taking any prescription medications, OTC drugs, or home remedies for your ears or for any other conditions? If so, which ones and how often?
(RATIONALE: Certain medications, such as aspirin, can affect hearing.)

Has anyone in your family had hearing problems?
(RATIONALE: Otosclerosis is a hereditary disorder that begins between ages 20 and 30 as unilateral conductive hearing loss and progresses to bilateral mixed hearing loss.)

Developmental considerations for pediatric patients

When assessing a child, try to involve the parent or guardian and the child in the interview. However, keep in mind that a child with an ear infection may be irritable from a high fever and severe pain. To assess the child, ask these questions:

Does the infant react to loud or unusual noises? If over age 6 months, does the infant babble? If over age 15 months, has the toddler at least attempted to speak? Is the toddler speaking appropriately for his or her age?
(RATIONALE: These questions explore critical hearing and language developmental milestones. The answer to each question should be positive. A negative response to any question necessitates referral to a pediatric hearing and speech specialist.)

Have you noticed the child tugging at either ear?
(RATIONALE: This is often a sign of ear infection. Otitis media is a major health problem in children. By age 3, about two-thirds of all children have had at least one episode of otitis media, and one-third of these have had more than three episodes.)

Have you noticed any coordination problems?
(RATIONALE: Inner ear infections can affect equilibrium.)

Has the child had meningitis, recurrent otitis media, mumps, or encephalitis?
(RATIONALE: These conditions can cause hearing loss.)

Developmental considerations for elderly patients
When assessing an elderly patient, ask these additional questions:

Have you noticed a recent change in your hearing?
(RATIONALE: Elderly patients commonly develop presbycusis—a physiologic hearing loss that usually occurs after age 50.)

Do you wear a hearing aid? If so, for how long? How do you care for it?
(RATIONALE: If the patient wears a hearing aid, be sure to speak clearly and directly. Also, some patients who hear poorly refuse to wear a hearing aid because they do not want to accept that they have a hearing problem.)

Health promotion and protection patterns
To continue the health history, ask the following questions to explore the patient's personal health habits and occupational health patterns related to the ear:

When was your last ear examination or hearing test? What were the results?
(RATIONALE: The answers to these questions could suggest the importance of preventive health care to the patient. Determining the last examination date also helps assess recent changes.)

Do you work near loud machinery? If so, do you wear ear protectors?
(RATIONALE: Working near loud machinery for long periods can cause hearing loss. However, the patient can prevent such loss by using ear guards.)

Role and relationship patterns
Ear disorders, especially hearing loss, can affect role and relationship patterns. To discover the extent of this influence, ask the patient the following questions:

Does your hearing problem affect your relationships with other people? If so, how?
(RATIONALE: The spouse or friends of a patient with hearing loss may become impatient with the hearing-impaired person. The patient may feel left out of conversations, especially if background noise makes hearing even more difficult.)

Does your hearing loss prevent you from working, driving, or taking care of your daily needs?
(RATIONALE: Hearing loss may cause problems keeping a job or caring for family and self.)

Physical assessment: The ear

Physical assessment of the ear includes inspection, palpation, hearing screening, and otoscopic examination. Although the structures of the middle and inner ear cannot be inspected, the nurse can assess their functioning through hearing screening. Equipment required for a basic ear assessment includes an otoscope, a tuning fork, and a watch.

Auditory function screening

The most common causes of hearing loss are conduction problems, neural problems, and problems with the auditory center caused by injury or damage. Conduction deafness results from interference with the functioning of external and middle ear structures. For example, a cerumen plug in the canal, otitis media, membrane rupture, or sclerosis of the ossicles can prevent the tympanic membrane from vibrating, leading to conduction deafness.

Sensorineural deafness results from damage to inner ear structures, such as the organ of Corti, or from damage to cranial nerve VIII. Central deafness (also a sensorineural deafness) results from damage to the auditory area of the brain's temporal lobe, such as from a cerebrovascular accident or a central nervous system lesion.

Gross hearing screening

Perform these two tests: the whispered or spoken voice test and the watch tick test. For the voice test, have the patient occlude one ear with a finger. Test the other ear by standing 1' to 2' (30 to 60 cm) behind the patient and whispering a word or phrase. A patient with normal auditory acuity should be able to repeat what was whispered.

The watch tick test evaluates the patient's ability to hear high-frequency sounds. Gradually move a watch until the patient no longer can hear the ticking, which should occur when the watch is about 5" (13 cm) away. Because these testing methods are crude, they should be used with other forms of auditory screening.

Use the remaining auditory screening tests—Weber's test and the Rinne test—to evaluate the patient for conduction or sensorineural hearing loss.

Weber's test

This test evaluates bone conduction. Place a vibrating 500- to 1,000-cycle tuning fork on the top of the patient's head at midline or in the middle of the forehead. The patient should perceive the sound equally in both ears. If the patient has a conductive hearing loss, the sound will be heard in (lateralize to) the ear with the conductive loss because the sound is being conducted directly through the bone to the ear. If the patient has a sensorineural hearing loss in one ear, the sound will lateralize to the unimpaired ear because nerve damage in the impaired ear prevents hearing. Document a normal Weber's test by recording a negative lateralization of sound.

Rinne test

This test compares bone conduction to air conduction in both ears. Assess bone conduction by placing the base of a vibrating tuning fork on the mastoid process, noting how many seconds pass before the patient can no longer hear it. Then quickly place the still-vibrating tuning fork with the tines parallel to the patient's auricle, near the ear canal (to test air conduction). Note how many seconds the patient can hear the tone. Then repeat the test on the other ear.

Because sound traveling through air remains audible twice as long (a 2:1 ratio) as sound traveling through bone, a sound heard for 10 seconds by bone conduction should be heard for 20 seconds by air conduction. A patient who reports hearing the sound longer through bone conduction has a conductive loss. With sensorineural loss, the patient reports hearing the sound longer through air conduction, but may hear poorly with either method.

Inspection

Although inspection and palpation usually are performed simultaneously, this section describes each separately to clarify the techniques used in each procedure. Prepare for the assessment by observing universal precautions. Then seat the adult patient and begin inspecting the external ear structures. The auricle should cross a line approximated from the outer canthus of the eye to the protuberance of the occiput. Ear position should be almost vertical, with no more than a 10-degree lateral-posterior slant.

Next, inspect the ears for color and size. The ears should be similarly shaped, colored the same as the face, and sized in proportion to the head. (Keep in mind, though, that ear size and shape vary greatly within the population.) Check behind the ear for inflammation, masses, or lesions, and observe the ear canal for signs of drainage.

Abnormal findings. A deviation in the alignment of the auricle, such as ears below the lateral angle of the eye (low-set ears), suggests a renal disorder or chromosomal abnormality, such as Down's syndrome. For this reason, carefully observe ear position and alignment in neonates and infants. Purulent drainage from the otic canal usually indicates an infection, whereas clear or bloody drainage could be cerebrospinal fluid leaking after head trauma.

Palpation

Palpate the external ear and mastoid process, checking for areas of tenderness, swelling, nodules, or lesions. Then gently pull the helix of the ear backward to determine the presence of pain or tenderness.

Abnormal findings. Tenderness on palpation can indicate infection. Pain with tragus pulling may indicate external otitis and usually is accompanied by otorrhea. Tenderness over the mastoid may indicate complicated otitis media.

Developmental considerations

Evaluate an infant's or a young child's responses to voices and a rattle to rule out a congenital hearing problem. When in doubt about the child's hearing ability, make an appropriate referral.

In elderly patients, the external structure of the ear, such as the auricle, may have lost adipose tissue and the cartilage may be harder. The skin and cerumen in the external auditory canal may be dry and flaky. Presbycusis, a sensorineural hearing loss of high-frequency tones that eventually leads to loss of all frequencies, also occurs with advancing age. Consonants become difficult to hear, making many words hard to understand. To minimize the effects of this handicap during the assessment, stand in front of the elderly patient when speaking so the patient can receive as much information as possible.

Otoscopic examination

The nurse uses an otoscope to examine the canal and tympanic membrane. Before starting this examination, become familiar with the function of the otoscope. The otoscopic examination is an advanced assessment skill and requires practice to master. The handles used for the otoscope and the ophthalmoscope are interchangeable.

Documentation: The ear

The following example illustrates how to document some normal physical assessment findings for the ear:

Hearing intact to watch tick and whispered voice test. Ears equal in size, appropriate position. No masses or tenderness in auricles or in postauricular or mastoid area. Weber's test—no lateralization; Rinne test—air conduction greater than bone conduction at 2:1 ratio. Canals clear, without irritation or excess cerumen.

The following example illustrates how to document some abnormal physical assessment findings for the ear:

Hearing diminished in right ear—unable to discern whispered voice at 1′ or to hear watch tick at 4″. Hearing in left ear within normal limits. Ear placement low, symmetrical. Tenderness and warmth noted over right mastoid area; left mastoid area nontender. Weber's test—lateralizes to the right; Rinne test—within normal limits.

STUDY ACTIVITIES

Matching related elements

Match the assessment findings on the left with the description on the right.

1. _B_ Nystagmus
2. _C_ Lid lag
3. _A_ Mydriasis
4. _E_ Otorrhea
5. _D_ Tinnitus

A. Pupillary enlargement
B. Involuntary oscillations of the eye
C. Unequal eyelid position
D. Ringing in the ears
E. Drainage from the ear

Short answer

6. Which two eye complaints constitute emergencies and necessitate immediate referral to an ophthalmologist?

_____

7. When assessing health promotion patterns, the nurse should ask the patient the date of the last eye examination. For optimal eye health, how often should the eyes be examined by an optometrist or ophthalmologist?

_____

8. Which of the following disorders are common age-related eye changes seen in elderly patients?
   A. Eye dryness
   B. Bacterial conjunctivitis
   C. Problems with glare
   D. Macular degeneration
   E. Strabismus

_____

9. Which physical assessment findings suggest bacterial conjunctivitis?

_____

10. The nurse is assessing William Russano, age 58, a construction worker. Based on his occupation, which question related to eye health should the nurse ask him during the health history interview?

_____

11. When testing Mr. Russano's vision using the Snellen alphabet chart, the nurse finds that without his eyeglasses, he can see with his right eye at 20′ what the person with normal vision can see at 100′. With his left eye, he can see at 20′ what the person with normal vision can see at 40′. Using both eyes, he can see at 20′ what the person with normal vision can see at 60′. With his eyeglasses, his vision is normal. How should the nurse record these findings?

_____

12. The nurse is performing a comprehensive assessment of Jason, age 2, during a well-child visit. What questions should the nurse ask his parent to investigate Jason's hearing?

_____

True or false

13. In a patient with a conductive hearing loss, Weber's test will reveal that sound lateralizes to the side with the conductive loss.
☑ True   ☐ False

14. In a normal Rinne test, the nurse should expect bone conduction to exceed air conduction.
☐ True   ☑ False

15. A patient with a renal or chromosomal abnormality may have low-set ears.
☐ True   ☐ False

16. Mastoid tenderness is a typical finding in uncomplicated otitis media.
☐ True   ☐ False

Fill in the blank

17. If the patient has a history of hypertension or diabetes, the nurse should stay alert for _____ , an ophthalmologic disorder that can lead to blindness.

18. _____ is an eye disorder in which central vision deteriorates but peripheral vision remains intact.

19. Physiologic hearing loss after age 50 is known as _____

ANSWERS

Matching related elements

1. B
2. C
3. A
4. E
5. D

Short answer

6. A complaint of a sudden change in the ability to see and a complaint of eye pain are emergencies that call for immediate referral to an ophthalmologist.

7. The eyes should be examined an optometrist or ophthalmologist at least every 2 years.

8. Eye dryness, glare, and macular degeneration are common findings in elderly patients.

9. Yellow or green purulent drainage accompanied by conjunctival vessel engorgement suggests bacterial conjunctivitis.

10. The nurse should ask Mr. Russano if he wears protective goggles at work because his occupation carries a significant risk for eye injury.

11. The nurse should record the findings as follows:

Snellen alphabet chart demonstrates visual acuity of 20/100 in right eye, 20/40 in left eye, and 20/60 using both eyes without corrective lenses; 20/20 using both eyes with corrective lenses.

12. The nurse should ask the parent if Jason reacted to loud sounds as an infant, if he babbled by age 6 months, if he attempted to speak by age 15 months, and if he now speaks as well as other children his own age.

True or false
13. True.
14. False. The nurse should expect air conduction to exceed bone conduction in a patient with normal hearing because sound traveling through air remains audible twice as long as sound traveling through bone.
15. True.
16. False. Mastoid tenderness may indicate complicated otitis media.

Fill in the blank
17. retinopathy
18. Macular degeneration
19. presbycusis

CHAPTER 9

Respiratory system

OBJECTIVES

After studying this chapter, the reader should be able to:

1. Identify the anatomic structures of the respiratory system.

2. Explain external and internal respiration

3. Gather appropriate health history information for a patient with a respiratory disorder.

4. Demonstrate how to inspect, palpate, percuss, and auscultate respiratory system structures.

5. Describe the normal assessment findings detected by inspection, palpation, percussion, and auscultation of the respiratory system.

6. Describe the most common abnormal findings detected by physical assessment of the respiratory system.

7. Describe tactile fremitus palpation, diaphragmatic excursion measurement, and voice resonance auscultation.

8. Document respiratory assessment findings.

OVERVIEW OF CONCEPTS

The respiratory system functions primarily to maintain the exchange of oxygen and carbon dioxide in the lungs and tissues and to regulate the body's acid-base balance (the stable concentration of hydrogen ions in body fluids). Because any change in the respiratory system affects every other body system, swift and accurate assessment is vital.

The respiratory system consists of the upper and lower airways and the thoracic cage. The nose, mouth, nasopharynx, oropharynx, laryngopharynx, and larynx (voice box) compose the upper airways. The bronchi, lungs, trachea, bronchioles, and alveoli compose the lower airways. (For illustrations, see *Upper and lower airways.*)

Composed of bone and cartilage, the thoracic cage supports and protects the lungs and allows for lung expansion and contraction. The vertebral column and twelve pairs of ribs form the thoracic cage and provide anatomical landmarks for respiratory assessment.

Breathing involves two actions: inspiration, an active process, and expiration, a relatively passive one. Both actions rely on the functioning of the muscles of respiration and the effects of pressure differences in the lungs.

Upper and lower airways

The respiratory system consists of the upper and lower airways and the thoracic cage. The structures work together to effect the vital exchange of oxygen and carbon dioxide.

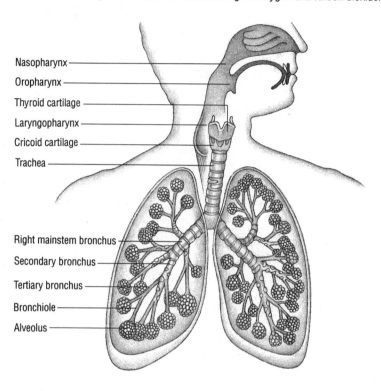

Nasopharynx

Oropharynx

Thyroid cartilage

Laryngopharynx

Cricoid cartilage

Trachea

Right mainstem bronchus

Secondary bronchus

Tertiary bronchus

Bronchiole

Alveolus

Effective respiration requires gas exchange in the lungs (external respiration) and in the tissues (internal respiration). External respiration occurs through ventilation (gas distribution into and out of the pulmonary airways), pulmonary perfusion (blood flow from the right side of the heart, through the pulmonary circulation, and into the left side of the heart), and diffusion. Internal respiration also relies on diffusion, which occurs when oxygen and carbon dioxide move between the alveoli and capillaries. These processes are vital in maintaining adequate oxygenation and acid-base balance.

Health history   Before beginning the health history, quickly assess the patient for signs of acute respiratory distress, such as restlessness, anxiety, inability to follow conversation, or noisy or labored respirations. If the patient displays these signs, obtain help and, if possible, question the patient's family about the current problem. Then, when the patient is breathing comfortably, proceed with the full health history.

Health and illness patterns

The most common signs and symptoms related to the respiratory system include dyspnea, cough, sputum production, and chest pain or discomfort. Using the PQRST method, thoroughly investigate all of these complaints. (For an explanation of this method, see *Symptom analysis,* page 15.)

Current health status

During this part of the health history, find out as much as possible about the patient's chief complaint by posing the following questions:

Do you have shortness of breath? If so, is it constant or intermittent? Does a position change, medication, or relaxation relieve the symptom? Do your lips or nail beds ever turn blue? Does body position, time of day, or a particular activity affect your breathing? How many stairs can you climb, or blocks can you walk, before you feel short of breath?
(RATIONALE: A distressing symptom, dyspnea can result from various respiratory disorders. Although dyspnea may begin suddenly in relation to a specific activity, it usually arises gradually and insidiously. Unconsciously, the patient may have made lifestyle changes to compensate for dyspnea, making the exact time of onset hard to determine. Intermittent attacks of dyspnea may result from asthma, whereas dyspnea that occurs during sleep [paroxysmal nocturnal dyspnea] or dyspnea that requires the patient to sit or stand to breathe normally [orthopnea] may indicate chronic lung disease or cardiac dysfunction. Dyspnea aggravated by activity suggests poor ventilation and perfusion or inefficient breathing mechanisms.)

Do you have a cough? If so, does it sound dry, hacking, barking, or congested? Does it usually occur at a certain time of day?
(RATIONALE: Cough, whether productive or nonproductive, usually indicates a respiratory disorder. Severe cough may disrupt activities of daily living, cause chest pain, or induce acute respiratory distress. Early-morning cough may result from chronic airway inflammation caused by smoking; late-afternoon cough may reflect exposure to irritants at work; and evening cough may suggest chronic postnasal drip, sinusitis, or gastric reflux with nocturnal aspiration. Dry cough may signal a cardiac condition; barking cough, croup or influenza; hacking cough, pneumonia; and congested cough, a cold, pneumonia, or bronchitis.)

Do you cough up sputum? If so, how much do you cough up each day? What color is it? How does it smell? Is it thick or thin? What time of day do you cough up the most sputum?
(RATIONALE: Sputum production accompanies a cough when the hairlike processes of the mucous membranes [cilia] attempt to clear airway debris by a wavelike, upward motion. In small amounts and with

sufficient fluidity, sputum production maintains airway hygiene and patency. Normal mucus is thin, clear to white, tasteless, odorless, and scant. Mucoid sputum may suggest tracheobronchitis or asthma; yellow or green sputum, bacterial infection; rust-colored sputum, pneumonia, pulmonary infarction, or tuberculosis [TB]; pink and frothy sputum, pulmonary edema.)

Do you have chest pain? If so, is it constant or intermittent? Is it localized? Does any activity produce this pain? Does pain occur when you breathe normally or when you breathe deeply?
(RATIONALE: Chest pain may have a cardiac, respiratory, or musculoskeletal origin. Pain characteristics help determine the probable origin.)

Past health status
Questions related to previous illnesses, injuries, and surgeries provide clues to assessment findings.

Have you had any lung problems, such as asthma or tuberculosis? When was the problem first diagnosed? What treatment did you receive?
(RATIONALE: Some respiratory problems, such as asthma and tuberculosis, may recur.)

Have you been exposed to anyone who has had a respiratory disease?
(RATIONALE: Certain respiratory disorders, such as influenza, pneumonia, and other infections, are highly contagious.)

Have you had chest surgery or any diagnostic study of the pulmonary system? If so, what type, and why did you have it?
(RATIONALE: Previous diagnostic studies—such as bronchoscopy, arterial blood gas analysis, and sputum cultures—or a thoracotomy or other chest surgery can reveal a history of, or predisposition to, respiratory disorders.)

How many pillows do you sleep on? Does this number represent a change from your previous number?
(RATIONALE: The need for more than one pillow could indicate nocturnal dyspnea or orthopnea that has developed over time. The patient may not realize that using more than one pillow relates to a breathing problem.)

Do you have allergies that flare up in different seasons? If so, what causes them? Do they cause runny nose, itching eyes, congestion, or other symptoms? How do you relieve these symptoms?
(RATIONALE: A patient with allergies may use over-the-counter [OTC] drugs and inhalers, which could interact with prescribed medications. Answers to these questions also reveal the use of common household remedies and whether they are successful.)

Do you smoke tobacco? If so, for how long, and how much?
(RATIONALE: Cigarette, cigar, or pipe smoking can predispose a smoker to various respiratory disorders. Information about pack-years [the

number of packs smoked per day multiplied by the number of years of smoking] can indicate the severity of the problem.)

Do you take any over-the-counter or prescription medications for your respiratory problems? If so, which ones? How often do you take them? When did you last take them?
(RATIONALE: Medications taken by the patient provide important clues to specific respiratory disorders. Breathing problems are often self-treated, so inquire about prescription and OTC drugs. Also ask about drugs that may be used as part of respiratory therapy because the patient may not identify these as medications. Many patients with chronic respiratory problems use inhalational products, such as nebulizer or metered-dose inhaler bronchodilators and anti-inflammatory agents.)

What other medications do you take? How often do you take them?
(RATIONALE: Many drugs can cause respiratory depression and other adverse respiratory reactions.)

Do you use oxygen at home? If so, do you use a cannula or mask? Do you use it continuously or intermittently? What is the liter flow rate at rest and with activity?
(RATIONALE: Use of oxygen therapy at home may indicate a chronic respiratory disorder. Learn the patient's maintenance amount as a baseline for future adjustments, and determine the patient's awareness of necessary precautions.)

How long have you been on home oxygen? Who is your supplier? Does your insurance cover the cost of oxygen therapy?
(RATIONALE: Economics may prevent the patient from complying with ordered treatments, necessitating referral to social service assistance.)

Have you ever been vaccinated against the flu or pneumonia?
(RATIONALE: Expect the very young, very old, and those with chronic respiratory disease to have been vaccinated. If such a patient has not been vaccinated, plan to teach the patient about the protection that vaccinations provide.)

Family health status
Obtain a family history of respiratory illness as well as an overview of family structure and support systems. A patient with a chronic respiratory disease eventually may need a good deal of family assistance. Also ask the following question:

Has any member of your family had emphysema, asthma, respiratory allergies, or tuberculosis?
(RATIONALE: A familial predisposition to emphysema and allergies may exist. If a family member has had TB, find out when the patient may have been exposed, to determine the need for a tuberculin skin test.)

Status of physiologic systems

When gathering information about a patient with a respiratory problem, look at other body systems that may show symptoms related to the primary problem.

In the last 1 to 2 months, have you had a fever, chills, fatigue, or night sweats?
(RATIONALE: These symptoms are associated with TB.)

Have you ever had a blood test that showed you had anemia? If so, when?
(RATIONALE: Anemia decreases the ability of the blood to carry oxygen because of reduced red blood cells and hemoglobin. This, in turn, leads to fatigue, dyspnea, and orthopnea.)

Do you suffer from ankle edema or shortness of breath at night?
(RATIONALE: These effects may be related to congestive heart failure.)

Have you noticed any weight change recently?
(RATIONALE: Weight gain could indicate fluid accumulation from congestive heart failure, whereas weight loss could mean generalized body wasting associated with a disease, such as lung cancer.)

Do you ever feel confused, restless, or faint?
(RATIONALE: These symptoms could result from inadequate oxygen to the brain, as seen in the patient with chronic obstructive pulmonary disease [COPD] who has an elevated plasma carbon dioxide level and a decreased plasma oxygen level.)

Developmental considerations for pediatric patients

Ask the parent or guardian the following questions:

Did the mother have any pregnancy-related problems? Was the pregnancy carried to full term? If not, what care did the infant require?
(RATIONALE: A premature infant may have had an underdeveloped respiratory system at birth.)

Did the infant have respiratory problems at birth? If so, how were they treated?
(RATIONALE: The nurse should know if problems were temporary, which the parent may forget about unless asked, or if residual respiratory difficulty continues and how it is treated.)

Does the infant suffer from frequent congestion, runny nose, or colds?
(RATIONALE: If yes, ask about the parents' smoking habits. Secondhand smoke can cause frequent congestion and other respiratory problems in infants.)

Does shortness of breath interfere with the infant's ability to suck a bottle or breast?
(RATIONALE: If yes, the infant will require referral to a physician or nurse practitioner.)

Does the child cough at night? If so, does the cough awaken the child?
(RATIONALE: A hacking cough could mean tracheobronchitis with epiglottitis, which could lead to airway obstruction.)

Does coughing or shortness of breath interfere with the child's play or school activities?
(RATIONALE: Asthma and dyspnea may interfere with the child's usual activities.)

Developmental considerations for elderly patients
When assessing an elderly patient, ask these questions:

Are you aware of any changes in your breathing patterns? Do you become easily fatigued when climbing stairs? Do you have trouble breathing when lying down? Do you seem to have more colds that last longer?
(RATIONALE: Elderly patients are susceptible to breathing problems because of their limited chest wall and respiratory muscle strength. Their altered immune systems may increase their susceptibility to colds and respiratory infections.)

Health promotion and protection patterns
Ask the following questions about the patient's occupation, home remedies, sleep and activity patterns, and stress. Also ask about home and work environments, which may contain irritants that trigger or aggravate breathing problems.

When was your last chest X-ray? Tuberculosis test?
(RATIONALE: Preventive and screening behaviors provide information about the patient's self-care patterns and possible teaching opportunities.)

Which home remedies do you use for respiratory problems?
(RATIONALE: Incorporating the patient's beliefs into the care plan aids compliance and healing. For example, a patient's plan of care could include a simple, traditional home remedy, such as herbal tea with honey.)

Have your sleep patterns changed because of breathing problems?
(RATIONALE: Changes in sleep patterns could lead to fatigue. In a patient with COPD, such changes could make breathing even more tiring.)

Does your breathing problem affect your daily activities? Which activities can you manage without assistance? Which ones can you manage with assistance? Which ones are you unable to manage? What or who provides assistance when you need it? How do your current activities compare with those before your breathing problems?
(RATIONALE: These questions uncover the patient's perceived need for help and provide information that might suggest the need for follow-up care and services.)

Do you have any hobbies that expose you to respiratory irritants, such as glues, paints, or sprays?
(RATIONALE: The patient who engages in such hobbies may need to increase room ventilation when working with these agents or may need to wear a protective mask.)

Do you have any difficulty breathing when eating? Do you eat three large meals or several small meals a day?
(RATIONALE: Many patients with chronic respiratory disorders eat small, frequent meals to reduce dyspnea and altered breathing.)

Does stress at home or work affect your breathing? If so, do you use any special measures for stress management? What are they?
(RATIONALE: Asthmatic and other patients may be able to identify an action reaction cycle that includes stress and dyspnea. Established stress-reduction measures should be incorporated into the care plan. If the patient uses none, explore the topic further and teach the patient an appropriate stress-reduction exercise.)

Can you afford the medication, equipment, and oxygen required for your health?
(RATIONALE: Noncompliance may occur for economic reasons, not lack of interest or understanding.)

How many people live with you? Do you have pets? If so, does the fur or feathers bother you? What type of home heating do you have? Is anything in your home a respiratory irritant, such as fresh paint, cleaning sprays, or heavy cigarette smoke?
(RATIONALE: The home environment is especially important to a patient with a respiratory problem. Data gathered from these questions can help the nurse and patient plan positive changes in the environment.)

What is your current occupation? What were your previous occupations? Are you exposed to any known respiratory irritants at work? Do you use safety measures during exposure?
(RATIONALE: Certain occupations, such as mining or chemical manufacturing, and working in a smoke-filled office can expose a patient to respiratory irritants.)

Role and relationship patterns
Ask these questions to explore role and relationship patterns:

What impact has your disease had on you and on your family? Are you able to meet family responsibilities? If not, is this a problem?
(RATIONALE: If the patient cannot meet expected role responsibilities, additional stress and family conflict may result.)

How have family members reacted to your respiratory illness? Whom among family and friends can you count on in your time of need?
(RATIONALE: Many patients with chronic respiratory illness need a great deal of assistance and may require outside help. Patients with

chronic breathing problems may feel depressed and isolated from their families.)

How has your breathing problem affected your sexual activity? Have you found ways to decrease the effects of breathing problems on sexual activity? Would you care to discuss them?
(RATIONALE: A patient with a breathing problem may be dyspneic during sexual activity, possibly avoiding sexual encounters.)

Physical assessment

Before assessing the respiratory system, the nurse must inspect the patient's skin as well as the upper and lower extremities (arms and legs). This provides an overview of the patient's clinical status and permits assessment of peripheral oxygenation. A dusky or bluish tint (cyanosis) may indicate decreased arterial oxygen content.

Be sure to differentiate between central cyanosis and peripheral cyanosis. Central cyanosis results from prolonged hypoxia and affects all body organs. It may appear in patients with right-to-left cardiac shunting or a pulmonary disease that causes hypoxemia, such as chronic bronchitis. Cyanosis appears on the buccal mucosa, tongue, and lips or in other highly vascular areas, such as the nail beds. Assessing for cyanosis in dark-skinned patients may be more difficult. In these patients, the most accurate areas to inspect are the oral mucous membranes and lips; in a dark-skinned patient with central cyanosis, these areas appear ashen gray, not bluish as in light-skinned patients. Facial skin may be pale gray or ashen in a cyanotic black-skinned patient and yellowish-brown in a cyanotic brown-skinned patient.

Peripheral cyanosis results from vasoconstriction, vascular occlusion, or reduced cardiac output. Often seen in patients after exposure to the cold, peripheral cyanosis appears in the nail beds and sometimes the lips. It does not affect the mucous membranes.

For all patients, the nurse then assesses the fingertips and toes for abnormal enlargement. Called clubbing, this condition results from chronic tissue hypoxia. Nail thinning accompanied by an abnormal alteration of the angle of the finger and toe bases characterizes clubbing.

Preparation for respiratory assessment

After gaining an overview of the patient's oxygenation, proceed with assessment of the respiratory system. Physical assessment of the respiratory system requires a quiet, well-lit environment and specific equipment, such as a stethoscope with a diaphragm.

For a basic assessment of the chest and lungs, use inspection, palpation, percussion, and auscultation. (For information about assessing the upper airways, see Chapter 7, Head and neck.)

If possible, have the patient sit in a position that allows access to the anterior and posterior thorax. Provide a gown that offers easy access to the chest and back without requiring unnecessary exposure. Make sure the patient is not cold, because shivering may alter breathing patterns. If the patient cannot sit up, use the semi-Fowler's position to assess the anterior chest wall and the side-lying position to assess the posterior thorax. However, be aware that these positions may distort findings.

Inspection

Basic assessment of respiratory function requires evaluation of the rate, rhythm, and quality of respirations as well as inspection of chest configuration, chest symmetry, skin condition, and accessory muscle use. Also assess for nasal flaring. To accomplish these steps, inspect the patient's breathing and the anterior and posterior thorax, noting any abnormal findings.

Respiration

Because respiratory rates vary with age, be aware of the patient's normal rate range. If the patient is eupneic, the respiratory rate is within the normal range for the patient's age group. (For specific ranges, see *How age affects vital signs,* page 39.)

When assessing respiratory rate, count the number of respirations—one respiration is composed of an inspiration and an expiration—for 1 full minute. For a patient with periodic or irregular breathing, monitor respirations for more than 1 minute to determine the rate accurately. Assess the duration of any periods lacking spontaneous respiration (apnea). Also note any abnormal respiratory patterns, such as tachypnea (persistently rapid, shallow breathing) or bradypnea (abnormally decreased respiratory rate); report alterations in respiration to the nurse practitioner or physician. (For more information, see *Respiratory patterns,* page 42).

Assess the quality of respiration by observing the type and depth of breathing. Assess the method of ventilation by having the patient lie in a supine position to expose the chest and abdominal walls. Adult females commonly exhibit thoracic breathing, which involves an upward and outward motion of the chest; infants, males, and sleeping patients most often exhibit abdominal breathing, using the abdominal muscles. Patients with COPD may use pursed-lip breathing, which prevents small airway collapse during exhalation. Forced inspiration or expiration may alter assessment findings; therefore, ask the patient to breathe quietly.

Anterior thorax

After assessing the patient's respirations, inspect the thorax for structural deformities, such as a concave or convex curvature of the anterior chest wall over the sternum. Inspect between and around the ribs for visible sinking of soft tissues (retractions). Assess the patient's respiratory pattern, checking for symmetry, and look for abnormalities in skin color or changes in muscle tone. For future documentation, note the location of any abnormalities according to regions delineated by imaginary lines in the thorax.

Initially inspect the chest wall to identify the shape of the thoracic cage. In an adult, the thorax should have a greater diameter laterally (from side to side) than anteroposteriorly (from front to back).

Note the angle between the ribs and sternum at the point immediately above the xiphoid process. Called the costal angle, this angle should be less than 90 degrees in an adult; it widens if the chest wall is chronically expanded, such as COPD.

To inspect the anterior chest for symmetry of movement, have the patient lie in a supine position with the head elevated as needed for comfort. Stand at the foot of the bed and carefully observe the patient's quiet, deep breathing for equal expansion of the chest wall. At the same time, be alert for abnormal collapse of part of the chest wall during inspiration along with abnormal expansion of the same area during expiration (paradoxical movement).

Next, check for accessory muscle use by observing the sternocleidomastoid, scalenus, and trapezius muscles in the shoulders and neck. During normal inhalation and exhalation, the diaphragm and external intercostal muscles alone should easily maintain breathing. Hypertrophy of any accessory muscle may indicate frequent use, especially in an elderly patient, but may be normal in a well-conditioned athlete. Also observe the position the patient assumes to breathe. A patient depending on accessory muscles may assume a "tripod" position, resting the arms on the knees or the sides of a chair.

Observe the patient's skin on the anterior chest for unusual color, lumps, or lesions, and note the location of any abnormality. Unless the patient has been exposed to significant sun or heat, skin on the chest should match the rest of the complexion.

Posterior thorax

To inspect the posterior chest, observe the patient's breathing again. A patient who cannot sit in a backless chair or lean forward against a supporting structure can lie in a lateral position. However, this may distort thoracic expansion.

Assess the posterior chest wall for the same characteristics as the anterior chest wall: chest structure, respiratory pattern, symmetry of expansion, skin color and muscle tone, and accessory muscle use.

Abnormal findings

Note all abnormal inspection findings. For example, unilateral absence of chest movement may indicate previous surgical removal of that lung, bronchial obstruction, or a collapsed lung caused by air or fluid in the pleural space. Delayed chest movement may indicate congestion or consolidation of the underlying lung. Paradoxical movement often follows trauma or incorrectly performed chest compression during cardiopulmonary resuscitation.

Inspection also may reveal structural deformities of the chest wall resulting from defects of the sternum, rib cage, or vertebral column. These deformities have many variations and may be congenital, acute, or progressive. A concave sternal depression—called a funnel chest (pectus excavatum)—or a convex deformity—called a pigeon chest (pectus carinatum)—are sternal defects that can hinder breathing by preventing full chest expansion. Also, COPD may cause a rounded chest wall (barrel chest).

Other structural deformities of the posterior thorax that may alter ventilation include anterior curvature of the lumbar spine (lordosis), lateral curvature of the spine (scoliosis), exaggeration of the anteroposterior spine (kyphosis), and lateral and anteroposterior curvature of the spine (kyphoscoliosis). These deformities can compress one lung while allowing overexpansion of the opposite lung, eventually leading to respiratory dysfunction. Acute changes in the thoracic wall resulting from trauma, such as fractured ribs or flail chest (fractures of two or more ribs in two or more places), alter ventilation by allowing uneven chest expansion. Pain caused by these deformities leads to shallow breathing, which increases respiratory distress.

Palpation
Palpation of the trachea and thorax can detect structural and skin abnormalities, areas of pain, and chest asymmetry.

Trachea and anterior thorax
First, palpate the trachea for position, which should be midline. Observe the patient to detect any use of accessory neck muscles to breathe.

Next, palpate the suprasternal notch. In most patients, the arch of the aorta lies close to the surface just behind the suprasternal notch. Using the fingertips, gently evaluate the strength and regularity of aortic pulsations there.

Then palpate the thorax to assess the skin and underlying tissues. Gentle palpation should not cause pain; assess any complaints of pain for localization, radiation, and severity. Be especially careful to palpate any areas that looked abnormal during inspection. If necessary, support the patient with one hand during the procedure while using the other hand to palpate one side at a time, continuing to compare sides. Note any unusual findings, such as masses, crepitus, skin irregularities, or painful areas.

Palpate any painful areas while attempting to determine the cause of pain. Certain disorders—such as musculoskeletal pain, irritation of the nerves covering the xiphoid process, or inflammation of the cartilage connecting the bony ribs to the sternum (costochondritis)—cause increased pain during palpation. These disorders also may produce pain during inspiration, causing the patient to breathe shallowly to decrease discomfort. On the other hand, palpation does not increase pain caused by cardiac or pulmonary disorders, such as angina or pleurisy.

To assess the anterior thorax for symmetrical chest movement, use a technique called respiratory excursion. Performed anteriorly and pos-

Respiratory excursion

To assess respiratory excursion, the nurse should follow these steps.

Stand behind the patient and place the thumbs in the infrascapular area on either side of the spine at the level of the tenth rib. Grasp the lateral rib cage and rest the palms gently over the latero-posterior surface (Step 1). To prevent restricting the patient's breathing, do not apply excessive pressure.

As the patient inhales, the posterior chest should move upward and outward and the thumbs should move apart (Step 2). When the patient exhales, the thumbs should return to midline and again touch.

Repeat the procedure after placing the thumbs equally lateral to the vertebral column in the interscapular area, with the fingers extending into the axillary area. Instruct the patient to take a deep breath, then watch for simultaneous, equal separation of the thumbs.

Step 1

Step 2

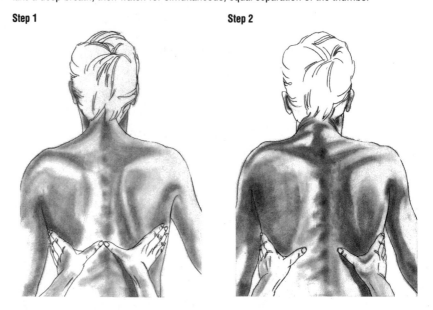

teriorly, respiratory excursion provides information about chest wall expansion during inspiration and chest wall contraction during expiration. (For an illustrated procedure, see *Respiratory excursion*.)

Posterior thorax

Palpate the posterior thorax in a similar manner, using the palmar surface of the fingertips of one or both hands. During the process, identify bony structures, such as the vertebrae and scapulae. To determine the location of any abnormalities, identify the first thoracic vertebra (with the patient's head tipped forward) and count the number of spinous processes from this landmark to the abnormal finding. Use this reference point for documentation. Also identify the inferior scapular tips and medial borders of both bones to define the margins of the upper and lower lung lobes posteriorly. Locate and describe all abnormalities in relation to these landmarks. Next, assess posterior respiratory excursion in a manner similar to that used for the anterior respiratory excursion.

Abnormal findings

Palpation may show that the trachea is not midline. This could result from a mass in the neck or from thyroid enlargement.

Tenderness upon palpation of the anterior chest could indicate musculoskeletal inflammation, especially if the patient complains of chest pain of unknown origin.

Palpation producing a crackly sound similar to the noise of crumpling cellophane paper suggests crepitus. Report this sign to the physician immediately, because crepitus indicates air leakage into the subcutaneous tissue from a rupture somewhere in the respiratory system.

Absence of or delay in chest movement during respiratory excursion may indicate previous surgical lung removal, complete or partial obstruction of the airway or underlying lung, or diaphragmatic dysfunction on the affected side.

Percussion

Percussion helps determine lung boundaries and the amount of gas, liquid, or solid in the lungs.

The most frequently used percussion technique is mediate percussion, which involves striking one finger with another. To percuss correctly, follow these guidelines. Ensure a quiet environment. Proceed systematically, percussing the anterior, lateral, and posterior chest over the intercostal spaces. Avoid percussing over bones, such as the manubrium, sternum, xiphoid, clavicles, ribs, vertebrae, or scapulae. Because of their denseness, bones produce a dull sound on percussion and therefore yield no useful information. Percussion over a healthy lung elicits a resonant sound—hollow and loud, with a low pitch and long duration.

To percuss the anterior chest, have the patient sit facing forward, hands resting at the sides of the body. Following the anterior percussion sequence, percuss and compare sound variations from one side to the other. Anterior chest percussion should produce resonance from below the clavicle to the fifth intercostal space on the right (where dullness occurs close to the liver) and to the third intercostal space on the left (where dullness occurs near the heart). (For more information, see *Percussion and auscultation sites,* page 152.)

Next, percuss the lateral chest to obtain information about the lung lobes. Position the patient's left arm on the patient's head. Repeat the same sequence on the right side. Lateral chest percussion should produce resonance to the sixth or eighth intercostal space.

Finally, percuss the posterior thorax according to the percussion sequence. Posterior percussion should sound resonant to the level of thoracic vertebra ten.

Percussion and auscultation sites

These illustrations show the proper sites for percussion and auscultation of the posterior thorax, lateral thorax, and anterior thorax. Because the lungs are paired organs, the nurse should think of percussion and auscultation sites as pairs, as shown by the numbers on each illustration.

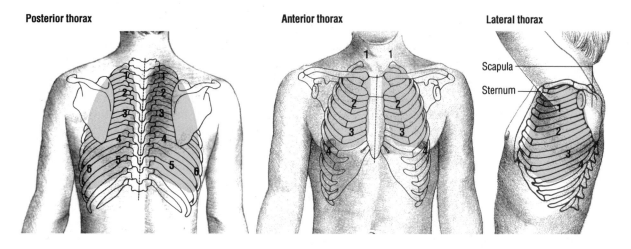

Posterior thorax

Anterior thorax

Lateral thorax

Scapula

Sternum

Abnormal findings

Hyperresonance and dullness are the most common abnormal percussion findings. Hyperresonance may result from air in the pleural space, which may be caused by pneumothorax or lung overinflation (such as with COPD). Dullness may result from consolidation of fluid or tissue, which may occur with pneumonia or atelectasis.

Auscultation

Auscultate the anterior, lateral, and posterior thorax to detect normal and abnormal breath sounds. To auscultate the thorax of an adult, warm the stethoscope between the hands and place the diaphragm of the stethoscope directly on the patient's skin. Clothing or linen interferes with accurate auscultation. If the patient has significant hair growth over the areas to be auscultated, wet the hair to decrease sound blurring. Instruct the patient to take deep breaths through the mouth (nose breathing may alter findings). To prevent light-headedness or dizziness, caution the patient against breathing too deeply or too rapidly.

Anterior and lateral thorax

Systematically assess the anterior and lateral thorax for normal as well as abnormal breath sounds, following the same sequence as that used for percussion. Begin at the upper lobes, and move from side to side and down.

Normal breath sounds

When auscultating the thorax, the nurse systematically assesses breath sounds. This chart describes normal breath sounds.

BREATH SOUND	DESCRIPTION	CAUSE
Bronchial (tracheal)	• Loud, high-pitched • Heard best over the trachea • Inspiration-expiration ratio 1:2	Air passing through the trachea
Bronchovesicular	• Soft • Medium-pitched, compared to bronchial sounds • Heard near mainstem bronchi in first and second intercostal spaces anteriorly, and between scapulae posteriorly • Inspiration-expiration ratio 1:1	Air traveling through branches and convergences of smaller bronchi and bronchioles
Vesicular	• Soft • Lower-pitched than bronchovesicular sounds • Heard best in periphery but inaudible over scapulae • Inspiration-expiration ratio 3:1	Air traveling through alveolar ducts and alveoli

Auscultate a point first on one side of the chest, and then auscultate the same point on the other side, comparing findings. Always assess one full breath (inspiration and expiration) at each point.

During auscultation, first identify normal breath sounds and then assess and identify abnormal (adventitious) sounds. Specific breath sounds occur normally only in certain locations; the same sound heard anywhere else in the lung field constitutes an important abnormality requiring intervention.

To assess the right middle lung lobe, auscultate breath sounds laterally at the level of the fourth to the sixth intercostal spaces. Follow the lateral auscultation sequence, which is the same as the lateral percussion sequence. Although the right middle lobe is hard to assess, especially in a female patient with large breasts, it requires special attention because it is a frequent site of aspiration pneumonia.

Normal breath sounds include bronchial (tracheal), bronchovesicular, and vesicular sounds. (For more details on these sounds, see *Normal breath sounds.*)

Classify normal and abnormal breath sounds by location, intensity (amplitude), characteristic sound, pitch (tone), and duration during the inspiratory and expiratory phases. When assessing duration, time the inspiratory and expiratory phases to determine the ratio between them. When describing specific sounds, identify the quality using specific terms, such as high-pitched or harsh.

Abnormal breath sounds

The nurse can use this chart as a guide to assessing and documenting abnormal (adventitious) breath sounds.

ABNORMAL SOUND	LOCATION	DESCRIPTION	CAUSE
Crackles (rales)	Lung periphery	High-pitched, crackling; heard on inspiration	Air passing through fluid in small airways, as in pneumonia or congestive heart failure
Rhonchi (rattling or snoring sound)	Under clavicle anteriorly, between scapulae posteriorly	Loud, coarse, low-pitched; heard during inspiration or expiration	Air passing through fluid in larger airways, as in bronchitis or chronic obstructive pulmonary disease
Wheezes	Under clavicle anteriorly, between scapulae posteriorly	Squeaky, high- to low-pitched, heard on expiration progressing to inspiration	Air passing through narrowed airways, such as in asthma
Friction rub	Any place in thorax	Rubbing, grating; heard on inspiration and expiration	Inflamed parietal and visceral pleural linings rubbing together, as in pleurisy
Stridor	Over trachea	High-pitched, grating; heard on inspiration	Air attempting to pass through obstruction in upper airway, as in croup or epiglottitis

Posterior thorax

The auscultation sequence for the posterior thorax follows the same pattern as the percussion sequence. During auscultation, be aware of the patient's breathing pattern. Breathing too rapidly or deeply causes excessive carbon dioxide loss and may lead to vertigo or syncope. In a normal adult, adolescent, or older child, bronchovesicular breath sounds (the sound of air moving through bronchial airways) should occur over the interscapular area; vesicular breath sounds (the sound of air moving through alveoli) should occur in the suprascapular and infrascapular areas. Note any absent, decreased, or abnormal breath sounds.

Abnormal findings

Abnormal or adventitious breath sounds are extra sounds, indicating a disease or disorder. Crackles and rhonchi also are adventitious; if these occur, instruct the patient to cough, and then listen again. Adventitious sounds may indicate alveolar fluid, opening of compressed alveoli, secretions in small or large airways, narrowed airways, or pleural membrane inflammation. Certain adventitious sounds, including crackles, wheezes, rhonchi, and pleural friction rubs, may appear in any lung lobe. Also, abnormal placement of a normal sound may be adventitious, such as bronchial breath sounds in the periphery over an area of pneumonia. (For more information, see *Abnormal breath sounds*.)

Adventitious sounds are classified by location, timing (whether heard during inspiration or expiration), and pitch. Document adventitious sounds by labeling the sound or describing its characteristics. (Although either method is correct, most nurses currently use a description of the sound with or without a label.)

When assessing the patient, note all abnormal findings. By the end of the assessment, a cluster of signs and symptoms may point to a particular disorder.

Developmental considerations for pediatric patients

For the most effective assessment, have a parent hold the child in the arms or on the examination table. If the patient is an infant or a small child, seat the child on the parent's lap. Using a stethoscope with a pediatric diaphragm, auscultate the child's lungs first, before performing any other assessment procedure, to avoid having the child cry. Crying increases the respiratory rate and creates noise that interferes with clear auscultation. To increase the child's cooperativeness, demonstrate equipment on the parent or a doll first.

Before inspecting an infant's respiratory system, inspect the skin. Infants have a thin layer of subcutaneous tissue, making cyanosis a more reliable sign of respiratory distress in them than in adults. Inspect the chest wall to gain further information about respiratory status. More cartilage than bone composes a child's thoracic cage and, because less subcutaneous tissue is present to mask findings, chest wall movement should be more visible during breathing. Infants and children often exhibit abdominal or paradoxical breathing. Paradoxical breathing, which occurs when the chest and abdomen do not work together to expand and contract during inspiration and expiration, results from the child's immature respiratory center and weak chest muscles.

Next, observe for changes in thoracic structures, which also are easier to evaluate in an infant or child than in an adult. Assess an infant's chest circumference by snugly wrapping a tape measure around the chest at the nipple line. Mean chest circumference at birth is about 13″ (33 cm), usually ¾″ to 1⅛″ (2 to 3 cm) smaller than the head circumference, and about 18½″ (47 cm) at 1 year. Normally, infants have a round thoracic structure.

Infants and children do not use accessory muscles when in respiratory distress. However, they may exhibit bulging or retractions during inspiration and expiration—a sign of breathing difficulty. The intercostal muscles often bulge during infant respiratory distress, while the suprasternal, substernal, and abdominal muscles retract. These findings also may appear in adults, especially small or thin patients. Infants commonly use only the abdominal muscles to breathe until age 6; girls then become thoracic breathers while boys remain abdominal breathers.

Infants and toddlers have small chest surfaces; therefore, palpation is of little use. Chest palpation becomes appropriate at about age 4 or 5.

Percussion usually is unreliable because of the disproportionate size between an infant's chest and an adult's fingers.

To auscultate a child, use a stethoscope with an appropriately sized diaphragm. A child's small chest size means fewer auscultation sites. An infant's thinner, more resonant chest produces breath sounds that are louder and harsher than an adult's; bronchovesicular sounds in the periphery are common.

Developmental considerations for pregnant patients

This patient normally has an increased costal angle—up to 103 degrees by the third trimester. As a result, the lower rib cage appears to flare out. Internal organs become crowded, causing deeper respirations, increased sighing, and greater dyspnea. During the second and third trimesters, respiratory rate and depth may increase to meet the growing oxygenation and ventilation needs of the mother and fetus.

Developmental considerations for elderly patients

With age, the thoracic structure typically becomes rounder and the anteroposterior chest increases in relation to the lateral diameter because of changes in the thoracic and lumbar spine. Calcification of the rib articulations may cause the elderly patient to use accessory muscles to breathe. Percussion may produce hyperresonant sounds because lung tissue is less distensible. A decreased cough reflex increases the risk of aspiration for this age group.

Documentation

The following example illustrates proper documentation of normal respiratory findings during physical assessment:

Weight: 165 lb

Height: 5'10"

Vital signs: Temperature 98.6° F, pulse 70 and regular, respirations 18 and unlabored, blood pressure 120/80.

Additional notes: Well-developed male, who looks to be his stated age of 42, sits quietly during interview. Alert and cooperative. Skin color appropriate for race; skin warm and dry. Chest symmetrical with equal expansion, no retractions noted, costal angle 90 degrees. Palpation of anterior, posterior, and lateral chest walls reveals no areas of pain, swelling, lesions, or crepitus. Percussion resonant throughout peripheral lung lobes. Auscultation reveals vesicular breath sounds in peripheral lung lobes and bronchovesicular breath sounds anteriorly and posteriorly over the central airways.

The following example illustrates proper documentation of abnormal respiratory findings:

Height: 5'6"

Weight: 124 lb

Vital signs: Temperature 99.2° F, pulse 104 and regular, respirations 36 and labored, blood pressure 168/96.

Additional notes: Thin, barrel-chested male appearing older than his stated age of 56, using accessory muscles and pursed-lip breathing. Chest expansion symmetrical, but limited. Percussion over all chest walls reveals hyperresonance. Breath sounds decreased over entire thorax, with prolonged expiratory phase.

STUDY ACTIVITIES

Short answer

1. What are the four most common signs and symptoms of respiratory dysfunction?

_____

2. Provide an accurate definition of orthopnea.

_____

3. Loretta Zeller, age 68, a patient with COPD, exhibits dyspnea during minimal exertion. Identify two questions the nurse should ask Ms. Zeller during the health history to assess how dyspnea might be affecting her nutritional status.

_____

4. While percussing Richard Lincoln's anterior thorax, the nurse notes dullness at the level of the fifth intercostal space on his right side. Should the nurse consider this a normal or abnormal finding?

_____

5. Sam Casey, age 4, is brought to the emergency department by his parents. They tell the nurse that Sam has had a fever with a congested cough for the past 3 days and has been coughing up yellow sputum. The nurse conducts a rapid assessment, which uncovers abdominal breathing, retraction at the intercostal spaces, and crackles in peripheral lung fields. Which of these findings should the nurse consider abnormal?

_____

6. Adventitious breath sounds, including rhonchi, wheezes, and stridor, are common in patients with certain pulmonary conditions. Name at least one disease or disorder that can cause each of those adventitious sounds.

_____

Matching related elements

Match the normal breath sound on the left with its best location for auscultation on the right.

7. ___ Bronchial sound   **A.** Over peripheral lung fields

8. ___ Bronchovesicular   **B.** Over the trachea
       sounds

9. ___ Vesicular   **C.** Under the clavicles anteriorly, between the scapula posteriorly

ANSWERS

Short answer

1. The four most common signs of respiratory dysfunction are cough, dyspnea, sputum production, and chest pain or discomfort.

2. Orthopnea is the need to sit or stand to breathe normally.

3. The nurse should ask Ms. Zeller the following questions: *Do you have difficulty breathing when eating?* (Ms. Zeller may not be meeting her nutritional needs because of dyspnea when eating.) *Do you eat three meals a day or many small meals?* (Ms. Zeller may be eating small, frequent meals to reduce dyspnea.)

4. Because the nurse is percussing at the level of the liver, dullness is considered a normal finding.

5. Retraction at the intercostal spaces is an abnormal finding indicating difficulty breathing. Crackles in peripheral lung fields also are abnormal, indicating that air is moving through fluid-filled airways. Abdominal breathing is normal for a child under age 6.

6. Bronchitis and COPD may cause rhonchi, asthma may cause wheezing, and epiglottitis and croup may cause stridor.

Matching related elements

7. B

8. C

9. A

CHAPTER 10

Cardiovascular system

OBJECTIVES   After studying this chapter, the reader should be able to:
1. Identify the major structures of the heart.
2. Trace blood flow through the heart.
3. Explain the events of cardiac conduction.
4. Write interview questions that help evaluate cardiovascular health.
5. Identify risk factors for cardiovascular diseases.
6. Differentiate between normal and abnormal findings during inspection and palpation of the cardiovascular system.
7. Demonstrate auscultation of the aortic, pulmonic, tricuspid, and mitral (or apical) areas, and describe the heart sounds normally heard at each one.
8. Document cardiovascular assessment appropriately.

OVERVIEW OF   The nurse's assessment of the cardiovascular system is important
CONCEPTS   because cardiovascular disease is the most prevalent health care problem—and the most common cause of death—in the United States. Every year, 25,000 children are born with congenital heart disease and more than 1.5 million adults have myocardial infarctions (MIs), which are commonly known as heart attacks.

The cardiovascular system consists of the heart and blood vessels. The heart, a strong pump, and the blood vessels, which are long conduits, deliver blood—and the oxygen, nutrients, metabolites, and hormones that it carries—to the body's cells. The blood picks up waste products in the cells and delivers them to target organs for detoxification and excretion.

A four-chambered muscle, the heart is roughly cone-shaped and about the size of a closed fist. It lies substernally in the mediastinum, between the second and sixth ribs. About one third of the heart lies to the right of the midsternal line; the remainder, to the left. Because the heart is hollow, blood can flow through its chambers and valves. When the heart muscle contracts, it pumps blood through arteries. (For illustrations of the chambers, valves, and blood flow, see *Cardiac anatomy and normal blood flow*, page 160.)

Cardiac anatomy and normal blood flow

The large illustration below depicts the major structures of the heart; the arrows show how blood flows through the heart. The small illustration shows the anatomy of the heart wall.

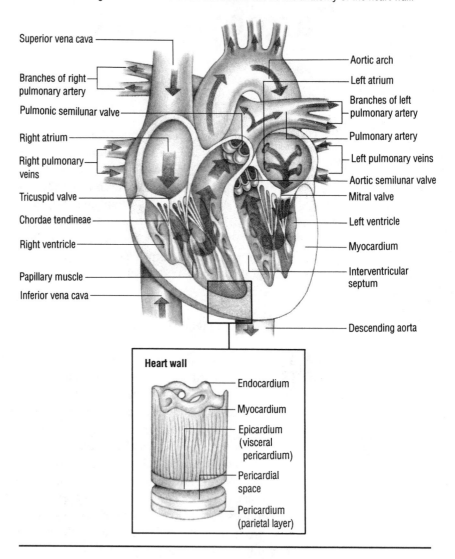

A vast network of vessels—about 60,000 miles (96,558 km) of arteries, arterioles, capillaries, venules, and veins—keeps blood circulating to and from every functioning cell in the body. This network has two basic branches: the pulmonary circulation and the systemic circulation. Through the pulmonary circulation, blood travels to the lungs to pick up oxygen and liberate carbon dioxide. Through the systemic circulation, blood carries oxygen and other nutrients to body cells and transports waste products for excretion. The coronary circulation, a

Cardiac conduction

This illustration shows the major structures of the cardiac conduction system and the path of electrical impulses through the heart.

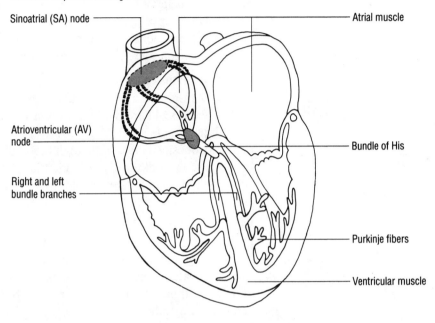

specialized part of the systemic circulation, supplies blood to the heart itself.

An electrical conduction system regulates myocardial contraction, thereby initiating the heartbeat and coordinating chamber contraction. Myocardial muscle cells, which provide strength during contraction, also have specialized pacemaker cells that allow conduction of an electrical impulse. This impulse spreads quickly throughout the muscle cell network, causing a generalized contraction.

Normally, the sinoatrial (SA) node serves as the driving pacemaker of the heart. Each impulse travels from the SA node via intranodal pathways to the right and left atria, causing atrial contraction. The impulse slows momentarily as it passes through the atrioventricular (AV) node to the bundle of His. Then it travels down the right and left bundle branches to Purkinje fibers, which stimulate ventricular contraction. (For an illustration, see *Cardiac conduction*.)

These electrical and mechanical events combine in the cardiac cycle (the period from the beginning of one heartbeat to the beginning of the next). To provide adequate blood flow to all parts of the body, these events must occur in the proper order and to the proper degree. The amount of blood the heart pumps in 1 minute (cardiac output) is determined by the stroke volume—the amount of blood ejected with each beat multiplied by the number of beats per minute.

Health history   The cardiovascular health history should focus on patient risk factors and signs and symptoms of heart disease. The history also should assess patient behaviors that promote or jeopardize cardiovascular health. This part of the health history can uncover the need for teaching the patient about behaviors that should be changed or may offer a chance to encourage the patient to continue healthful behaviors.

Health and illness patterns

When obtaining the cardiovascular health history, carefully evaluate for risk factors of cardiovascular disease, such as family history of cardiac disease, male gender, age, (over age 60 in males or over age 70 in females), obesity, consistently high blood pressure (above 140/90 mm Hg), cigarette smoking, hyperlipidemia (elevated cholesterol level), diabetes mellitus, and left ventricular hypertrophy. Also note factors that reduce the risk of heart disease, such as proper diet and exercise.

Current health status

Because current health is foremost in the patient's mind, the nurse should begin the interview by exploring this topic. The questions below can help evaluate the patient's cardiovascular system. Using the PQRST method, ask the patient to describe completely the chief complaint and any others. (For a detailed explanation of this method, see *Symptom analysis,* page 15.)

Do you ever have chest pain or discomfort? If so, how would you describe it? Where in your chest do you feel the pain? Does it radiate to any other area? How long have you been having the pain? How long does an attack last? How many times per day or week or month do you have the pain?
(RATIONALE: Chest pain can result from many cardiac disorders, such as angina, MI, and pericarditis [pericardial inflammation]. It also can result from pulmonary and gastroesophageal disorders. The patient's answers to these questions should help determine the source of pain.)

Do you ever experience shortness of breath or cough?
(RATIONALE: Shortness of breath (dyspnea) commonly results from congestive heart failure. As heart failure worsens, lung congestion occurs, leading to dyspnea and coughing. Dyspnea also may result from pulmonary disorders as well as other cardiovascular disorders, such as coronary artery disease, myocardial ischemia, and MI.)

Do you ever have dizzy spells?
(RATIONALE: Syncope develops when reduced cardiac output or vascular insufficiency deprives the brain of blood. It can accompany various cardiovascular problems, such as aortic stenosis [valve narrowing], mitral stenosis, certain arrhythmias, and pacemaker failure.)

Do your shoes or rings feel tight? Do your ankles or feet feel swollen? If so, how long have you felt this way?
(RATIONALE: Swelling in the extremities signals edema, a common sign of cardiac disease. Edema indicates interstitial fluid collection and can occur when the heart fails to pump blood adequately, as in congestive heart failure [CHF].)

Does your heart ever feel like it is pounding, racing, or skipping beats?
(RATIONALE: Palpitations may result from an arrhythmia or vigorous exercise.)

Do you tire more easily than you used to? What type of activity causes you to feel fatigued? How long can you perform this activity before you feel fatigued? Does rest relieve the fatigue?
(RATIONALE: Fatigue and weakness resulting from mild exertion, especially if relieved by rest, may indicate early CHF. In this disorder, the heart cannot provide enough blood to meet the cells' slightly increased metabolic needs.)

Do you have ulcers or sores on your legs? If so, are they healing? Have you noticed any change in the feeling in your legs?
(RATIONALE: Decreased circulation to the lower extremities can cause ulcers that do not heal and can decrease sensation.)

Past health status
Ask the following questions to explore the patient's medical history for additional information related to the cardiovascular system:

Were you born with a heart problem? If so, when and how was it treated?
(RATIONALE: Problems related to certain congenital heart disorders, such as tetralogy of Fallot and ventricular septal defect, may persist even after treatment or surgical correction.)

Have you had rheumatic fever? If so, when? Have any heart problems resulted from the rheumatic fever?
(RATIONALE: Rheumatic fever can lead to rheumatic heart disease, eventually causing valvular stenosis or insufficiency.)

Have you ever had a heart murmur? If so, who told you about it and when?
(RATIONALE: Many people have innocent, or functional, murmurs that are unrelated to structural heart disease. Others have murmurs that are caused by permanent structural problems.)

For a female patient, ask the following question:

Do you take oral contraceptives?
(RATIONALE: Women who take oral contraceptives, paticularly smokers, have an increased risk for MI and pulmonary embolism [blood clot in the lung].)

Family health status

Next, investigate the cardiovascular status of the patient's family by asking the following questions:

Has anyone in your family been treated for heart disease?
(RATIONALE: Certain types of heart disease, such as coronary artery disease, have a familial tendency.)

Has anyone in your family died suddenly of an unknown cause?
(RATIONALE: The family member may have died from cardiac arrest due to heart disease. This may place the patient at higher risk for this problem.)

Does anyone in your family have high blood pressure, high cholesterol, or diabetes mellitus?
(RATIONALE: These heart disease risk factors tend to run in families.)

Developmental considerations for pediatric patients

Whenever possible, involve the child in the interview. Ask the following questions:

Has the child experienced any growth delay?
(RATIONALE: Slow growth may result from impaired cardiac output.)

Does the child turn blue when crying or have difficulty feeding?
(RATIONALE: Bluish skin color [cyanosis] and feeding difficulty may indicate a congenital heart disease. In such a child, the heart cannot increase its work load enough to provide the extra energy required by crying or eating.)

Does the child tire easily or sleep excessively?
(RATIONALE: Poor exercise tolerance and fatigue may indicate congenital heart disease or CHF.)

Developmental considerations for pregnant patients

Pregnancy causes many physiologic changes. The following additional questions help assess for these effects:

During this pregnancy, has any health care professional said that you have a heart murmur?
(RATIONALE: The increased blood volume associated with pregnancy can cause an innocent, physiologic murmur. However, any murmur requires further study to exclude a pathologic cause.)

Has your blood pressure been elevated during this pregnancy?
(RATIONALE: Blood pressure elevation can signal toxemia of pregnancy, an abnormal and potentially fatal condition characterized in its early stages by hypertension, proteinuria, and edema.)

Have you noticed any swelling in your feet or ankles? Have you developed varicose veins in your legs or genitals? Have you developed hemorrhoids?
(RATIONALE: During pregnancy, increased venous pressure and venous pooling can result in edema and varicosities, including hemorrhoids.)

Developmental considerations for elderly patients

With age, the cardiovascular system undergoes many physiologic changes that make it more susceptible to disorders. To uncover potential problems in an elderly patient, ask the following questions:

Do you ever feel dizzy when changing position or exerting yourself? Does your heart beat rapidly at times?

(RATIONALE: Tortuous carotid arteries, a thickened endothelium, and a fibrotic conduction system can reduce blood supply to the brain, causing syncope. As the heart loses elasticity, it may beat rapidly in response to stress or exertion.)

Do you suffer from shortness of breath? If so, is it ever accompanied by coughing or wheezing?

(RATIONALE: In an elderly patient, an MI or an ischemic episode may cause dyspnea, but no pain. A nonproductive cough or wheezing may accompany dyspnea.)

Health promotion and protection patterns

To determine how the patient provides for or maintains health, investigate health promotion and protection behaviors.

Personal habits

Personal habits can affect health positively or negatively. To assess the patient's personal habits, pose the following questions:

Do you smoke cigarettes, cigars, or a pipe or chew tobacco? If so, how long have you smoked? How many cigarettes, cigars, or pipes of tobacco do you smoke per day? Did you ever stop smoking? If so, for how long? What method did you use to stop?

(RATIONALE: Smoking, especially cigarette smoking, is a major risk factor for cardiac disease. Report the patient's smoking history in pack-years by multiplying the number of years of smoking by the number of packs smoked per day.)

Do you drink alcohol? If so, what type? How often do you drink? How many drinks?

(RATIONALE: Alcohol can be habit-forming or addictive and can cause cardiomyopathy as well as problems in other body systems.)

Sleep and waking patterns

Cardiovascular problems can interfere with sleep and rest. The following questions investigate such problems:

How long do you sleep each night? Do you feel rested after sleeping? Do you nap?

(RATIONALE: Abnormally long sleep, feeling poorly rested, or the need for abnormally frequent naps may indicate a cardiovascular problem, such as cardiomyopathy. To determine if the amount of sleep is abnormal for the patient's age, see Chapter 4, Activities of daily living and sleep patterns.)

Do you awaken during the night to urinate?
(RATIONALE: Nocturia may occur in a patient with CHF.)

Do you experience episodes of shortness of breath or coughing during the night? If so, when do these episodes occur? How frequently do they occur? How long do they last?
(RATIONALE: Episodes of dyspnea and coughing at night are signs of paroxysmal nocturnal dyspnea, which results from CHF and interstitial pulmonary congestion.)

Do you become short of breath when you lie flat? How many pillows do you use at night? Has this number changed recently?
(RATIONALE: Orthopnea, or shortness of breath that occurs when supine, may result from the pulmonary congestion that accompanies CHF.)

Exercise and activity patterns

Although aerobic exercise is the best cardiac conditioner, any regular exercise or activity can help prevent cardiovascular problems. The following questions investigate the patient's exercise and activity levels:

Do you exercise routinely? If so, what exercises do you perform? How would you describe the frequency, intensity, and length of time that you exercise?
(RATIONALE: With activity or exercise, the body's need for oxygen and other nutrients increases. The heart meets this need by increasing the cardiac output. The degree of exercise tolerance reveals the patient's cardiovascular response to increased metabolic demands.)

Have you noticed any change in your ability to care for yourself?
(RATIONALE: For an elderly or sedentary patient, inability to perform activities of daily living may be the first sign that cardiac output cannot meet the metabolic demands caused by low-energy activities.)

When you walk or exercise, do you experience leg pain?
(RATIONALE: Leg pain may result from narrowed arteries that cannot provide the increased blood and oxygen needed.)

Nutritional patterns

Because diet is important to cardiovascular health, investigate this area by asking the following questions:

What have you eaten during the past 24 hours? Do you follow any special diet?
(RATIONALE: A diet recall may reveal dietary patterns that contribute to the risk of cardiac disease. It also may reveal any dietary patterns the patient adheres to for health, ethnic, or religious reasons.)

Have you gained or lost weight recently?
(RATIONALE: A weight gain of 2 to 3 lb [.9 to 1.3 kg] in 48 hours may signal fluid retention, which can lead to CHF. Rapid weight loss may demonstrate an appropriate response to diuretic therapy.)

Stress and coping patterns

Examining stress and coping patterns provides information about the patient's personality type and aids in planning nursing interventions. The following questions investigate these concerns:

What causes you to feel stressed? How often does this occur? What physical feelings do you have when you experience stress?
(RATIONALE: Stress raises the heart rate and blood pressure and, if chronic, can lead to progressive changes in the heart and vessels, thereby increasing the risk of cardiac disease. In a patient with coronary artery disease, stress can lead to chest pain and dyspnea—symptoms of myocardial ischemia.)

Other health promotion and protection patterns

Other factors can affect a patient's health, such as economic influences, environmental and occupational health patterns, and daily activities. To assess these factors, ask the following questions:

Do your financial resources and insurance adequately cover your health care needs?
(RATIONALE: Without adequate health insurance and financial resources, the patient may be unable to obtain necessary health care services and prescribed medications.)

How is your house or apartment laid out physically? Must you climb steps to get inside, or to get from room to room? On which level are the bathroom, bedroom, and kitchen?
(RATIONALE: The physical layout of the patient's house or apartment can provide an estimate of the energy needed to get around it. If the patient has significant heart disease, the layout may need to be modified.)

What is your occupation?
(RATIONALE: The patient may be unable to perform occupational responsibilities because of cardiovascular limitations.)

Role and relationship patterns

Cardiovascular disorders can affect many role and relationship patterns. To discover the extent of this effect, ask these questions:

Do you think of yourself as a healthy person or sick person?
(RATIONALE: A cardiovascular dysfunction can negatively affect the patient's sense of identity and self-esteem.)

Has your usual pattern of sexual activity changed in any way? If so, how would you describe this change? How do you feel about it?
(RATIONALE: Some patients with cardiac disease, or their spouses, may avoid sexual activity because they incorrectly fear it will cause further heart damage. Other patients may experience decreased desire or impotence caused by fear or adverse drug reactions.)

Physical assessment
Before assessing the patient's cardiovascular system, the nurse should evaluate various patient factors that may reflect cardiovascular function, including general appearance, body weight, vital signs, and related body structures.

Physical assessment of the cardiovascular system involves the basic techniques of inspection, palpation, and auscultation. (Percussion yields little information and is seldom performed.) However, the assessment need not be performed in this exact order. As appropriate, combine parts of the assessment to conserve time and the patient's energy.

General appearance, body weight, and vital signs

To begin the physical assessment, observe the patient's general appearance, particularly noting weight and muscle composition. Document any departures from the norm.

Body weight

Accurately measure and record the patient's height and weight. A weight increase or decrease may be significant, especially if extreme. A gain of several pounds overnight commonly occurs in a patient who is developing CHF.

Vital signs

An elevated body temperature can indicate cardiovascular inflammation or infection, or an infection from another source. Whatever the cause, temperature elevation speeds the metabolism, which increases the cardiac workload. Generally, the heart rate increases 10 beats per minute for every degree (°F) of fever.

Next, assess the patient's blood pressure. Elevated blood pressure may result from hypertension or emotional stress associated with the physical assessment. If the patient's blood pressure is elevated, allow the patient to relax, then repeat the measurement in 5 to 10 minutes to determine if the elevation is stress-related. Hypertension is present when blood pressure is elevated above 140/90 mm Hg on several successive readings. (The diagnosis is not made on one reading alone.)

After measuring blood pressure, calculate pulse pressure (the difference between the higher, systolic pressure and the lower, diastolic pressure). Pulse pressure, which reflects arterial pressure during the resting phase of the cardiac cycle, normally ranges from 30 to 50 mm Hg. Pulse pressure increases when stroke volume increases, as in exercise, anxiety, or bradycardia. It also increases aortic insufficiency in anemia, hyperthyroidism, fever, hypertension, aortic coarctation, and aging. Pulse pressure declines when a mechanical obstruction exists, such as mitral or aortic stenosis; when peripheral vessels constrict, as in shock; or when stroke volume decreases, as in heart failure, hypovolemia, or tachycardia.

When obtaining vital signs, assess the radial pulse to determine the heart rate. For a patient with suspected cardiac disease, be sure to palpate for a full minute to detect any arrhythmias. Normally, an adult's pulse ranges from 60 to 100 beats/minute, with a regular rhythm.

Count the patient's respirations, observing for eupnea—a regular, unlabored, and bilaterally equal breathing pattern. Tachypnea (rapid respirations) may indicate a low cardiac output. Dyspnea, which may signal CHF, may not be evident at rest but may occur when the patient speaks.

Assessment of related body structures

Because the cardiovascular system affects many other body systems, a patient with a cardiovascular disorder may exhibit signs of illness in other parts of the body. The nurse should include these areas in the physical inspection.

Skin, hair, and nails

Inspect the skin color, particularly noting any cyanosis. (For more information, see Chapter 9, Respiratory system). Examine the underside of the tongue, buccal mucosa, and conjunctivae for signs of central cyanosis. (This is helpful regardless of the patient's skin color.) Inspect the skin of the extremities and nail beds for signs of peripheral cyanosis. Also inspect the mucous membranes. (For more information on mucous membrane assessment, see Chapter 7, Head and neck).

When evaluating the patient's skin color, observe for flushing (a reddish discoloration caused by vasodilation) and pallor (unusual paleness or absence of skin color), which may result from anemia or peripheral vascular disease.

Touch the patient's skin, which should feel warm and dry. Cool, clammy skin results from vasoconstriction, which occurs when cardiac output is low, as in shock. Observe the skin for signs of edema (swelling caused by abnormal fluid accumulation in the interstitial spaces). Edema can result from CHF or venous insufficiency, which may be caused by varicosities or thrombophlebitis. Because edema usually affects lower or dependent areas of the body first, be especially alert when assessing the arms, hands, legs, feet, and ankles of an ambulatory patient or the buttocks and sacrum of a bedridden patient. If edema is present, determine its type (pitting or nonpitting), location, extent, and symmetry (unilateral or symmetrical). If the patient has pitting edema, assess the degree of pitting. (For details on assessing pitting edema, see Chapter 13, Urinary system.)

While inspecting the extremities, note any lesions consistent with cardiovascular disease. Dry, open lesions on the lower extremities accompanied by pallor and cool skin signify arterial insufficiency, as seen with peripheral arterial disease. Wet, open lesions with red or purplish edges that appear on the legs may result from the venous stasis associated with peripheral venous disease.

Assess capillary refill in the fingernails to estimate the rate of peripheral blood flow. To do this, apply pressure to the patient's fingernail for 5 seconds; the area under pressure should blanch. Then remove the pressure and observe how rapidly the normal color returns to the nail. In a patient with a good arterial supply, the color should return briskly, in less than 3 seconds. Note any delays, which may signify decreased circulation to the area.

Eyes

The eyes should be clear and bright, and the eyelids free of lesions. Inspect the eyelids for xanthelasmas—small, slightly raised, yellowish plaques that usually appear around the inner canthus. Because these plaques result from lipid deposits, they may signal severe hyperlipidemia, a risk factor for cardiac disease.

Observe scleral color, which normally is white. Yellowish sclerae may be the first sign of jaundice, which typically results from a liver disorder but also may reflect liver congestion caused by CHF. Inspect the eyes for arcus senilis—a thin, grayish ring around the edge of the cornea. Although common in the elderly, it can indicate hyperlipidemia in a younger person. The retinal vessels can be examined by using an ophthalmoscope.

Inspection and palpation

Assess the cardiovascular system first by inspection and then by palpation. Expose the patient's anterior chest and observe its general appearance. Normally, the lateral diameter is twice the anteroposterior diameter. Note any deviations from the typical chest shape, such as barrel chest (a rounded thoracic rib cage caused by chronic obstructive pulmonary disease), pectus excavatum (a depressed sternum), scoliosis (lateral curvature of the spine), or kyphosis (convex curvature of the thoracic spine). If severe, these conditions can impair cardiac output by preventing chest expansion and inhibiting heart muscle movement. If breathing is affected by a cardiac condition, such as heart failure, the patient may use accessory muscles to breathe. (For more information, see Chapter 9, Respiratory system.)

Jugular veins

Inspect the neck for jugular vein distention. Normally, neck veins protrude when the patient is supine and lie flat when the patient stands. When the patient sits at a 45-degree angle in semi-Fowler's position, the jugular vein appears distended only if the patient has right-sided heart dysfunction. To check for jugular vein distention, place the patient in semi-Fowler's position with the head turned slightly away from the side being examined. (For an illustration, see *Patient positioning for jugular vein assessment*.) For better visualization of pulse wave movement, use tangential lighting (lighting from the side) to cast small shadows along the neck.

If distention is present, classify it as mild, moderate, or severe. Determine the level of distention in fingerbreadths above the clavicle or in relation to the jaw or clavicle. Also, note the amount of distention in

Patient positioning for jugular vein assessment

The illustration below shows the correct patient positioning and key anatomical landmarks used for assessing jugular vein distention.

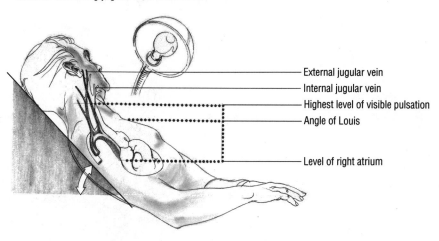

- External jugular vein
- Internal jugular vein
- Highest level of visible pulsation
- Angle of Louis
- Level of right atrium

relation to head elevation. Jugular vein distention occurs when right atrial pressure is above normal and reflects increased fluid volume caused by right-sided heart dysfunction.

Precordium

Before inspecting the precordium (the area over the heart), place the patient supine with the head flat or elevated for respiratory comfort. Stand to the right of the patient. Then identify the necessary anatomic landmarks.

Using tangential lighting to cast shadows across the chest, watch for chest wall movement, visible pulsations, and exaggerated lifts or heaves (strong outward thrusts palpated over the chest during systole) in these six areas of the precordium:

- aortic area, located in the second intercostal space on the right sternal border
- pulmonic area, located in the second intercostal space on the left sternal border
- right ventricular area, located at the left sternal border at the fifth rib
- left ventricular (apical) area, located at the fifth intercostal space, at the midclavicular line (also called the point of maximum impulse [PMI])
- epigastric area, located at the base of the sternum (For an illustration of the six precordial areas, see *Precordium inspection and palpation,* page 172.)
- Erb's point, located in the third intercostal space just left of the sternum.

Precordium inspection and palpation

This illustration shows the six areas the nurse should inspect and palpate to detect normal and abnormal pulsations over the precordium.

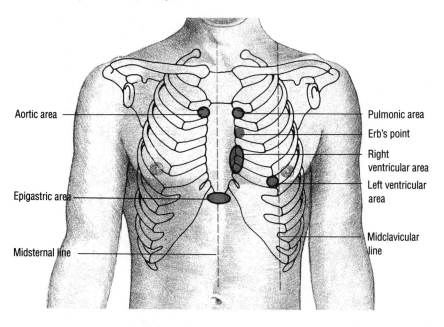

Inspection may reveal pulsations at the PMI of the apical impulse. Consider any other pulsations abnormal.

When palpating the precordium, use the pads of the fingers because they are especially sensitive to vibrations and can effectively assess large pulse sites. Follow a systematic palpation sequence that covers the aortic, pulmonic, right ventricular, left ventricular, and epigastric areas.

The PMI is the place where pulsations are felt; in fact, the apical area is commonly the only place on the precordium where pulsations are palpable. At the PMI, light palpation should reveal a tap with each heartbeat over a space that is roughly $\frac{3}{4}''$ (2 cm), or one intercostal space.

A displaced or diffused PMI may indicate left ventricular hypertrophy. A pulsation in the aortic, pulmonic, or right ventricular area can result from chamber enlargement or valvular disease. A pulsation in the epigastric area or sternoclavicular area (located at the top of the sternum, at the junction of the clavicles) suggests an aortic aneurysm.

Pulses

While assessing the patient's vital signs, the nurse palpates the radial pulse to assess the heart rate quickly. To assess blood flow to the tissues, now palpate the other major pulse points: the carotid, brachial, radial, femoral, popliteal, dorsalis pedis, and posterior tibial pulses.

Be sure to press gently over the pulse sites; excess pressure can obliterate the pulsation, making the pulse seem absent when it is not. Also, palpate only one carotid artery at a time; simultaneous palpation can slow the pulse or decrease the blood pressure, causing the patient to faint. Identify the pulse rate, rhythm, symmetry, contour, and strength at each site, using the pulse rating scale required by the health care facility.

A weak pulse indicates low cardiac output or increased peripheral vascular resistance, as in arterial atherosclerotic disease. A strong, bounding pulse results from hypertension or a high cardiac output state, such as exercise, pregnancy, anemia, or thyrotoxicosis.

Auscultation

To complete the basic cardiovascular assessment, auscultate the precordium to detect heart sounds, and auscultate the central and peripheral arteries to detect vascular sounds.

Precordium

The cardiovascular system requires more auscultation than any other body system. To develop the requisite skill, practice auscultating and identifying heart sounds in the precordium. Be aware that the nurse can detect abnormal heart sounds only after becoming proficient at identifying normal ones.

Auscultating heart sounds can be difficult. Increased distance between the source of the sound and the outer chest wall can affect which sounds are heard. Thus, if a patient is obese or has a muscular chest wall or hyperinflated lungs, the sounds may seem more distant and difficult to hear. To improve auscultation results, reduce noise from equipment and other sources.

To prepare for auscultation, select a stethoscope with a chest piece that is sized appropriately for the patient's chest. Use the diaphragm of the stethoscope to detect high-pitched heart sounds, such as the normal first heart sound (S_1) and second heart sound (S_2). Use the bell of the stethoscope to identify low-pitched sounds. Also, make sure the stethoscope tubing is not excessively long.

After explaining the procedure, help the patient into a comfortable position. For best results, a right-handed nurse should stand at the patient's right side to auscultate.

Do not try to auscultate through clothing or surgical dressings; these will muffle heart sounds or make them inaudible. Drape the patient as appropriate. Instruct the patient to breathe normally, inhaling through the nose and exhaling through the mouth.

Listen at each cardiac auscultation site: aortic, pulmonic, mitral valve, and tricuspid valve areas. Because the opening and closing of valves creates most normal heart sounds, auscultation sites lie close together, behind or to the left of the sternum. These sites do not lie directly over valves, but rather over the pathways blood takes as it flows through chambers and valves.

To assess heart sounds, listen for a few cycles to become accustomed to the rate and rhythm of the sounds. The two sounds that normally occur—S_1 and S_2—are separated by a silent period.

The first heart sound—the *lub* of *lub-dub*—marks the beginning of systole. It occurs as the mitral and tricuspid valves close. This event immediately precedes the increase in ventricular pressure, aortic and pulmonic valve opening, and blood ejection into the circulation. These events all occur within one third of a second. S_1 is louder in the mitral and tricuspid listening areas (LUB-dub) and softer in the aortic and pulmonic areas (lub-DUB).

The second heart sound—the *dub* of *lub-dub*—occurs at the beginning of diastole. Because closing of the aortic and pulmonic valves produces S2, this sound is louder in the aortic and pulmonic areas. At these sites, the sequence sounds like lub-DUB. S2 coincides with the pulse downstroke. At normal rates, the diastolic pause between S2 and the next S1 exceeds the systolic pause between S1 and S2.

To help differentiate systole from diastole, carefully compare the loudness of the normal heart sounds at each site. Identifying the phases of the cardiac cycle is necessary to time any abnormal sounds that occur. S_2 also can be identified by palpating the carotid pulse during auscultation. The pulse upstroke occurs almost simultaneously with S_1.

During auscultation, S_2 may have a split sound (similar to the difference between "split" and "spit"). Occurring when the aortic and pulmonic valves do not close at exactly the same time, this split is common in healthy children and younger adults.

At each auscultation site, use the diaphragm of the stethoscope to listen to heart sounds. Then, auscultate again, using the bell of the stethoscope. The systolic and diastolic periods should be silent. If any sounds are audible during these periods or if any variations in S_1 or S_2 occur, document the characteristics of the sound, noting the auscultation site and the part of the cardiac cycle in which it occurred.

Murmurs. A nurse who gains skill in auscultating the heart may notice that in certain patients, diastole is not silent, as it is normally. Instead, auscultation reveals a murmur—a vibrating, blowing, or rumbling noise caused by turbulent blood flow.

Heart murmurs usually are identified by the following characteristics, which help determine the cause of the murmur.

Location. Murmurs can occur in any cardiac auscultation site and usually are identified by the area in which they are best heard.

Timing. When timing a murmur, determine if it occurs during diastole or systole. A murmur that occurs between S_1 and S_2 is a systolic murmur; between S_2 and the next S_1, a diastolic murmur. Additional identification may place the murmur in the early, middle, or late part of the cardiac cycle. Some murmurs are continuous.

Pitch. The rate and pressure of blood flow determine the pitch of a heart murmur. The pitch may be high, medium, or low. Low-pitched murmurs are best heard with the bell; high-pitched murmurs, with the diaphragm.

Quality. Many factors affect the quality of a murmur, including blood flow volume, the force of contraction, and the degree of valve compromise. Heart murmur quality can be described as musical, blowing, harsh, rasping, rumbling, or machine-like.

Intensity. Use a standard, six-level grading scale (I to VI) to describe the intensity of the murmur (from barely audible to extremely loud with a palpable thrill).

A murmur can be innocent (nonpathologic) or a sign of a cardiac problem (pathologic). An innocent, or functional, murmur may appear in a patient without heart disease. It may affect up to 25% of all children but usually disappears by adolescence. An innocent murmur occurs early in systole, seldom exceeds grade II in intensity, and usually is heard best in the pulmonic area. When the patient changes from a supine to a sitting position, this type of murmur may disappear. Any murmur may become more intense with an increase in cardiac output, as from fever, exercise, anemia, anxiety, or pregnancy.

Arteries

Auscultate the carotid, femoral, and popliteal arteries as well as the abdominal aorta. No sounds should be heard over the vessels, although bowel sounds may be heard in the distance when auscultating over the abdomen.

Abnormal findings

Auscultation may detect first and second heart sounds that are accentuated, diminished, or inaudible. These abnormalities may result from pressure changes, valvular dysfunctions, or conduction defects. Auscultation also may reveal a prolonged, persistent, or reversed split sound, which may result from a mechanical or electrical problem.

Two additional heart sounds, S_3 and S_4, may occur in a patient with cardiovascular disease. Because these sounds are high-pitched, the nurse must use the bell of the stethoscope to auscultate them. S_3, heard in early diastole, indicates overdistension of the ventricles and is common in patients with CHF. S_4, heard in late diastole, signals resistance to ventricular filling and is common in patients with a recent MI or hypertension.

Both S_3 and S_4 may occur in a patient who has suffered a recent MI and has CHF. Usually, such a patient has tachycardia. Because diastole shortens as the heart rate increases, S_3 and S_4 are so close together that they seem to be one sound. This is called a summation gallop.

Auscultation also may reveal three other abnormal sounds: a click, snap, or rub. A click—a high-pitched sound auscultated at the apex during mid- to late-systole—is caused by abnormal billowing of the mitral valve into the left atrium. It is best heard medial to or at the apex. The click usually precedes a late systolic murmur caused by regurgitation of blood from the left ventricle into the left atrium. To enhance the sound, change the patient's position to sitting or standing. Mitral valve prolapse and these classic auscultatory findings occur in about 5% to 10% of adults, and affect more women than men.

A snap is a very early diastolic sound, heard immediately after S_2. A high-pitched sound, it is best heard medial to the apex along the lower left sternal border. A snap results from a stenotic valve (most commonly the mitral valve) attempting to open.

A friction rub is a harsh, scratchy, scraping, or squeaking sound. To detect a rub, use the diaphragm of the stethoscope and listen for a squeaking sound at the third left intercostal space along the lower left sternal border. To enhance the sound, have the patient sit upright and lean forward or exhale. A friction rub usually results from pericarditis, an inflammation of the pericardial sac. The sound arises from the pericardial layers grating against one another; therefore, it may be heard throughout systole, diastole, or both.

A sound heard over a vessel may represent a bruit—a continuous vibrating, blowing, or rumbling noise caused by turbulent blood flow. A bruit over the carotid artery usually indicates atherosclerosis; over the abdominal aorta, an aneurysm (a weakness in the arterial wall that allows a sac to form).

Pathologic murmurs can occur during systole or diastole and can affect any heart valve. They may result from valvular stenosis (inability of the valves to open properly), valvular insufficiency (inability of the valves to close properly, allowing blood regurgitation), or a septal defect (a defect in the septal wall separating two heart chambers).

Developmental considerations for pediatric patients
A child's pulse rate may range from 70 to 190—much faster than an adult's. As the child ages, the pulse rate gradually decreases to adult levels. A neonate's blood pressure normally is much lower than that of a child. (For more information, see *The effect of age on vital signs,* page 39.)

Developmental considerations for pregnant patients
In this patient, heart sounds may be loud and the PMI may be shifted slightly to the left. These normal physiologic findings occur as the enlarged uterus displaces the heart. Palpation of the patient's pulse may reveal edema and varicosities, especially in the legs.

Developmental considerations for elderly patients
With age, the heart rate slows and the normal blood pressure may increase. Although both systolic and diastolic pressures increase, the sys-

tolic rise is greater because of the increased rigidity of the vascular tree. Superficial vessels of the forehead, neck, and extremities may feel prominent and ropelike on palpation.

Documentation The following example shows how to document some normal physical assessment findings:

Weight: 165 lb

Height: 5′9″

Vital signs: Blood pressure 126/72 right arm and 120/76 left arm, with a 4 mm Hg systolic drop when moving from a supine to standing position; temperature 98.4° F; pulse 64 and regular; respirations 14 and regular.

Additional notes: Muscles well-defined. Muscle strength and gait normal. Skin color within normal limits (WNL). Mucous membranes pink and moist. Skin turgor WNL. Lower extremities exhibit brisk capillary refill. No neck veins visible with patient at 45-degree angle. All pulses palpated, bilaterally equal +2. PMI at fifth intercostal space at mid-clavicular line. No thrills or heaves palpated. S_1 and S_2 with no murmurs, gallops, clicks, snaps, rubs, or bruits.

The following example shows how to document some abnormal physical assessment findings:

Weight: 102 lb

Height: 5′6″

Vital signs: Blood pressure 100/80 in both arms with a 10 mm Hg systolic and diastolic drop when moving from supine to sitting position; temperature 99.5° F; pulse 104 and irregular; respirations 28 and labored with an audible inspiratory wheeze.

Additional notes: Generalized pallor with purplish discoloration from toes to 3″ above ankles and 2-cm-diameter lesion on right inner aspect of left ankle. Lower extremity perfusion delayed with color return in 20 seconds. Skin turgor poor. No hair growth bilaterally below knees. +3 pedal edema bilaterally at ankles diminishes to +1 just below knee. Capillary refill sluggish. Neck veins distended 6 cm with patient at 45-degree angle. Pedal and popliteal pulses +1; all other pulses bilaterally equal +2. PMI palpated in fifth intercostal space at anterior axillary line. Auscultation reveals third heart sound, bilateral carotid bruits, and Grade III holosystolic murmur heard best in aortic area with radiation to the neck.

STUDY ACTIVITIES **Fill in the blank**

1. The heart has _____ chambers and lies between the _____ and the _____ ribs.

2. Normally, the _____ serves as the driving pacemaker of the heart.

3. Cardiac output equals the _____ multiplied by the

_____.

Short answer

4. Donald Williamson, age 72, comes to the emergency department complaining of recent chest pain. He states that he is "not in that much pain" right now, but his wife insisted he come to the hospital. When questioning Mr. Williamson about his chest pain, which method should the nurse use to analyze his symptom? What are some examples of questions the nurse might ask to investigate each major aspect of his symptom?

_____

_____

5. The nurse obtains the following information from Mr. Williamson and his previous emergency department records: a 20-year history of hypertension, currently under treatment; total cholesterol level 260 mg/dl; height 5'8"; weight 230 lb; and left ventricular hypertrophy as determined by electrocardiogram. Based on these data and the patient description in the previous question, the nurse determines that Mr. Williamson has six risk factors for cardiovascular disease. What are these risk factors?

_____

6. The nurse has completed Mr. Williamson's health history and is ready to begin the physical assessment. Describe the order in which the nurse should conduct the assessment.

_____

7. Angela Parish, age 51, reports that her anginal symptoms have gotten worse. She has a history of coronary artery disease and angina. The nurse proceeds with the comprehensive health history. What components of the health history are vital to developing an appropriate care plan for Ms. Parish?

_____

_____

8. What technique should the nurse use to assess Ms. Parish's carotid pulses?

_____

9. During auscultation, the nurse finds that Ms. Parish has a regular heart rate at 72 beats/minute and an extra heart sound in late diastole. What is this extra sound and what does it signify?

_____

10. John Regalto, age 74, has CHF and is receiving care at home from a visiting nurse. On today's visit, he tells the nurse he has been feeling increasingly short of breath. The nurse suspects his heart failure is worsening. What other subjective information should the nurse obtain to ensure a thorough assessment?

---

11. When weighing Mr. Regalto, the nurse discovers he has gained 3 lb in the last 24 hours. The nurse then proceeds with a thorough physical assessment. Identify the findings the nurse should expect when assessing Mr. Regalto's heart rate, heart sounds, jugular veins, and general appearance.

True or false

12. An overnight weight gain of more than two pounds is common in patients developing CHF and results from fluid overload.
☐ True ☐ False

13. Normal pulse pressure (the difference between systolic and diastolic blood pressure) ranges from 30 to 50 mm Hg.
☐ True ☐ False

14. When the patient sits at a 45-degree angle in semi-Fowler's position, the jugular vein appears distended only in the presence of CHF.
☐ True ☐ False

15. The PMI normally is located at the sixth intercostal space, at the anterior axillary line.
☐ True ☐ False

ANSWERS ### Fill in the blank
   1. four, second, sixth
   2. sinoatrial (SA) node
   3. stroke volume, number of beats per minute

Short answer
   4. The nurse should use the PQRST method to analyze the patient's symptom. Examples of questions the nurse might ask to investigate each major aspect of the symptom include:
   • *P*rovocative or palliative: What causes the chest pain? What makes it better? What makes it worse?
   • *Q*uantity or quality: How does the chest pain feel? How much pain are you experiencing now?
   • *R*egion or radiation: Where is the chest pain located? Has it spread?
   • *S*everity: How would you rate the chest pain on a scale of 1 to 10, with 10 being the most extreme?

• *Timing*: When did the chest pain begin? How often does it occur? Was its onset gradual or sudden?

5. Mr. Williamson's risk factors for cardiovascular disease include his age (over 60), male gender, obesity, high blood pressure, hyperlipidemia, and left ventricular hypertrophy.

6. The nurse should begin the assessment by observing the patient's general appearance, measuring weight, and obtaining vital signs. Then the nurse conducts a survey of the skin, hair, nails, and eyes. Next, the nurse inspects and palpates the jugular veins, precordium, and pulses. Finally, the nurse auscultates the precordium and arteries.

7. Components of the health history that are vital to developing the plan of care for Ms. Parish include:

• current health status (using the PQRST method to analyze her angina)

• medications, including all prescription and nonprescription products, the reasons for taking them, and any adverse effects and lost doses

• past health status, including congenital, valvular, or other cardiac disorders

• health promotion and protection patterns, including personal habits, sleep and waking, exercise and activity, nutrition, stress and coping, occupation, and roles and relationships.

8. The nurse should assess one carotid pulse at a time, using light palpation. Simultaneous palpation may significantly reduce cerebral blood flow and cause fainting.

9. This extra heart sound, called S4, signifies resistance to ventricular filling.

10. The nurse should use the PQRST method to obtain further subjective information about Mr. Regalto's dyspnea. This information will provide the physician or nurse practitioner with a complete analysis of his symptom and allow further testing and intervention.

11. The nurse may find tachycardia from an increased cardiac work load; S3, S4, an occasional summation gallop, and murmur of mitral regurgitation (insufficiency); distended jugular veins; and dependent and generalized edema in the person with CHF.

True or false

12. True.
13. True.
14. True.
15. False. The PMI normally is located at the fifth intercostal space, at the midclavicular line.

CHAPTER 11

Female and male breasts

OBJECTIVES After studying this chapter, the reader should be able to:

1. Locate the parts of the human breast and surrounding lymph nodes.

2. Identify specific questions the nurse should ask when obtaining the patient's breast health history.

3. Describe and demonstrate the technique the nurse should use to inspect and palpate the breast, axilla, and surrounding lymph nodes.

4. Teach breast self-examination to a female patient.

5. Differentiate between normal and abnormal findings during physical assessment of the breast.

6. Document breast assessment findings appropriately.

OVERVIEW OF CONCEPTS Many women have questions and concerns surrounding the breasts—largely because of the fear of breast cancer, which affects about 10% of American women and is the second leading cause of death in this group. Most breast tumors and changes are not cancerous, but they require careful assessment to rule out malignancy. The nurse is in an ideal position to promote breast care and provide education, teaching patients how to perform breast self-examination and encouraging regular health examinations and mammography when appropriate.

Normally occurring in pairs, the breasts are located vertically between the second or third and the sixth or seventh ribs on the anterior chest wall over the pectoralis major and the serratus anterior muscles. Horizontally, they lie between the sternal border and the midaxillary line.

The breasts are similar in both sexes until puberty, when the ovaries secrete the hormones estrogen and progesterone, causing breast enlargement in females. (For illustration of the breast structures, see *The female breast,* page 182.) Unstimulated by hormones, the male breast retains preadolescent characteristics. Estrogen secretion causes duct tissue growth and fat deposits; progesterone stimulates glandular development.

The female breast

This illustration shows a lateral cross section of the female breast.

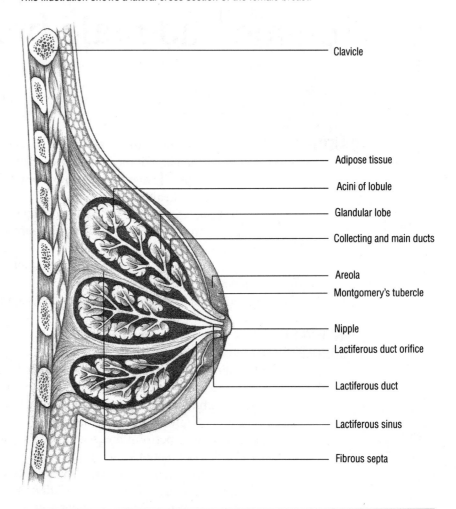

- Clavicle
- Adipose tissue
- Acini of lobule
- Glandular lobe
- Collecting and main ducts
- Areola
- Montgomery's tubercle
- Nipple
- Lactiferous duct orifice
- Lactiferous duct
- Lactiferous sinus
- Fibrous septa

In females and males, each breast contains a lymphatic network, which drains lymph from the breast and returns it to the blood. (For an illustration of the lymph nodes, see *Lymph nodes of the breast*.)

Health history Discussing the breasts may be embarrassing and difficult for a female patient, so the nurse should ensure a comfortable environment that offers privacy and freedom from interruptions. Perform the interview before the physical examination, while the patient is sitting up and dressed or covered with a gown. Most of the questions in this section relate to women, because few breast disorders occur in men. As applicable, ask questions that relate to male breast history.

Lymph nodes of the breast

In males and females, the lymph nodes illustrated drain lymph from the breast.

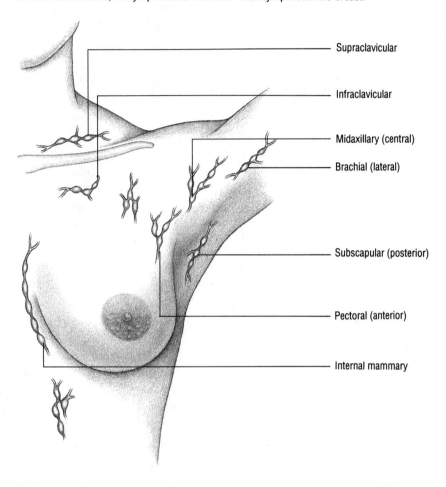

Supraclavicular

Infraclavicular

Midaxillary (central)

Brachial (lateral)

Subscapular (posterior)

Pectoral (anterior)

Internal mammary

Health and illness patterns

Explore the patient's current, past, and family health status, as well as developmental considerations.

Current health status

A woman about to undergo breast assessment probably will be concerned about her current health status, especially if she has noticed a change or lump in her breast. If she has, carefully document the chief complaint in the patient's own words. Using the PQRST method, ask the patient to describe completely this complaint and any others. (For a detailed explanation of the PQRST method, see *Symptom analysis*, page 15.) Ask the following questions to learn more about the patient's current health status:

How old are you?
(RATIONALE: Age is an important factor in breast assessment because certain findings are more common in particular age groups. Approximately 80% of breast cancers occur in women over age 40. Fibroadenomas affect women ages 15 to 35; fibrocystic breast disorders primarily occur in premenopausal women.)

Have you noticed any breast lumps or breast changes?
(RATIONALE: Breast lumps and changes may result from various causes, including fibrocystic disease, fibroadenomas, and malignant tumors. Also note any skin changes, such as dimpling, swelling, increasing venous prominence, or a newly acquired inverted nipple; these may indicate cancer.)

If you have noticed a change, how long ago did you first notice it?
(RATIONALE: Some changes relate to the menstrual cycle and come and go. Others, such as those related to cancer, do not vary. A change also could relate to muscle strain from strenuous chest movement, such as playing tennis.)

Do you have any breast pain or tenderness?
(RATIONALE: Breast pain or tenderness may be related to the menstrual cycle or may result from breast trauma. Breast cancer usually is painless.)

Have you noticed any nipple discharge?
(RATIONALE: Data about the discharge, such as color and consistency, the number of ducts involved, and whether the discharge occurs spontaneously or manually or from one or both nipples, can help diagnose the problem. A spontaneous discharge unrelated to childbirth or lactation calls for evaluation—especially when bloody and associated with a breast mass in a patient over age 50.)

Do you have any rash or eczema on either nipple?
(RATIONALE: Paget's disease, a cancer of the nipple and areola, may look like exzema and is associated with cancer in deeper breast structures.)

Do you currently take any medications, including contraceptives or hormone replacements? If so, which ones and how often do you take them?
(RATIONALE: Some medications, such as antidepressants, can cause breast engorgement and galactorrhea in females and gynecomastia in males.)

Past health status
Ask the following questions to explore the patient's medical history for breast-related information:

Have you ever had breast cancer?
(RATIONALE: A history of breast cancer increases the risk for subsequent breast cancer fivefold.)

Have you ever had breast surgery?
(RATIONALE: Previous breast surgery, for benign or malignant conditions, should be noted. Also, previous surgeries could have caused skin and tissue changes.)

At what age did you start to menstruate? If applicable: At what age did you go through menopause?
(RATIONALE: Onset of menses before age 12 and late menopause [after age 55] slightly increase the risk of breast cancer by prolonging exposure to estrogen.)

Did you go through menopause before age 35, either naturally or by surgery?
(RATIONALE: Early menopause reduces the risk of breast cancer.)

Do you have children? If so, at what age did you bear them?
(RATIONALE: Childlessness or bearing a first child after age 30 increases the risk of breast cancer.)

Have you been exposed to radiation, such as radiation therapy for cancer?
(RATIONALE: Depending on the location and dose of radiation, the patient may have an increased risk of breast cancer.)

Have you ever had a breast implant?
(RATIONALE: Silicone breast implants may cause breast problems.)

Family health status
Investigate the patient's family history of breast disease by asking these questions:

Have your mother or any siblings had breast cancer?
(RATIONALE: The breast cancer risk increases if the patient's mother or sibling had breast cancer, especially if the cancer developed before menopause.)

If your mother or sibling had breast cancer, was it in one or both breasts?
(RATIONALE: The risk of breast cancer increases further for a patient whose mother or sibling had bilateral breast cancer.)

Developmental considerations for pediatric patients
If the child is over age 10, ask the following question:

How do you think your breasts will change as you get older?
(RATIONALE: The premenarchal child needs to know what growth and development to expect so that changes will not be frightening. To help alleviate the child's potential fears, present an illustrated, matter-of-fact introduction to expected changes.)

Developmental considerations for pregnant patients
Help alleviate the pregnant patient's concerns by asking:

Do you wear a supportive brassiere?
(RATIONALE: Wearing a well-fitting, supportive brassiere can help prevent breast tone loss and reduce discomfort caused by the enlarging breast.)

Do you plan to breast-feed?
(RATIONALE: The patient should start thinking about infant feeding methods before delivery. If she plans to breast-feed, she may need education on breast preparation to toughen the nipple.)

Do you have concerns about breast-feeding?
(RATIONALE: Many women are afraid their breasts will be smaller when they stop breast-feeding. Reassure the patient that the size decrease after breast-feeding seems great only because the lactating breast enlarges so dramatically. Also, the patient may need to know that breast-feeding does not increase the risk of breast cancer.)

Developmental considerations for elderly patients
The elderly patient also needs breast-care assessment. Ask the patient:

Do you wear a well-fitting, supportive brassiere?
(RATIONALE: Because breasts tend to sag with age, a good supportive brassiere can prevent breast pain and discomfort.)

Health promotion and protection patterns
Ask the following questions to assess the patient's personal health habits:

Do you perform breast self-examination? If so, how often?
(RATIONALE: The answer reveals the patient's knowledge about breast care. If the patient does not examine her breasts monthly, explain that breast self-examination is important for early cancer detection. For teaching guidelines, see *Teaching breast self-examination.*)

Would you please demonstrate how you perform breast self-examination?
(RATIONALE: A demonstration ensures that the patient knows the correct technique, which is essential for maximum effectiveness. The nurse also can demonstrate the proper technique during the physical assessment.)

When do you perform breast self-examination?
(RATIONALE: The patient should perform breast self-examination on the 5th to 7th day after the first day of the menstrual period, when the hormonal effect, which can cause breast tenderness or lumpiness, is reduced. A postmenopausal patient should choose a regular time each month to examine her breasts. If the patient is on cyclical estrogen therapy, the last day the patient is off the medication is best for self-examination.)

When was your last mammogram?
(RATIONALE: The American Cancer Society recommends a baseline mammography screening between ages 35 and 40, then a mammo-

Teaching breast self-examination

Breast self-examination (BSE) is one of the most important health habits to teach the patient. The nurse can teach BSE during the palpation phase of assessment. (If the patient already performs BSE, check to make sure her technique is correct.) Follow the steps below.

1. First, teach the patient how to look at herself in a mirror and, with her arms at her sides, check for any visible abnormalities. She should observe for dimpling, retraction, or breast flattening as she first elevates her arms slowly, then presses her hands against her hips, and finally, bends forward.

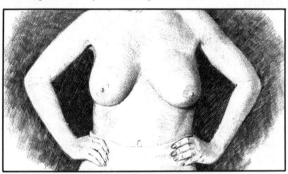

2. Next, place one hand over the patient's and show her how to use the pads of the middle three fingers of the opposite hand to palpate the breast systematically by compressing the breast tissue against the chest wall. She should palpate all portions of the breast, areola, nipple, tail of Spence, and axilla when she is in the shower or standing before a mirror. She can choose either the circle (A), the up and down (B), or the wedge (C). She

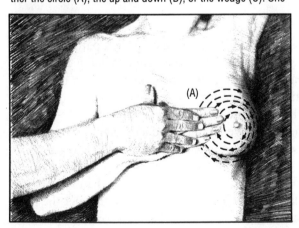

should repeat the procedure lying down with a pillow or folded towel under the shoulder of the side she is examining.

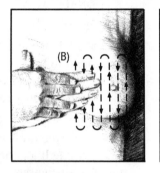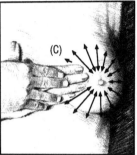

3. Next, show the patient how to compress the nipple gently between the thumb and index finger as she observes for discharge.

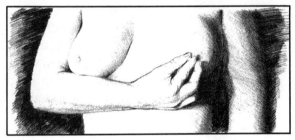

4. Finally, explain that she should report any redness or inflammation, swelling, masses, flattening, puckering, dimpling, retraction, sunken areas, asymmetrical nipple direction, discharge, bleeding, lesions, or eczematous nipple changes to her primary care provider.

gram every 1 to 2 years between ages 40 and 49 and once a year after age 50. After age 75, mammograms should be done at the discretion of the patient and health care provider. A patient with a family history of breast cancer may need more frequent mammograms, as determined by the primary health care provider.)

How much fat do you consume in your diet?
(RATIONALE: A high-fat diet may increase the breast cancer risk.)

How much alcohol do you drink?
(RATIONALE: Moderate to heavy alcohol intake may increase the risk of breast cancer.)

Role and relationship patterns

Any threat to the breast can threaten a woman's body image and feelings of personal worth, directly affecting relationships with others, especially men. When assessing role and relationship patterns, ask these questions:

How important are your breasts to a positive view of yourself?
(RATIONALE: If a patient has a breast lump that may need surgery, she may fear disfigurement and the threat of cancer. This question will help the patient express her fears and her feelings about the impending breast assessment.)

If you have breast tenderness or discomfort related to fibrocystic breast changes, does it affect your sex life?
(RATIONALE: If breast tenderness caused by fibrocystic disease affects a patient's activity level or sexual relationships, suggest treatments to help relieve discomfort. Such treatments include mild analgesics, warm compresses, or sleeping bras; a low-salt diet, especially in the latter half of the menstrual cycle; caffeine restrictions; vitamin E supplements; and diuretics.)

Physical assessment

Because a breast assessment may be embarrassing for a patient, take care to ensure privacy. To ease anxiety, use a gentle technique and warm hands, and explain the examination in advance. With a male patient, help him understand the need for breast assessment.

To prepare for a thorough breast assessment, obtain a flashlight; a small pillow, folded sheet, or towel; a ruler; and a cytologic fixative and slide for nipple discharge. Plan to use both inspection and palpation techniques.

Ensure adequate lighting to help detect subtle skin changes. For a supine examination, place a small pillow or folded towel under the patient's back on the side being assessed. This allows the breast tissue to spread more evenly across the chest wall. During inspection of suspicious-looking lesions, use a ruler to measure lesions and a flashlight to augment lighting.

Inspection

Begin the assessment with the patient seated, disrobed to the waist, and with arms resting at each side. First inspect the breasts for size and symmetry, keeping in mind that one breast usually is smaller than the other. Look for obvious masses, flattening of the breast on one side, and signs of retraction, such as dimpling (a depression in a localized breast surface area). To check for hidden dimpling, ask the patient to place her hands against her hips and then raise her arms slowly over her head. Inspect for equal and free breast movement without signs of dimpling or abnormal breast contours. Repeat if necessary.

Ask a patient with large or pendulous breasts to stand and lean forward with her arms outstretched. Support the patient's arms by the back of a chair or with the examiner's hands. Next, evaluate breast skin, including color, texture, and venous pattern. The skin should be smooth and soft, with a similar venous pattern bilaterally.

Inspect the skin carefully for lesions. Examine recent changes closely. Purple striations, which turn silver with time, may appear if the patient has been pregnant or has gained weight.

Inspect the nipples and areolae for size, shape, and color. They should be similarly round or oval, of equal size, and free of rashes, fissures, and ulcerations. The nipples usually point in the same direction; note any nipple inversion. Inspect the nipples for discharge; if present, note its appearance and obtain a specimen for cytologic examination. Montgomery's tubercles (sebaceous glands that secrete a waxy substance) normally appear on the areolae.

Check the axillae for rashes, hair growth, signs of infection, and unusual pigmentation. The axillae should be free of rashes and lesions and should have hair growth if the patient is past puberty. However, hair growth diminishes with aging.

Abnormal findings

Masses, dimpling, or flattening may indicate an abnormality, possibly cancer. Dimpling results from a tumor shortening fibrotic breast areas or immobilizing Cooper's ligaments. Edema, skin thickening, and an orange peel appearance (peau d'orange) may result from a cancer that blocks lymph drainage.

A reddish color may signify infection and inflammation. A red, scaly, eczemalike area over one nipple and areola could indicate Paget's disease. A unilateral venous pattern may indicate dilated veins caused by an underlying disease. Although some women normally have bilaterally inverted nipples, one inverted nipple (unless long present) should arouse suspicion. View any eczematous lesion as possible cancer and assess further.

A few women have an extra nipple, an extra breast with a nipple, or extra breast tissue along the milk lines—embryonic ridges that extend from the axilla to the groin. Called supernumerary breasts or nipples, these congenital anomalies are small, visible, palpable masses.

Milk lines normally atrophy during fetal development. In some women, however, the ridges persist in part or in their entirety.

Malignant acanthosis nigricans, a rare cancer, is associated with dark pigmentation and velvety skin texture in the axillae.

Palpation

For breast palpation, have the patient lie supine; for axillary palpation, have the patient sit up. (For an illustrated description of the palpation procedure, see *Palpating the axillae and breasts*.)

To describe the location of breast abnormalities, mentally divide the breast into four quadrants and a fifth segment, the tail of Spence. Alternatively, view the breast as a clock with the nipple in the center, and describe lesions by the "time" and distance in centimeters from the nipple.

Abnormal findings

Any palpable mass, induration, tenderness, or sign of inflammation in the breast is abnormal and should be carefully documented. Cancerous nodules typically are hard, irregularly shaped, fixed, not tender, and poorly circumscribed. If a mass is palpated, note the size in centimeters, the shape (oval, round, or irregular), consistency (firm, soft, hard, or rubbery), circumscription (delineation from surrounding tissue), mobility (whether fixed to the underlying tissue or freely movable), tenderness, and location. Abnormal findings call for further evaluation using specific diagnostic tests and procedures, such as mammography, ultrasound, biopsy, and aspiration.

Because spontaneous nipple discharge may indicate cancer (especially when unilateral), refer the patient to a physician for further evaluation. Other abnormal findings requiring referral include skin breakdown and masses in the areolae.

Developmental considerations for pediatric patients

The adolescent female may exhibit asymmetrical breast development. Reassure her that the breasts will become fairly symmetrical with full development. Gynecomastia is common in young adolescent males and usually disappears within 1 year.

Developmental considerations for pregnant patients

Tingling, fullness, and tenderness are common during pregnancy. Darkened nipples and areolae are normal; purplish linear streaks may develop on the breasts as they increase in size. Striae also may appear on the abdomen. Colostrum may flow and dry on the nipple after the 16th week of gestation. The breasts may feel nodular from alveolar enlargement.

In a lactating patient, examine the breasts for engorgement. Engorged breasts feel hard and warm, and the skin appears red and shiny; the patient usually complains of pain. If the patient is breast-feeding, check the nipples for irritation, such as cracks, fissures, bleeding, redness, tenderness, or blisters.

Palpating the axillae and breasts

Palpate the male or female axillae with the patient sitting or lying down. The sitting position, however, provides easier access.

1. Begin with the patient's right axilla. Ask the patient to relax the right arm while you use your left hand to support the patient's elbow or wrist. With the right middle three fingers cupped, reach high into the central axilla. Sweep the fingers downward and against the ribs and serratus anterior to try to feel the central nodes. Palpating one or two small, nontender, freely movable nodes is normal.

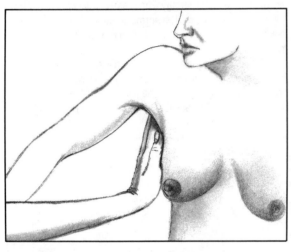

2. Assess the anterior nodes by palpating along the anterior axillary fold.

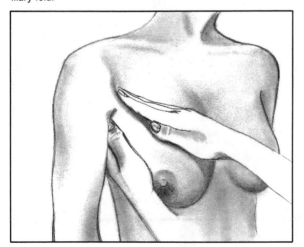

3. Assess the posterior nodes by palpating along the posterior axillary fold.

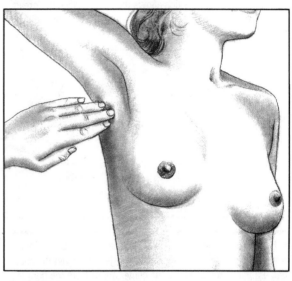

4. Palpate the lateral nodes by pressing the fingers along the upper inner arm, trying to compress these nodes against the humerus. Repeat the assessment on the patient's left side. If any axillary node findings appear abnormal, assess the infraclavicular and supraclavicular nodes.

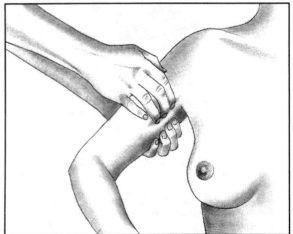

Palpating the axillae and breasts (continued)

5. To palpate the breast, ask the patient to lie supine with a small pad or pillow placed under the shoulder of the side being examined and with the arm on that same side placed above the patient's head. This position allows the breast tissue to spread out evenly. Palpate a woman with large breasts in the supine and seated positions.

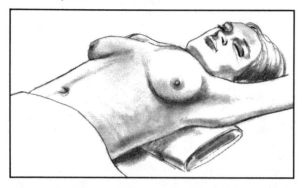

6. Using the middle three finger pads, palpate the breast in a systematic pattern, rotating the fingers gently against the chest wall. Palpate circularly from the center out or from the periphery in, making sure to palpate the tail of Spence.

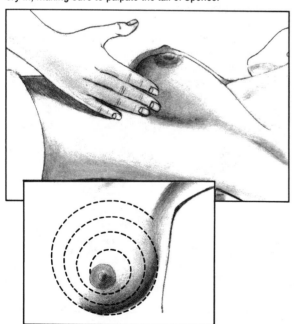

7. Choosing to palpate across or down the breast also is satisfactory, especially on a patient with pendulous breasts. This is best done with the patient seated.

While palpating, feel for masses or areas of induration (hardness). If a mass is suspected, move or compress the breast gently to look for dimpling. Also palpate for consistency and elasticity. The youthful breast is firmly elastic, with glandular tissue that feels like small lobules. The mature breast may feel more granular or stringy. The premenstrual breast may be fuller and more nodular. The normal inframammary ridge at the lower edge of the breast is firm and may be mistaken for a tumor.

Also assess for tenderness, which varies with the time in the menstrual cycle when assessment is performed. The breasts commonly are tender the week before the menstrual period. Note where the patient is in the menstrual cycle when the breast exam is complete.

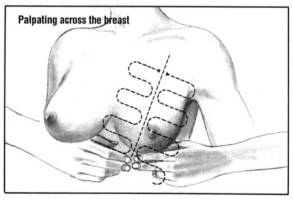

Palpating across the breast

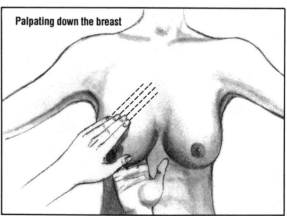

Palpating down the breast

Palpating the axillae and breasts *(continued)*

8. Palpate the areola and nipple of male and female patients alike. Palpate the nipple by gently compressing it between the thumb and index finger. The nipple will become erect and the areola will pucker normally from tactile stimulation.

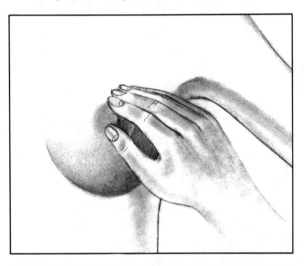

9. Gently milk the nipple for discharge by compressing it between the thumb and index finger. If discharge occurs, note the duct or ducts through which it appears.

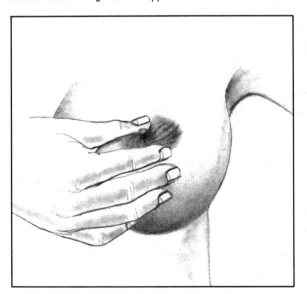

10. Make a cytologic smear of any discharge not explained by pregnancy or lactation. Place a glass slide over the nipple, smear the discharge on it, and spray with fixative immediately.

Some experts no longer check for discharge by squeezing the nipples because many women normally have benign discharge on palpation. However, spontaneous discharge is significant and warrants physician referral.

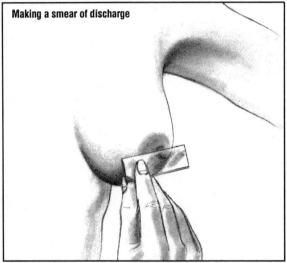

Making a smear of discharge

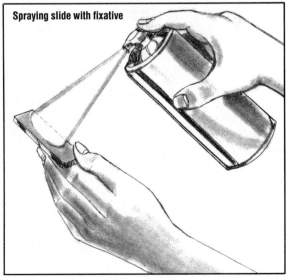

Spraying slide with fixative

Developmental considerations for elderly patients

The breasts of an elderly female normally feel more granular and the tissue is less firm and elastic. The inframammary ridge (cartilage below the breast) thickens as a woman matures; do not mistake it for a mass.

In an elderly male, gynecomastia may occur; it may be bilateral (the result of an estrogen-secreting tumor or estrogen treatment for cancer) or unilateral (most commonly caused by drugs, such as prednisone, phenothiazines, or cardiac glycosides). Unilateral gynecomastia may indicate cancer.

Documentation

The following example shows how to document normal physical assessment findings for the breast:

Breasts and nipples symmetrical in shape. No dimpling, retractions, skin lesions, nodules, inflammation, or tenderness. Nipples erect and point in same direction. Breasts move symmetrically when patient raises arms. No nipple discharge spontaneously or on palpation. Axillae have no masses, tenderness, unusual pigmentation, or lesions.

The following example shows how to document abnormal physical assessment findings for the breast:

Left breast has no dimpling, retractions, skin lesions, nodules, inflammation, or tenderness. Right breast has area of irregular thickening, tenderness, and inflammation in upper outer quadrant at 10 o'clock that is 5 to 6 cm in diameter and 3 cm long. Area is warm to touch and slightly elevated. Three nodes in right anterior axillary area are tender and enlarged (about 1.5 cm). Nodes are firm, oval, and mobile.

STUDY ACTIVITIES

Matching related elements

Match the assessment finding on the left with its possible cause on the right.

1. ___ Nipple rash   **A.** Fibrocystic disease

2. ___ Galactorrhea   **B.** Breast cancer

3. ___ Breast tenderness   **C.** Antidepressant use
     with lumpiness

4. ___ Peau d'orange   **D.** Congenital anomaly

5. ___ Extra nipple   **E.** Paget's disease

Short answer

6. Alice Rogers, age 68, comes to the clinic after noticing a lump in her breast. What are some pertinent questions the nurse should ask this patient to investigate her current and past health status?

_____

_____

7. Jimmy Allen, age 12, is seeking evaluation for enlarged breasts. The nurse's assessment reveals bilateral swelling under the areolae with no other findings. What should the nurse tell Jimmy and his parents about his condition?

_____

8. Identify at least four breast changes that occur during pregnancy and one change that occurs during the immediate postpartal period.

_____

9. Name at least three risk factors for breast cancer.

_____

10. Describe typical breast assessment findings in an adolescent female and in a postmenopausal female.

_____

11. Discuss the technique the nurse should use to detect abnormalities in a patient with large or pendulous breasts.

_____

12. Identify breast inspection and palpation findings that suggest cancer and warrant further evaluation.

_____

13. How often and at what time of the month should a premenopausal woman perform breast self-examination?

_____

14. According to the American Cancer Society, how often should a woman have a mammogram?

_____

ANSWERS

Matching related elements

1. E

2. C

3. A

4. B

5. D

Short answer

6. Examples of pertinent questions the nurse should ask Ms. Rogers to explore her current health status include: When did you first notice the lump? What did the lump feel like? Have you noticed any breast or nipple skin changes or any nipple discharge? Do you take any medications?

Examples of questions the nurse should ask to investigate the patient's past health status include: Do you have a family history of breast cancer? Have you had children? If so, how old were you when you bore them? How many years did you menstruate?

7. The nurse should assure Jimmy and his parents that temporary gynecomastia occurs in two of three adolescent males and should resolve on its own when testosterone's effect overcomes estrogen's influence.

8. Breast changes during pregnancy include increased breast size, colostrum production, nipple and areolae darkening, and striae. During the immediate postpartal period, the breasts become engorged.

9. Risk factors for breast cancer include a mother or sibling who had breast cancer (especially if it developed before menopause), childlessness, childbearing after age 30, and previous breast cancer. Factors that slightly increase the risk of breast cancer include a high alcohol or dietary fat intake, early onset of menses, and late menopause.

10. Typical breast findings in an adolescent female include asymmetrical breast development; in a postmenopausal woman, granular breast tissue that is less firm and elastic and a thickened inframammary ridge.

11. The nurse should ask the patient with large or pendulous breasts to stand and lean forward with her arms outstretched. The patient's arms are supported by the back of a chair or the examiner's hands.

12. Breast inspection findings that suggest cancer include signs of retraction, such as nipple deviation or skin dimpling, increased venous prominence, and edema or eczema of the nipple. Abnormal breast palpation findings include a breast mass, lymph gland swelling, and bloody nipple discharge.

13. The premenopausal woman should perform breast self-examination every month, on the 5th to 7th day after the first day of the menstrual period.

14. Currently, the American Cancer Society recommends a baseline mammography screening between ages 35 and 40, then a mammogram every 1 to 2 years between ages 40 to 49 and once a year after age 50. After age 75, mammograms should be done at the discretion of the patient and health care provider.

CANCER INDICATORS

1. NIPPLE DEVIATION
2. DIMPLING
3. MASS
4. LYMPH NODE SWELL
5. BLOODY NIPPLE DISC
6. VENOUS PROM.
7. EDEMA OF NIPPLE

CHAPTER 12

Gastrointestinal system

OBJECTIVES   After studying this chapter, the reader should be able to:

1. Describe the organs of the gastrointestinal (GI) system.
2. Discuss important health history components that provide information about GI system status.
3. Demonstrate how to perform an abdominal assessment on an adult, a pediatric patient, a pregnant patient, and an elderly patient.
4. Differentiate between normal and abnormal findings detected during physical assessment of the GI system.
5. Document GI system assessment findings correctly.

OVERVIEW OF CONCEPTS   Virtually everyone experiences some type of GI system problem at one time or another. Besides being common, GI disorders have wide-ranging metabolic implications. For example, untreated vomiting and diarrhea can affect acid-base balance (the stable concentration of hydrogen ions in the body), and numerous disorders can interfere with nutritional status and normal body processes. For these reasons, the nurse should take a holistic approach to GI system assessment.

The GI system has two major components: the alimentary canal (or GI tract) and the accessory organs. The alimentary canal consists primarily of a hollow muscular tube starting in the mouth and extending to the anus. Accessory organs that aid GI function include the liver, biliary duct system (gallbladder and bile ducts), and pancreas. (For an illustration, see *Gastrointestinal system,* page 198.)

Together, the alimentary canal and accessory organs serve two major functions: digestion, the breaking down of food and fluid into simple chemicals that can be absorbed into the bloodstream and transported throughout the body; and elimination of waste products from the body through excretion of feces. The accessory organs also aid digestion and perform other functions to enhance the body's nutritional status. For example, the pancreas functions as an endocrine gland and an exocrine gland. (For information about the pancreas's endocrine functions, see Chapter 19, Endocrine system.) Exocrine functions involve secretion of pancreatic digestive enzymes, which aid intestinal absorption of proteins, fats, and carbohydrates.

Gastrointestinal system

The GI system consists of the alimentary canal and accessory organs, shown in this illustration.

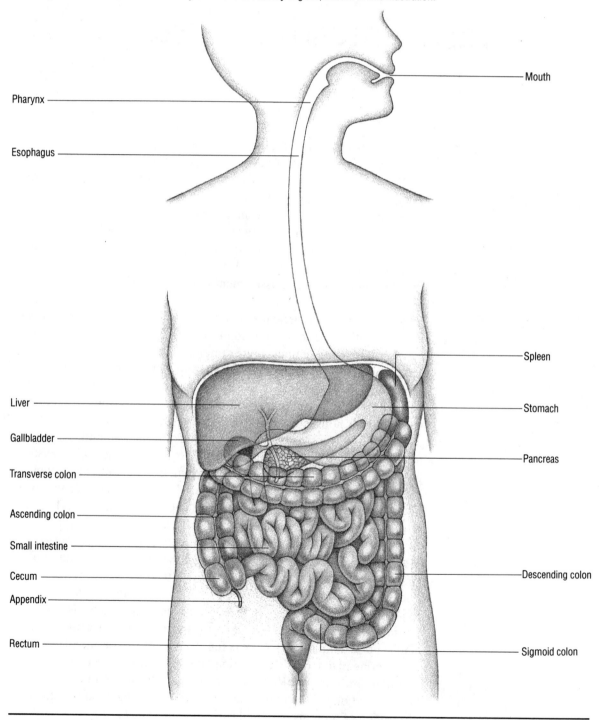

Health history   A complete and accurate GI system assessment depends on the nurse asking the right health history questions, then relating the patient's responses to physical assessment findings. Whether or not the patient has an overt GI problem, questions should cover dietary intake, appetite, digestion, bowel elimination patterns, medication use, and history of past and present GI disorders. (For health history questions on dietary intake and appetite, see Chapter 5, Nutritional status.)

Fully explore all GI complaints, even vague or seemingly mild ones, such as "heartburn," "upset stomach," and "too much gas." Although the patient may dismiss such complaints as unimportant, they may signal a serious underlying problem. Also, ask only those detailed questions that apply to the patient's condition. For example, ask a patient with abdominal pain detailed questions about the pain and related symptoms. If the patient does not report vomiting, skip the detailed questions about this symptom.

Health and illness patterns

Use the following questions to explore the patient's current, past, and family health status, as well as the patient's developmental status.

Current health status

Because current health status is foremost in the patient's mind, begin the interview by exploring this topic. Carefully document the chief complaint in the patient's own words. Using the PQRST method, ask the patient to describe this complaint and any others completely. (For a detailed explanation of this method, see *Symptom analysis,* page 15.) To investigate the patient's current health status further, ask the following questions about GI function:

Do you have any pain in your mouth, throat, abdomen, or rectum? If so, how would you describe it?
(RATIONALE: Pain is one of the most common GI symptoms; abdominal pain may signal a serious GI problem. GI pain usually is described as burning, squeezing, or dull or as a sensation of the stomach being tied in knots.)

Were you drinking alcohol before the stomach pain began?
(RATIONALE: Bouts of pancreatitis, gastritis, or peptic ulcer disease may occur after consumption of a large amount of alcohol.)

What, if anything, reduces the pain?
(RATIONALE: Ulcer pain is often relieved by ingesting food or antacids.)

Exactly where does the pain occur? Is it confined to one area or can you feel it in other parts of your abdomen?
(RATIONALE: Pain in an abdominal organ may be felt in other areas. For more information, see *Understanding referred pain,* page 200.)

Understanding referred pain

Referred pain—pain felt at a site different from that of the injured or diseased organ—occurs because some nerves that supply the organ also supply the body surface. These nerves transmit pain impulses along common pathways. The pain may occur relatively near the affected organ or some distance from it. Organ pain usually feels more diffuse than surface pain. This chart identifies common areas to which specific organ pain is referred.

ORGAN	REFERRED PAIN AREA
Gallbladder	• Right upper quadrant • Right posterior infrascapular area
Diaphragm	• Posterior neck • Posterior shoulder area
Duodenum	• Midline of abdominal wall just above umbilicus (usually)
Appendix	• Umbilicus • Parietal peritoneal involvement, right lower quadrant
Ureter	• Inguinal region • Either side of spinal column above hip bones

If you have abdominal pain, when does it occur in relation to eating?
(RATIONALE: Peptic ulcer pain usually begins 2 hours after meals or when the stomach is empty. Insufficient blood flow to the bowel usually causes pain within 30 minutes after a meal.)

Do you have indigestion? Do you ever experience heartburn or excessive gas?
(RATIONALE: Indigestion, a common complaint, typically refers to GI distress associated with eating. This term may be applied to many different symptoms, including heartburn, excessive gas, and cramping. Heartburn usually refers to reflux of gastric acid into the esophagus and often is precipitated by eating a heavy meal, lying down, or bending forward. Alcohol, caffeine, citrus or tomato products, fatty or spicy foods, and aspirin may cause heartburn. Excessive gas manifests as frequent belching, abdominal bloating, or flatus. Ask the patient about specific foods that produce these symptoms, including milk products especially if the patient lacks the intestinal lactase required to break down milk.)

Have you had nausea, vomiting, or diarrhea in addition to the pain?
(RATIONALE: Nausea and vomiting may indicate appendicitis; diarrhea along with these symptoms may indicate gastroenteritis.)

Did you notice any blood or fecal matter in the vomited material?
(RATIONALE: Hematemesis [vomiting of bright red blood] may indicate a bleeding ulcer or esophageal bleeding. A fecal odor may indicate an obstruction in the small intestine.)

Is the pain related to constipation and swelling in the abdomen?
(RATIONALE: Such findings may indicate intestinal obstruction.)

Have you had other problems, such as fever, at the same time?
(RATIONALE: Fever commonly accompanies such serious abdominal problems as appendicitis and pancreatitis.)

Do you have any difficulty swallowing (dysphagia)? If so, what seems to trigger the problem?
(RATIONALE: Dysphagia results from disorders of the pharynx or esophagus that interfere with swallowing. Dysphagia with solid foods but not liquids suggests esophageal narrowing, possibly from a tumor. Dysphagia related to swallowing hot or cold liquids suggests esophageal spasm.)

When did you last have a bowel movement or pass gas?
(RATIONALE: Inability to pass feces or gas [flatus] may indicate an obstruction. Diarrhea may indicate infection or inflammation.)

How often do you have bowel movements? Have you noticed any change in your normal bowel movement pattern?
(RATIONALE: Normal bowel movement frequency ranges from three times a day to three times a week. A change in pattern could result from bowel cancer, infection, or another disorder and should be explored.)

Are your stools formed or loose? If formed, are they soft or hard?
(RATIONALE: Hard stools may indicate constipation; loose or frequent liquid stools indicate diarrhea.)

What color are your stools? Have you seen any red blood in the stools?
(RATIONALE: Clay-colored or very lightly pigmented stools may indicate a liver or biliary tract problem. Black stools may indicate GI bleeding or use of iron supplements. Red blood in stools may indicate cancer of the colon, diverticula, an inflammatory condition, hemorrhoids, or anal fissures. Green stools may result from eating green vegetables.)

Have you recently had an unintentional weight loss, appetite loss, unexplained fatigue, or recurrent fever?
(RATIONALE: These symptoms may indicate malabsorption, GI cancer, or GI infection or inflammation.)

Have you felt depressed or anxious recently?
(RATIONALE: Emotional distress can cause symptoms of GI distress, such as diarrhea, constipation, bloating, nausea, and anorexia.)

Past health status

Ask the following questions to explore the patient's medical history for additional GI information:

Have you ever had surgery on your mouth, throat, abdomen, or rectum?
(RATIONALE: Surgery may cause adhesions that can lead to strictures and altered GI function.)

Do you have any allergies, such as to milk products?
(RATIONALE: Allergic reactions to foods or medications may cause various GI symptoms.)

Do you use laxatives or enemas? If so, how often?
(RATIONALE: Laxatives and frequent enemas affect intestinal motility. Chronic use may cause constipation or diarrhea.)

Do you take any prescription or over-the-counter medications? If so, which ones and at what dosages?
(RATIONALE: Many medications alter GI function or produce adverse GI reactions.)

Family health status

Next, investigate the GI history of the patient's family by asking the following questions:

Has anyone in your family had colorectal cancer or polyps?
(RATIONALE: A family history of either disorder increases the patient's risk for developing colorectal cancer.)

Has anyone in your family had colitis?
(RATIONALE: A family history of colitis increases the patient's risk for colitis.)

Developmental considerations for pediatric patients

Try to involve both the child and the parent in the interview. If the child can speak, encourage participation in the interview and use age-appropriate words. To help assess a child thoroughly, direct the following questions to the parent:

What is the color, consistency, and number of your newborn's stools?
(RATIONALE: During the first 5 to 6 days after birth, the neonate's stools normally change from greenish black to greenish yellow, then to pasty yellow for the formula-fed infant and mushy yellow for the breast-fed infant. The neonate typically passes 4 to 6 stools during the first 5 days, then only 1 or 2 stools a day.)

Does your infant continually want to eat despite bouts of projectile vomiting (forceful vomiting that is propelled away from the body)?
(RATIONALE: Projectile vomiting may indicate pyloric stenosis or gastroesophageal reflux. An infant with such a disorder is continually hungry but cannot retain food.)

At what age was your child toilet trained? Did any problems occur?
(RATIONALE: Achievement of independent toileting is a developmental milestone indicating a level of physical maturity.)

Does your child have more "accidental" bowel movements when ill?
(RATIONALE: Regression in bowel elimination habits is fairly common during a child's illness and hospitalization.)

Do you suspect your child sometimes deliberately holds back stool?
(RATIONALE: This may indicate the cause of constipation. A child may use bowel function as a weapon in power struggles with parents.)

Do your child's stools ever appear large, bulky, and frothy and float in the toilet bowl? Are they especially malodorous?
(RATIONALE: These signs may indicate a malabsorptive state, such as celiac disease or cystic fibrosis.)

Developmental considerations for pregnant patients

Be aware that pregnancy normally displaces the colon, thereby decreasing peristaltic activity. This commonly leads to such GI problems as constipation. Hemorrhoids result from pelvic vein compression caused by the expanding uterus. To assess the pregnant patient, ask the following questions:

Do you ever experience nausea and vomiting? If so, does it occur at a specific time or throughout the day?
(RATIONALE: "Morning sickness" with early-morning nausea and vomiting is common during the first trimester of pregnancy, although afternoon or evening episodes also may occur. However, continual nausea and vomiting throughout the day may indicate a more serious GI problem.)

How have your bowel habits changed since you became pregnant?
(RATIONALE: Constipation is common during pregnancy because of pressure on the bowel caused by the expanding uterus.)

Have you experienced abdominal pain?
(RATIONALE: Abdominal pain before the expected delivery date may indicate ectopic pregnancy, abruptio placentae, or uterine rupture. Conditions unrelated to pregnancy, such as appendicitis, sometimes occur.)

Have you experienced heartburn?
(RATIONALE: Heartburn, caused by abnormal gastroesophageal sphincter activity from diaphragmatic pressure from the expanded uterus, is common during pregnancy.)

How do you feel about your pregnancy?
(RATIONALE: Negative feelings, depression, fear, and anxiety can produce a wide variety of GI symptoms.)

Developmental considerations for elderly patients

Aging alters intestinal motility and liver size and decreases digestive enzyme secretions. These changes may reduce the patient's digestive function and increase food intolerance. Also, an elderly patient may metabolize certain drugs more poorly than a younger patient. To assess for these potential problems, ask the following questions:

Do you ever lose control of your bowels?
(RATIONALE: Fecal incontinence in an elderly patient may result from loss of sphincter tone or leakage of liquid stool around a fecal impaction.)

Do you experience constipation regularly? Does this represent a change in your normal bowel elimination habits?
(RATIONALE: Constipation may result from decreased intestinal motility associated with aging; however, sudden onset may herald colorectal cancer.)

Do you experience diarrhea after eating certain foods?
(RATIONALE: Diarrhea may result from a food intolerance, to which an elderly patient may have increased susceptibility.)

Do you need assistance at home to go to the bathroom?
(RATIONALE: Decreased mobility or other aging-related problems may hinder the patient's ability to use the bathroom, possibly leading to constipation or incontinence.)

Health promotion and protection patterns
Ask the following questions about health care habits, which may identify potential GI system problems:

Do you smoke? If so, how much and for how many years?
(RATIONALE: Heavy smoking can aggravate an ulcer and may predispose the patient to oral cancer.)

Do you drink alcohol? If so, how much and how often? How long have you maintained this pattern?
(RATIONALE: Alcohol irritates the stomach lining and can precipitate hepatic and pancreatic disease.)

Do you drink coffee, tea, or cola or use any other caffeine-containing products?
(RATIONALE: Caffeine irritates the stomach lining and increases intestinal motility.)

How do you care for your teeth and gums?
(RATIONALE: Poor dental hygiene can lead to gingivitis or other gum disease as well as tooth loss.)

Do you engage in a regular exercise program?
(RATIONALE: A sedentary lifestyle can contribute to constipation.)

What do you do for a living? How do you feel about your job?
(RATIONALE: The answers to these questions may identify unusual stressors or circumstances that may trigger GI problems.)

Role and relationship patterns

Inquire about role and relationship patterns affected by GI system problems by asking the following questions:

Have you lived in or traveled to a foreign country? If so, when and where?
(RATIONALE: A patient who has recently immigrated or returned from traveling abroad may have a GI ailment endemic to the foreign country, such as intestinal parasites.)

In your family, who does the food shopping and who prepares meals? Does the entire family usually eat together? Have these routines changed recently?
(RATIONALE: Illness can disrupt family roles and relationships, increasing stress and exacerbating GI symptoms.)

Have you recently lost a loved one, experienced the breakup of a relationship, or undergone a similar stressful event?
(RATIONALE: Depression, loss, and life changes can affect eating and elimination patterns and produce various GI symptoms.)

Physical assessment

Physical assessment of the GI system usually includes evaluation of the mouth, abdomen, and rectum. This section discusses abdominal and rectal assessment; for information on assessing the mouth, see Chapter 7, Head and neck.

To perform a thorough abdominal assessment, gather the following equipment: gloves (if necessary), stethoscope, flashlight, measuring tape, felt-tip pen, and a gown and drapes to cover the patient. Make sure the examination room is private, quiet, warm, and well lit.

Before beginning, explain the steps and reassure the patient that the assessment should not be painful, although it may be uncomfortable at times. Then, ask the patient to urinate, undress, put on a gown, and lie supine on the examination table with arms at the sides and the head supported comfortably on a pillow (to prevent abdominal muscle tensing). Drape the genital area and raise the gown to bare the abdomen, making sure to keep a female patient's breasts covered.

To assess the abdomen, perform the four basic steps in the following sequence: inspection, auscultation, percussion, and palpation. Unlike other body systems, the GI system requires abdominal auscultation before percussion and palpation, because these two assessment techniques can alter intestinal activity and bowel sounds.

To ensure more accurate assessment findings and consistent documentation of findings, mentally divide the patient's abdomen into regions, using either the quadrant or the nine regions method. (For illustrations, see *Identifying abdominal landmarks,* page 206.) When assessing a patient with abdominal pain, always auscultate, percuss, and palpate the painful quadrant last; touching the painful area first may cause the patient to tense the abdominal muscles, making assessment difficult.

Identifying abdominal landmarks

The diagrams below show how the underlying abdominal organs relate to the two methods of identifying abdominal landmarks—the quadrant method and the nine regions method.

QUADRANT METHOD

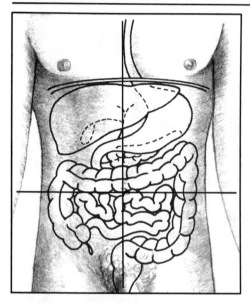

Right upper quadrant (RUQ)
Liver and gallbladder
Pylorus
Duodenum
Head of pancreas
Hepatic flexure of colon
Portions of ascending and
transverse colon

Left upper quadrant (LUQ)
Left liver lobe
Stomach
Body of pancreas
Splenic flexure of colon
Portions of transverse and
descending colon

Right lower quadrant (RLQ)
Cecum and appendix
Portion of ascending colon

Left lower quadrant (LLQ)
Sigmoid colon
Portion of descending colon

NINE REGIONS METHOD

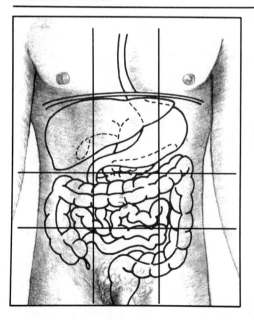

Right hypochondriac
Right liver lobe
Gallbladder

Epigastric
Pyloric end of stomach
Duodenum
Pancreas
Portion of liver

Left hypochondriac
Stomach
Tail of pancreas
Splenic flexure of colon

Right lumbar
Ascending colon
Portion of duodenum
and jejunum

Umbilical
Omentum
Mesentery
Lower part of duodenum
Jejunum and ileum

Left lumbar
Descending colon
Portions of jejunum
and ileum

Right inguinal
Cecum
Appendix
Lower end of ileum

**Suprapubic or
hypogastric**
Ileum

Left inguinal
Sigmoid colon

Inspection

Inspect the patient's entire abdomen, noting overall contour and skin integrity, appearance of the umbilicus, and any visible pulsations. Assess abdominal contour from the foot of the bed and the patient's side, stooping so the abdomen is at eye level. With the patient supine, the abdomen normally appears slightly rounded, with gently curved, symmetric lateral borders. Be aware of variations in contour depending on body type. Note any localized distention or irregular contours for further assessment.

Next, inspect the abdominal skin, which normally appears smooth and intact, with varying amounts of hair. Look for discolored areas, striae (lines resulting from rapid or prolonged skin stretching), rashes or other lesions, dilated veins, and scars. Document the location and character of these findings.

Observe the entire abdomen for movement caused by peristalsis or arterial pulsations. Normally, peristalsis is not visible. In some patients, aortic pulsations may be seen in the epigastric area.

To detect any umbilical or incisional hernias, have the patient raise the head and shoulders while remaining supine. True umbilical or incisional hernias may protrude during this maneuver. Finally, inspect the umbilicus for position, contour, and color. The umbilicus should be midline, concave, and consistent in color with the rest of the abdomen.

Abnormal findings

A concave (scaphoid) abdominal contour may indicate malnutrition. Abdominal distention may point to a tumor, excessive fluid or gas accumulation, or, less commonly, severe malnutrition.

Visible skin abnormalities often provide valuable clues to underlying abdominal problems. Bulging around old scars may indicate an incisional hernia. Striae commonly result from obesity or pregnancy, but also may signal an abdominal tumor or other disorder, such as Cushing's syndrome, which characteristically causes purplish striae. Recently developed striae usually appear pink or blue; older striae, white or silver. In a dark-skinned patient, striae may be lighter than the surrounding skin. Tense, glistening skin may indicate ascites. Dilated, tortuous superficial abdominal veins may point to inferior vena caval obstruction. Spider angiomas may indicate liver disease.

An everted umbilicus is normal in some patients; in others, however, it may indicate increased intra-abdominal pressure. A bluish tinge around the umbilicus may point to intra-abdominal bleeding.

Strong, visible peristaltic waves commonly indicate intestinal obstruction. Abdominal aortic pulsations may become more pronounced and obvious from increased intra-abdominal pressure, as from a tumor or ascites.

To help document assessment findings, draw a diagram of the patient's abdominal quadrants and record the location, size, and color of any abnormalities.

Auscultation sites for vascular sounds

Using the bell of the stethoscope, listen for vascular sounds at the sites shown here.

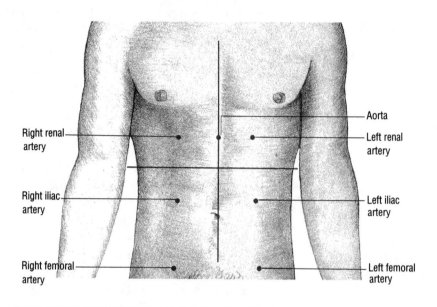

Right renal artery

Right iliac artery

Right femoral artery

Aorta

Left renal artery

Left iliac artery

Left femoral artery

Auscultation

Auscultation provides information on bowel motility and the underlying vessels and organs. After inspecting the patient's abdomen, use a stethoscope to auscultate for bowel and vascular sounds. To auscultate bowel sounds, lightly press the stethoscope diaphragm on the abdominal skin in all four quadrants. Normally, air and fluid moving through the bowel by peristalsis create soft, bubbling sounds with no regular pattern, often with soft clicks and gurgles interspersed, every 5 to 15 seconds. A hungry patient normally may have a familiar "stomach growl," a hyperperistaltic condition called borborygmi. Rapid, high-pitched, loud, gurgling bowel sounds are hyperactive, and may occur normally in a hungry patient. Sounds that occur at a rate of one every minute or longer are hypoactive and normally occur after bowel surgery or when the colon is filled with feces.

Before reporting absent bowel sounds, be sure the patient has an empty bladder; a full bladder may obscure the sounds. Gently pressing on the abdominal surface may initiate peristalsis and audible bowel sounds, as will having the patient eat or drink something.

Next, use the bell of the stethoscope to auscultate for vascular sounds. Normally, no vascular sounds are detected. (For illustrations of auscultation sites, see *Auscultation sites for vascular sounds.*)

DIAPHRAGM — Abdomen Sounds
Bell — Bruits (Vascular) Sounds

Abnormal abdominal sounds

This chart describes some abnormal abdominal sounds, lists the best places to listen for them, and explains what they may indicate.

SOUND AND DESCRIPTION	LOCATION	POSSIBLE INDICATION
Bowel sound alterations Sounds created by air and fluid movement through the bowel	All four quadrants	• Hyperactive sounds unrelated to hunger: diarrhea or early intestinal obstruction • Hypoactive, then absent, sounds: paralytic ileus or peritonitis • High-pitched "tinkling" sounds: intestinal fluid and air under tension in a dilated bowel • High-pitched "rushing" sounds coinciding with an abdominal cramp: intestinal obstruction
Systolic bruits Vascular "blowing" sounds resembling cardiac murmurs	• Abdominal aorta site • Renal artery sites • Iliac artery sites	• Partial arterial obstruction or turbulent blood flow, as in dissecting abdominal aneurysm • Renal artery stenosis • Hepatomegaly
Venous hum Continuous, medium-pitched tone created by blood flow in a large, engorged vascular organ, such as the liver	Epigastric and umbilical regions	• Increased collateral circulation between portal and systemic venous systems, as in hepatic cirrhosis
Friction rub Harsh, grating sound resembling two pieces of sandpaper rubbing together	Hepatic area	• Inflammation of the peritoneal surface of an organ, as from a liver tumor

Abnormal findings

Abdominal auscultation may reveal such abnormal sounds as bowel sound alterations, systolic bruits, venous hums, and friction rubs. (For more information on these sounds, see *Abnormal abdominal sounds*.)

Percussion

Abdominal percussion helps determine the size and location of abdominal organs and detects excessive accumulation of fluid and air in the abdomen. To perform this technique, percuss in all four quadrants, keeping approximate organ locations in mind. (For more information, see *Percussing the abdomen,* page 210.)

Percussion sounds vary with the density of underlying structures; usually, dull notes are detected over solids and tympanic notes over air. Tympany, the predominant abdominal percussion sound, is created by percussing over an air-filled stomach or intestine. Dull sounds normally occur over the liver and spleen, a lower intestine filled with feces, and a bladder filled with urine. In an obese patient, distinguishing abdominal percussion notes may be difficult.

Percussing the abdomen

Percuss the abdomen systematically, starting with the right upper quadrant and moving clockwise to the percussion sites in each quadrant. However, if the patient complains of pain in a particular quadrant, adjust the percussion sequence to percuss that quadrant last. When tapping, remember to move the right finger away quickly to avoid inhibiting vibrations.

Percussion sites

Right upper quadrant (RUQ)   Left upper quadrant (LUQ)

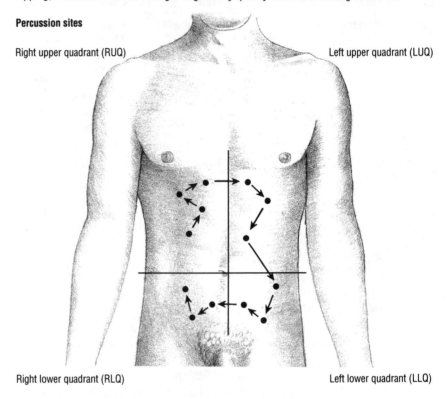

Right lower quadrant (RLQ)   Left lower quadrant (LLQ)

Keep in mind that abdominal percussion or palpation is contraindicated in patients with a suspected abdominal aortic aneurysm or those who have received abdominal organ transplants, and should be performed cautiously in patients with suspected appendicitis.

Abnormal findings

Abnormal percussion findings usually occur in patients with abdominal distention from air accumulation, ascites, or masses. Extremely high-pitched tympanic notes may indicate gaseous bowel distention. Ascites produces shifting dullness (a shift in the point where the percussion note changes from tympany to dullness when the patient changes position), caused by fluid shifting to dependent areas. Areas of dullness may indicate a mass or liver enlargement.

If the patient has abdominal distention, assess its progression by taking serial measurements of abdominal girth. Wrap a tape measure around the patient's abdomen at the umbilical level and record the measurement. To ensure that subsequent readings are taken at the same point, mark the point of measurement with a felt-tip pen.

Palpation

Abdominal palpation provides clues about the character of the abdominal wall; the size, condition, and consistency of abdominal organs; the presence and nature of any abdominal masses; and the presence, degree, and location of any abdominal pain. Commonly used techniques for abdominal palpation include light palpation, deep palpation, and ballottement.

To perform light palpation, gently press the fingertips about $\frac{1}{2}''$ to $\frac{3}{4}''$ (1 to 2 cm) into the abdominal wall. The light touch helps relax the patient. A patient who finds the sensation disagreeable or ticklish can place his or her hand atop the nurse's hand and follow along; this usually relaxes the patient and decreases involuntary muscle contractions in response to touch. To perform deep palpation, press the fingertips of both hands about $1\frac{1}{2}''$ (4 cm) into the abdominal wall. Move the hands in a slightly circular fashion, so that the abdominal wall moves over the underlying structures.

When palpating the abdomen, systematically cover all four quadrants, assessing for organ location, masses, and areas of tenderness or increased muscular resistance. If a mass is detected during light or deep palpation, note the location, size, shape, consistency, type of border, degree of tenderness, presence of pulsations, and degree of mobility (fixed or mobile). However, do not palpate a pulsating midline mass; it may be a dissecting aneurysm, which can rupture under the pressure of palpation. Report such a mass to the physician immediately.

Abnormal findings

Abnormal abdominal palpation findings include increased abdominal wall resistance, tenderness or guarding (flexion of the abdominal muscles), and masses. Tenderness, guarding, and complaints of abdominal pain may indicate appendicitis. Deep palpation may evoke rebound tenderness when the fingertips are withdrawn suddenly—a possible sign of peritoneal inflammation. Accurate evaluation of palpation findings may be difficult in a patient who complains of generalized tenderness. To assess tenderness accurately in such a patient, place your stethoscope on the abdomen and pretend to auscultate, but actually press into the abdomen with the stethoscope as you would with the hands and see if the patient still complains of pain.

Developmental considerations for pediatric patients

When preparing a child for an abdominal examination, explain the procedure in age-appropriate terms (for example, "I'll be checking your tummy"). Reassure the child that the parent can stay in the examination room throughout the assessment. To reduce anxiety, allow the child to touch the equipment and ask questions about what the nurse is doing. Demonstrate the techniques on a doll or stuffed toy.

Positioning for the assessment depends on the child's age and level of cooperation. An older child may lie supine on the examination table, as an adult would. When examining a young child or infant, place the child across a parent's lap, or lay the child's buttocks and legs across your lap and place the child's head on the parent's lap.

The assessment sequence for a pediatric patient also depends on the child's age and level of cooperation. The normal assessment sequence may need to be altered. For example, if the child has remained quiet for auscultation of heart and lung sounds, consider auscultating the abdomen at once. Because percussion and palpation involve touching the child, defer these until the end of the examination, when the child has developed some trust in the nurse and is more likely to cooperate.

Inspection of a child's abdomen resembles inspection of an adult's. However, keep in mind the differences in normal and abnormal findings among age groups. The contour of a child's abdomen may be the first clue to a possible GI disorder. In a child under age 4, a mild potbelly (distention) when the child stands or sits is normal. In a child between ages 4 and 13, a mildly protruding abdomen is normal only when the child stands. An extreme potbelly may result from visceral enlargement, ascites, neoplasm, abdominal wall defects, or starvation; a depressed or concave abdomen may indicate a diaphragmatic hernia, especially when accompanied by localized swelling. Note any scars or abdominal vascularity. Superficial veins normally are readily visible in an infant.

To inspect an infant's abdomen, stand at the foot of the table and direct a light across the abdomen from the infant's right side. Observe for peristaltic waves, which normally are invisible. Visible peristaltic waves may indicate intestinal obstruction. Reverse (left-to-right) peristaltic waves commonly point to pyloric stenosis; other possible causes include bowel malrotation, duodenal ulcer, and duodenal stenosis.

When inspecting a child's abdomen, keep in mind that a child's respiratory movements are primarily abdominal; costal respiratory movements may indicate peritonitis, obstruction, or accumulation of ascitic fluid. The transition from abdominal to costal respirations is gradual with age. Usually, a child breathes abdominally until age 6 or 7.

Also observe a young child for diastasis recti abdominis (separation of the two rectus abdominis muscles with a protrusion in the separation). This benign condition, especially common in black infants, usually disappears during the preschool years. At the same time, inspect for umbilical hernia. (For the best view, wait until the child cries, which increases intra-abdominal pressure and makes herniation more apparent.)

Auscultation of a child's abdomen also resembles that of an adult's. In a child with a disorder, auscultation may reveal an abnormal finding. For example, it may detect an abdominal murmur, suggesting coarctation of the aorta; a venous hum, suggesting portal hypertension; or a double "pistol shot" sound in the femoral artery, possibly signaling aortic insufficiency. Besides these vascular sounds, auscultation may reveal high-pitched bowel sounds, suggesting gastroenteritis or impending intestinal obstruction; absent bowel sounds, a sign of paralytic ileus or peritonitis; or a hepatic friction rub, which usually indicates inflammation.

A child's underdeveloped abdominal wall should make palpation easier than in an adult. However, this part of the abdominal examination is subjective and requires the child's cooperation in reporting symptoms truthfully. Because the child may be more ticklish and tense than an adult, distract the child during palpation, perhaps by starting a discussion or asking the child to count or recite the alphabet. Get a preschool child to cooperate by playing a game ("Let me feel your tummy and guess what you had for breakfast. A watermelon? A box of candy?"). Having an infant suck on a pacifier (not a bottle of milk, which may cause regurgitation) may help relax the abdomen and enhance palpation. To minimize ticklishness and give the child some sense of control over the situation, palpate the abdomen with the child's hand under the nurse's hand. (However, be aware that although this technique can identify localized pain, it is not sensitive enough to detect most palpable findings.)

To augment the child's verbal descriptions of pain, look for visible clues while palpating. A child may use abdominal guarding more than an adult in response to abdominal pain. Other clues to a child's pain include grimacing, sudden protective movement with an arm or leg, and a change in the pitch of the cry.

Palpation in a quadrant other than the painful one should reveal a soft, nontender abdomen. If not, the child is still tense. To avoid inaccurate findings, try to relax the child before proceeding. A slightly tender descending colon may be caused by stool. Tenderness in the right lower quadrant may indicate an inflamed appendix. Generalized tenderness and rigidity in the affected quadrant commonly points to peritoneal irritation. If these findings are present, ask the child to cough; a reduced or withheld cough may confirm peritoneal irritation. These findings contraindicate palpating for rebound tenderness, a potentially painful procedure for a child.

Palpate the infant's abdomen for umbilical hernia. (Commonly present at birth and often not visible, umbilical hernias usually enlarge until age 1 month, then gradually become smaller until about age 1.) Press down on the infant's umbilicus. If a fingertip can be inserted, the infant has a small hernia. Treatment usually consists of letting the hernia close by itself without surgery. Any hernia that is larger than $\frac{3}{4}''$

(2 cm) or increases in size after age 1 month requires further assessment.

Because a child commonly swallows air when eating and crying, percussion may reveal louder tympanic notes than those normally found in an adult. Tympany along with abdominal distention may result from ascites. In a neonate, ascites usually results from GI perforation; in an older child, from congestive heart failure, cirrhosis, or nephrosis.

Developmental considerations for pregnant patients

Vary the assessment position for a pregnant patient depending on the pregnancy stage. In the final weeks, for example, a patient may find the supine position uncomfortable because it can impair respiratory excursion and blood flow. To enhance comfort, place her in a side-lying or semi-Fowler's position.

When assessing a pregnant patient's abdomen, keep in mind the normal variations in assessment findings associated with pregnancy. Common findings include increased pigmentation of the abdominal midline (linea nigra), striae, upward displacement of the umbilicus, and diastasis recti abdominis.

Developmental considerations for elderly patients

Positioning of an elderly patient for abdominal assessment depends on the patient's physical condition. For example, an elderly patient with orthopnea (difficulty breathing while lying down) cannot recline. Position this patient with the head and trunk raised and knees slightly flexed to help relax the abdomen.

Abdominal assessment in an elderly patient follows the same pattern as that for any adult. Because the abdominal wall usually thins (from muscle wasting and fibroconnective tissue loss) and abdominal muscle tone relaxes with aging, abdominal palpation may be easier and the results more accurate in an elderly patient. For these same reasons, abdominal rigidity—an important sign of peritoneal inflammation in a younger patient—is far less common and abdominal distention more common in elderly patients.

Documentation

The following sample illustrates the proper way to document normal physical assessment findings in the GI system:

Weight: 148 lb

Height: 5′8″

Additional notes: Abdomen slightly convex, no skin lesions, no herniations, no pulsations. Normal bowel sounds auscultated every 10 seconds, all four quadrants. No bruits. No tenderness or masses. Percussion reveals liver edge at costal margin.

The following sample shows how to document abnormal physical assessment findings:

Weight: 204 lb

Height: 5′7″

Additional notes: Abdomen distended. Visible dilated vein over peri-umbilical area and abdominal wall. Protruding umbilicus. Abdominal girth 94 cm, measured at level of umbilicus. Normal bowel sounds auscultated every 6 seconds. No bruits or friction rubs detected. Diminished tympany over suprapubic area; shifting dullness present. Fluid wave present. No abdominal tenderness.

STUDY ACTIVITIES

Fill in the blank

1. The predominant abdominal percussion sound is ___DULL TYMPANY___.

2. A gallbladder disorder is likely to cause referred pain in the

___R.U___ quadrant.

3. Bowel sounds normally occur every ___5___ to ___15___ seconds.

Multiple choice

4. Which suspected or diagnosed GI disorder contraindicates abdominal palpation?
   (A) Aortic aneurysm
   B. Bowel obstruction
   C. Cirrhosis
   D. Umbilical hernia

5. Which aging-related change in the elderly patient helps make abdominal palpation easier and more accurate than in a younger patient?
   A. Abdominal wall thickening
   B. Abdominal guarding
   (C) Relaxed abdominal muscle tone
   D. Increased connective tissue

6. Which physical finding suggests pyloric stenosis?
   (A) Left-to-right peristaltic waves
   B. Abdominal distention
   C. Abdominal concavity
   D. Superficial abdominal veins

7. In a pregnant patient, which of the following is *not* a normal variation that may be detected during an abdominal assessment?
   A. Linea nigra
   (B) Diastasis recti abdominis
   C. Striae
   D. Downward displacement of the umbilicus

True or false

8. To assess for an umbilical or incisional hernia, the nurse should have the patient raise the head and shoulders while remaining supine.
   ☐ True   ☐ False

9. A systolic bruit is a harsh grating sound that resembles two pieces of sandpaper rubbing together.

☐ True ☐ False

10. During percussion of a urine-filled bladder, dullness is a normal sound.

☐ True ☐ False

11. Palpation is the first technique the nurse uses when assessing a patient's abdomen.

☐ True ☐ False

ANSWERS

Fill in the blank

1. tympany
2. right upper
3. 5, 15

Multiple choice

4. A. Abdominal palpation is contraindicated in a patient with a known or suspected aortic aneurysm because it may cause the aneurysm to rupture.

5. C. Because the abdominal wall usually thins and abdominal muscle tone relaxes with aging, abdominal palpation may be easier and the results more accurate in an elderly patient.

6. A. Left-to-right (reverse) peristaltic waves suggest pyloric stenosis.

7. D. During pregnancy, the umbilicus is displaced upward.

True or false

8. True.

9. False. A systolic bruit is a vascular "blowing" sound that resembles a cardiac murmur.

10. True.

11. False. Because percussion and palpation can alter bowel sounds, the nurse inspects and auscultates before percussing and palpating the abdomen.

CHAPTER 13

Urinary system

OBJECTIVES

After studying this chapter, the reader should be able to:

1. Locate the urinary system structures.

2. Discuss the main functions of the kidneys.

3. Describe normal urine characteristics.

4. Give examples of appropriate health history questions to ask the patient when assessing the urinary system.

5. Differentiate between normal and abnormal findings during physical assessment of the kidneys, bladder, and urethral meatus.

6. Document urinary system assessment findings properly.

OVERVIEW OF CONCEPTS

The kidneys play a vital role in many body functions, including waste excretion, maintenance of acid-base balance (the stable concentration of hydrogen ions in body fluids), and homeostasis (chemical and physical equilibrium of fluids in the body's internal environment). Therefore, a urinary system assessment may uncover clues to possible problems in any body system. Because a disorder in another system can disrupt urinary system function, the nurse always must assess for signs and symptoms of urinary system disorders even if the patient's chief complaint seems unrelated.

The urinary system consists of two kidneys, two ureters, one bladder, and one urethra. (For an illustration of urinary system structures, see *The urinary system,* page 218.)

The kidneys can vary the amount of substances reabsorbed and secreted in the nephrons—the functional units of the kidneys—changing the composition of excreted urine. Normal urine constituents include sodium, chloride, potassium, calcium, magnesium, sulfates, phosphates, bicarbonates, uric acid, ammonium ions, creatinine, urobilinogen, a few leukocytes and red blood cells (RBCs), and, in the male, possibly a few sperm.

Total daily urinary output varies with fluid intake and climate, averaging 720 to 2,400 ml. Usually, when fluid intake is high, urinary output increases; conversely, urinary output drops when fluid intake is reduced.

The urinary system

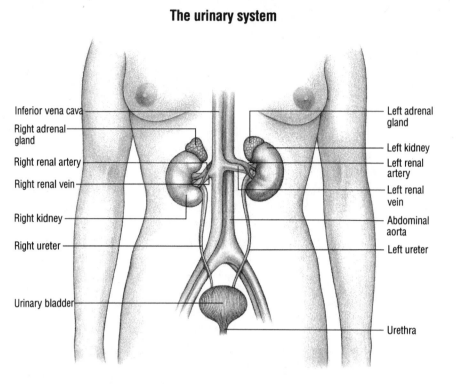

Inferior vena cava
Right adrenal gland
Right renal artery
Right renal vein
Right kidney
Right ureter
Urinary bladder

Left adrenal gland
Left kidney
Left renal artery
Left renal vein
Abdominal aorta
Left ureter
Urethra

Health history

When obtaining the health history of a patient with a urinary problem, document the chief complaint using the PQRST method. (For a detailed explanation of this method, see *Symptom analysis,* page 15.) To promote a conducive interview environment and minimize embarrassment, provide privacy. Use terms the patient understands, avoiding such terms as *void* or *catheter* unless the patient is familiar with them.

Health and illness patterns

Explore the patient's current, past, and family health status as well as the patient's developmental status using questions below.

Current health status

A patient with an indwelling urinary catheter is at high risk for urinary tract infection (UTI). Routinely evaluate such a patient for this problem. To investigate current health status in any patient, ask the following questions:

Do you ever feel a burning sensation or pain when you urinate? If so, how often?

(RATIONALE: A burning sensation during urination may result from a urinary tract infection or obstruction.)

Do you ever have urinary urgency—the feeling that you must urinate immediately?
(RATIONALE: Urinary urgency, with or without urination, suggests bladder dysfunction or UTI. Incontinence may accompany this sensation if the patient cannot make it to the bathroom quickly enough.)

Does your bladder feel full after you urinate?
(RATIONALE: A full sensation after voiding may indicate retention caused by bladder dysfunction or bladder irritation and spasm caused by infection.)

What color is your urine? Does it look clear? Does it have an odor? Is this a change?
(RATIONALE: Urine normally appears amber or straw-colored and is clear and relatively odorless. Abnormal colors, which range from dark yellow to black, may result from a urinary disorder, a change in fluid intake or diet, or use of certain drugs. Dehydration causes dark yellow to amber (concentrated) urine. A well-hydrated patient or one receiving diuretics produces dilute, straw-colored urine. Jaundice may cause dark orange-brown urine with a high bile content. A UTI commonly causes foul-smelling, cloudy urine.)

Do you have pain in your side that goes around to your back or into your lower abdomen?
(RATIONALE: Flank pain may indicate renal colic; lower abdominal pain may signal obstruction or infection.)

Do you have pain in your back, in the kidney region? (Point out the costovertebral angle [CVA] to the patient.)
(RATIONALE: CVA pain or tenderness commonly indicates upper UTI [pyelonephritis].)

Do you have discharge from your penis (if the patient is male) or vagina (if the patient is female)? If so, how does it look and smell? How much is there? Does your sexual partner have the same symptoms?
(RATIONALE: Urethral discharge frequently accompanies a sexually transmitted disease [STD], such as gonorrhea or chlamydia. Both infections can cause dysuria.)

Do you ever have trouble starting or maintaining a urine stream?
(RATIONALE: Urinary hesitancy, or difficulty starting a urine stream, may result from a urethral stricture, such as from an enlarged prostate gland or partial obstruction caused by a kidney stone.)

Have you noticed a change in the size of your urine stream? If so, can you describe it?
(RATIONALE: Decreased stream size may indicate a partial urethral obstruction, such as from a renal calculus that has descended into the urethra or an enlarged prostate.)

Do you ever leak urine when you laugh, cough, sneeze, or move quickly? Do you need to wear a pad or adult diaper to control this?
(RATIONALE: Stress incontinence is a common problem, often treatable with bladder training and exercise. Although more common in women, it also can be a problem in men. The patient may limit social activities out of fear of "wetting.")

Ask a male patient the following question:

Are you circumcised? If not, do you have any problems pulling back your foreskin?
(RATIONALE: Difficulty retracting the foreskin may lead to inadequate cleaning of the glans penis. Phimosis, or foreskin constriction over the glans, may result from infection and, when severe, can limit the ability to urinate.)

Ask a female patient the following question:

Have you ever been pregnant or given birth? If so, how many times? Have you ever injured the vaginal area during delivery?
(RATIONALE: Pregnancy and delivery can weaken pelvic floor muscles, impairing bladder control. Traumatic delivery can injure urinary and genital structures.)

Past health status

Ask the following questions to explore the patient's medical history for additional information related to the urinary system:

Have you ever had a kidney or bladder problem, such as a UTI? If so, please describe the problem and tell when it first occurred. How many times has it occurred since then? What kind of treatment did you receive?
(RATIONALE: A history of kidney or bladder problems increases the risk of recurrence or urinary system complications.)

Have you ever had kidney or bladder stones? If so, when? How were they treated?
(RATIONALE: Kidney or bladder stones [calculi] can recur. Determining how the problem was treated provides information that can help formulate the nursing care plan.)

Have you ever had a kidney or bladder injury? If so, when? How was it treated?
(RATIONALE: Trauma can alter kidney or bladder structure or function.)

Have you ever been catheterized? If so, why?
(RATIONALE: A history of catheterization usually indicates that the patient could not urinate or had urine retention or inhibited bladder emptying. However, catheterization occasionally is performed to collect a urine specimen.)

Do you currently take any prescribed or over-the-counter medications? If so, which ones and how frequently?
(RATIONALE: Some medications can affect urinary function or alter urine appearance.)

Are you allergic to any medications? If so, which ones? Can you describe your reaction?
(RATIONALE: Some allergic reactions can cause tubular damage; severe anaphylactic reactions can cause temporary renal failure and permanent tubular necrosis.)

Do you have diabetes or high blood pressure? If so, when was it diagnosed? How is it being controlled?
(RATIONALE: Diabetes mellitus can increase the risk of UTI; both diabetes mellitus and hypertension can lead to nephropathy and renal failure.)

Do you use anything to help control your urine, such as a drainage bag, pads, or diapers? If so, why?
(RATIONALE: The patient may have had urinary diversion surgery or incontinence. If surgery was performed, find out what type. If the patient is incontinent, investigate further and assess for possible causes. Incontinence may be reversible. Also, an incontinent patient may need assistance with skin management.)

Family health status
Next, investigate the history of the patient's family by asking the following questions:

Has anyone in your family had hypertension, diabetes mellitus, gout, or coronary artery disease?
(RATIONALE: These disorders, which may have a familial tendency, can alter renal function.)

Has anyone in your family ever been treated for kidney problems, such as polycystic kidney disease or nephritis?
(RATIONALE: These problems may be genetically transmitted.)

Has anyone in your family ever had kidney or bladder stones?
(RATIONALE: Kidney and bladder calculi have a familial tendency.)

Developmental considerations for pediatric patients
Try to involve the child in the interview whenever possible. To help perform a thorough urinary assessment of a pediatric patient, ask the following questions:

If the child has not been toilet trained, how many diapers does the child wet each day? Has this number changed recently?
(RATIONALE: A change in the number of diapers wet daily may indicate a urine volume change. For example, urine volume may decrease with fever and increased perspiration.)

Does the child have frequent or severe diaper rash?
(RATIONALE: Diaper rash may be caused by irritation from ammonia or a candidal infection [yeast diaper rash]. A rash caused by ammonia irritation usually responds to better hygiene practices. Candidal diaper

rash, characterized by reddish pink, raised, scattered lesions, requires an antifungal cream.)

Does the child cry when urinating? Has the child's urine changed in color or odor? Does the child have a fever?
(RATIONALE: Crying during urination may indicate pain or a burning sensation, suggesting a UTI. Urine changes and fever also suggest such an infection, which is a serious condition in children and warrants prompt intervention.)

Has the child recently had difficulty urinating or a urine stream change?
(RATIONALE: Difficulty urinating or a urine stream change suggests urinary obstruction.)

Has the child ever been sexually abused?
(RATIONALE: Children who are victims of sexual abuse and exploitation may contract the same STDs sexually active adults and may suffer severe genital trauma. Although this question may be uncomfortable for the nurse and parent or child, it is vital to holistic assessment of a child's environment and safety.)

For the toilet-trained child, ask these questions:

Does the child have a specific routine when urinating (for example, always urinating after a meal or before bedtime)?
(RATIONALE: Determining the child's routine and attempting to maintain it can help prevent urine retention or loss of bladder control in a strange environment, such as a hospital.)

Has the child's bladder control changed recently? For instance, has the child suddenly started to wet the bed?
(RATIONALE: Stress may cause a child's bladder control to regress. Enuresis [bed-wetting] may result from an emotional disturbance, small bladder capacity, or a UTI.)

Did the child learn to sit, stand, and talk at the expected times?
(RATIONALE: In a child who learned to sit, stand, and talk at the expected times, delayed toilet training may indicate a urinary system dysfunction.)

Developmental considerations for pregnant patients
When assessing a pregnant patient, be aware that pregnancy normally increases urine volume and frequency and decreases urine specific gravity. Ask the patient the following questions:

Do you ever have pain during urination or in the kidney area? (Point out this area to the patient.) Have you ever been diagnosed with a UTI?
(RATIONALE: Painful urination or pain in the kidney area may indicate UTI—the most common urinary problem during pregnancy. An untreated UTI can lead to preterm labor.)

Developmental considerations for elderly patients

Bladder muscles weaken with age, possibly causing incomplete bladder emptying and chronic urine retention. Consequently, the elderly patient is at increased risk for UTI, nocturia (excessive urination at night), and incontinence. To assess for these potential problems, ask the following questions:

How much and what types of liquid do you drink in the evening?
(RATIONALE: A high fluid intake in the evening may cause nocturia. On the other hand, a patient with nocturia, incontinence, or other urinary problem may limit fluid intake to decrease urinary output in an attempt to relieve the problem.)

Do you ever lose control of your bladder? If so, does this occur suddenly or do you feel a warning?
(RATIONALE: Bladder muscle weakening commonly impairs bladder control in the elderly patient, leading to incontinence. Many types of incontinence are treatable and should be thoroughly assessed.)

Health promotion and protection patterns

To continue the health history, determine the patient's personal habits, sleep and waking patterns, and typical daily activities. Ask the following questions to identify potential urinary system problems:

How many glasses of liquid do you drink daily?
(RATIONALE: A low fluid intake usually leads to a low urinary output; a high fluid intake, to a high output).

How many times do you urinate daily? Have you noticed any change in frequency?
(RATIONALE: Voiding pattern changes can result from a local urinary disorder, such as a bladder infection, or a systemic disorder, such as diabetes mellitus.)

Have you noticed any increase or decrease in the amount of urine you void each time?
(RATIONALE: A urine volume change may result from renal dysfunction, a fluid intake change, or a systemic disorder, such as diabetes insipidus or diabetes mellitus.)

How much salt do you use in cooking and on food? How often do you eat salty foods?
(RATIONALE: Salt contains sodium, which increases fluid retention and can decrease urine output.)

Does the need to urinate awaken you at night? If so, how often? Does this happen only when you drink large amounts of liquid in the evening?
(RATIONALE: Nonpathologic nocturia can result from a high intake of fluids—especially coffee, tea, or beer—in the evening. Pathologic nocturia can result from bladder cancer; UTI; renal disease, such as polycystic kidney disease or chronic interstitial nephritis; or congestive heart failure.)

What is your occupation?
(RATIONALE: Assembly-line workers, nurses, and other workers with limited access to lavatory facilities may develop urinary stasis and subsequent infection. Certain other workers also have a high risk of urinary dysfunction. For example, jackhammer operators may develop renal ptosis [kidney drop] from operating drills with a constant pounding movement.)

Role and relationship patterns
To discover the influence of a urinary system disorder on role and relationship patterns, ask the patient the following questions:

Can you get to and from the bathroom without help?
(RATIONALE: Determining whether a patient needs assistance with toileting can help the nurse plan appropriate interventions. Such planning can reduce the risk of incontinence or urine retention.)

If you have urinary frequency or get up often at night to urinate, does it affect any family members?
(RATIONALE: Frequent trips to the bathroom can disturb the sleep of a spouse or other family members, thus straining family relationships.)

Do you have any pain when you clean yourself after urinating? Do you ever have pain during sexual intercourse?
(RATIONALE: A bladder or urethral infection may cause perineal inflammation, leading to tenderness and dyspareunia [painful intercourse]. This, in turn, may impede the patient's sexual behavior. These complaints warrant further investigation.)

Physical assessment

Before assessing the patient's urinary system, gather the necessary equipment: stethoscope, sphygmomanometer with inflatable cuff, scale, gown and drapes to cover the patient, and specimen cup to collect a urine sample. Then evaluate various factors that may reflect the patient's renal function, including body weight, vital signs, and body position. Also evaluate the status of related body structures.

Physical assessment of the urinary system involves the basic techniques of inspection, palpation, percussion, and auscultation. However, percussing and palpating before auscultating may increase bowel motility, which interferes with sound transmission during renal artery auscultation. Therefore, when assessing the urinary system, perform inspection first, followed by auscultation, percussion, and palpation.

Before beginning the physical assessment, ask the patient to urinate into a specimen cup. Then assess the specimen for color, odor, and clarity. Provide a gown to prevent unnecessary exposure, and ask the patient to undress. Explain each assessment step beforehand and reassure the patient that drapes will be used appropriately throughout the assessment.

Body weight and vital signs

Begin the physical assessment by weighing the patient and comparing the result with baseline weight, if available. Be aware that a gain or loss of 2 to 3 lb (.9 to 1.4 kg) within 48 hours reflects a change in fluid status, not body mass. A rapid weight change may indicate fluid loss (such as from vomiting, diarrhea, fever, or restricted intake) or fluid gain (such as from fluid retention or edema).

To assess the fluid status of a hospitalized patient, measure weight at the same time daily using the same scale with the patient wearing the same amount of clothing. If these constants cannot be maintained, document the differences for each weigh-in. Instruct a patient to weigh self at home using the same procedure.

Measure and compare fluid intake and output daily. Because of insensible (immeasurable) fluid loss from the skin and lungs, output should equal only about two-thirds of intake over 24 hours. For an adult, hourly output normally ranges from 30 to 100 ml (1 to 3.3 oz); 24-hour output, from 720 to 2,400 ml (24 to 80 oz). When measuring output, be sure to consider fluid loss stemming from diarrhea, vomiting, fever, or wound drainage.

Next, obtain vital signs. Measure blood pressure in both arms for comparison, and take readings with the patient lying down and sitting up. Blood pressure should not drop more than 10 to 15 mm Hg with a position change; a drop of 20 mm Hg or more usually indicates fluid volume depletion, especially when accompanied by dizziness or other symptoms.

Hypotension (systolic pressure below 90 mm Hg) causes diminished renal blood flow and may precipitate acute renal failure. Hypertension, defined as several serial readings over 140/90 mm Hg, can lead to renal insufficiency. Hypertension may result from vascular damage caused by a primary renal disorder.

Assessing related body structures

Because the urinary system affects many body functions, chronic renal disease may make the patient appear seriously ill. Start by observing the patient's general appearance; then assess orientation to person, place, and time and evaluate memory of the immediate past. Renal dysfunction may cause poor concentration and loss of recent memory. Chronic, progressive renal failure can lead to toxin accumulation and electrolyte imbalance, producing such neurologic signs as lethargy, confusion, disorientation, stupor, somnolence, coma, and convulsions. The following guidelines apply to the remaining portions of the assessment.

Eyes

Using an ophthalmoscope, examine the internal eye, especially if the patient has hypertension. Various abnormal findings may indicate hypertension, a possible consequence or cause of renal disease. Check for retinal arteriolar narrowing, which may be accompanied by small areas of infarction or hemorrhage. With high blood pressure accompanied by cerebral edema, the patient may have blurred disk margins, caused by papilledema (optic nerve head swelling); cotton-wool patches; and dilated, tortuous veins.

Skin, hair, and nails

Inspect the patient's skin for pallor. Pallor typically stems from abnormally low hemoglobin concentration and hematocrit values, which worsen gradually as the kidneys fail. End-stage renal failure reduces erythropoietin production, thereby causing decreased RBC production. Also, uremic toxins shorten the RBC life span.

Inspect the patient's skin for large ecchymoses (bruises) and petechiae (tiny purple or red spots)—signs of clotting abnormalities and decreased platelet adhesion that may reflect chronic renal failure. Observe for uremic frost—white or yellow urate crystals on the skin—indicating late-stage renal failure. To assess the patient's hydration status, inspect mucous membranes in the mouth. Dryness may reflect mild dehydration or mouth breathing. Markedly dry mucous membranes and sunken eyes suggest severe dehydration. Inspect the skin for dryness and scratches; renal failure causes sweat and oil gland atrophy, leading to subcutaneous calcium deposits. Evaluate skin integrity, checking for cracks or tears with or without signs of infection. Chronic renal failure also can cause severe itching, which the patient may try to ease by scratching.

Evaluate skin turgor by gently pinching the patient's skin over the forehead or sternum with the thumb and index finger, then releasing it. (For details on this assessment technique, see Chapter 6, Skin, hair, and nails.) If the skin does not return to its normal position immediately, suspect severe dehydration.

Inspect the patient's neck veins for distention. (For a description of this technique, see Chapter 10, Cardiovascular system.) Also check for edema, the abnormal buildup of excess sodium and water within the interstitial spaces. Sometimes accompanying renal disease, edema may be systemic or local; local edema may be pitting (in which an indentation remains after edematous skin is pressed with a finger) or nonpitting.

To check for signs of systemic nonpitting edema, inspect the eyelids for swelling or puffiness—signs of periorbital edema. Auscultate the lungs for crackles, which may reflect pulmonary edema. Then inspect the abdomen for ascites (abnormal peritoneal fluid accumulation). To assess for local edema, inspect for swelling in the lowest (dependent) body portions, such as the ankles, sacrum, and scrotum.

Determine if local edema is pitting or nonpitting by applying pressure with the fingertip. Pitting edema commonly is graded on a four-point scale: +1 denotes a barely perceptible pit, with normal foot and leg contours; +2 indicates a deeper pit with fairly normal contours; +3 signifies a deep pit accompanied by leg and foot swelling; and + 4 denotes an even deeper pit accompanied by severe foot and leg swelling.

Inspection

Urinary system inspection includes examination of the abdomen and urethral meatus.

Abdomen

Help the patient assume a supine position with arms relaxed at the sides. Make sure the patient is comfortable and draped appropriately in this position. Then expose the abdomen from the xiphoid process to the symphysis pubis.

Inspect the abdomen for gross enlargements or fullness by comparing the left and right sides, noting any asymmetrical areas. In an adult, the abdomen should be smooth, flat or scaphoid (concave), and symmetrical. Abdominal skin should be free of scars, lesions, bruises, and discolorations. Note and inquire about any surgical scars not explained by the patient's history.

Extremely prominent veins may accompany other vascular signs associated with renal dysfunction, such as elevated blood pressure and renal artery bruits. Such abnormalities as distention, skin tightness and glistening, and striae (stretch marks) may signal fluid retention. Ascites may indicate nephrotic syndrome, a condition characterized by edema and increased urine protein and decreased serum albumin levels.

Urethral meatus

To put the patient at ease, explain beforehand how this area will be assessed. Be sure to observe universal precautions.

Position a female patient in the dorsal lithotomy position and drape her appropriately. Spread the labia with a gloved hand while looking at the urethral meatus. It will appear as a slit or a round opening at the midline, superior to the vagina and inferior to the clitoris. The meatus should be pink and free of swelling and discharge.

Drape the male patient so that only the penis is exposed. Compress the tip of the glans penis to open the urethral meatus. Normally, the meatus is centrally located and free of discharge.

In any patient, inflammation and discharge may signal urethral infection. Ulceration usually indicates an STD. In a male patient, a meatus deviating from the normal central location may represent hypospadias, a congenital defect.

Auscultation

Auscultate the renal arteries in the left and right upper abdominal quadrants by pressing the bell of the stethoscope lightly against the abdomen and instructing the patient to exhale deeply. (The renal arteries are located approximately 2″ to 3″ [5 to 7.5 cm] from the midline of the abdomen, at the costal [rib] margin.) Normally, no vascular sounds are audible. (For information on auscultating other abdominal areas, see Chapter 12, Gastrointestinal system.)

Percussing the urinary organs

The illustrations below show where the nurse should place the hands when percussing the kidney and bladder. When percussing the bladder, make sure to tap only the index and middle finger.

Kidney percussion

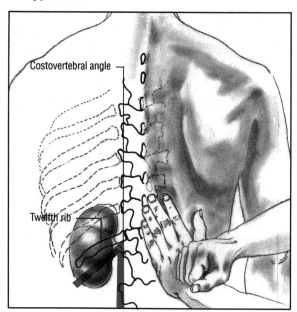

Costovertebral angle

Twelfth rib

Bladder percussion

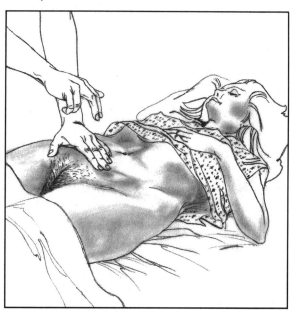

Abnormal auscultation findings include renal artery bruits. Produced by turbulent blood flow, such bruits suggest renal artery stenosis.

Percussion

For kidney percussion, have the patient sit upright, then percuss over each CVA. Place the left palm over the CVA and gently strike it with the right fist. Normally, the patient feels only a thudding sensation. A patient with glomerulonephritis may complain of tenderness or severe pain with this maneuver.

For bladder percussion, use mediate percussion over the bladder, starting 2″ (5 cm) above the symphysis pubis. Percussion normally produces a tympanic sound. Over a urine-filled bladder, it produces a dull sound. Be aware that percussing and palpating may trigger the urge to void. (For an illustration of proper hand placement for percussion, see *Percussing the urinary organs*.)

Palpation

In the average adult, the kidneys cannot be palpated because of their location deep within the abdomen. However, they may be palpable in a thin adult or a patient with reduced abdominal muscle mass. For opti-

Palpating the urinary organs

To palpate the urinary organs, stand at the patient's right side and proceed as follows:

With the patient supine, place your left hand under the back, midway between the lower costal margin and the iliac crest.

Next, place your right hand on the patient's abdomen, directly above the left hand. Angle this hand slightly toward the costal margin. To palpate the right lower edge of the kidney, press the fingertips of the right hand about 1½" to 2" (4 to 5 cm) above the iliac crest while pressing the fingertips of the left hand upward into the right costovertebral angle.

To assess the left kidney, move to the patient's left side and position the hands as described above, but with this change: place the right hand 2" above the left iliac crest. Then apply pressure with both hands as the patient inhales. If the left kidney can be palpated, compare it to the right kidney; it should be the same size. Repeat the procedure on the other side — but keep in mind that the right kidney may lie about 1" to 2" lower than the left.

Step 1

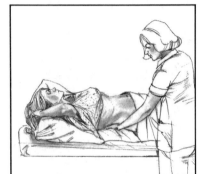

Step 2

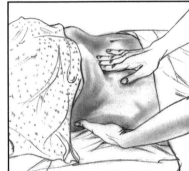

Step 3

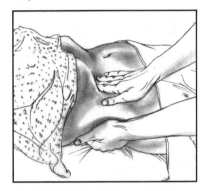

mal results, have the patient relax the abdomen by taking deep breaths. Instruct the patient to flex the knees slightly.

Before palpating the bladder, make sure the patient has voided. Then locate the symphysis pubis, and press firmly but gently with one hand about 1" to 2" (2.5 to 5 cm) above this landmark. The bladder usually is not palpable when empty. Note any tenderness or masses. (For an illustrated palpation procedure, see *Palpating the urinary organs*.)

Abnormal kidney palpation findings may signify various problems. A lump, a mass, or tenderness may indicate a tumor or cyst. A soft kidney may reflect chronic renal disease; a tender kidney, acute infection. Unequal kidney size may reflect hydronephrosis, a cyst, a tumor, or another disorder. Bilateral kidney enlargement suggests polycystic disease.

Abnormal bladder palpation findings include a mass, possibly indicating a tumor or cyst, or tenderness, which may indicate infection. A bladder that is palpable after urination may indicate urinary retention.

Developmental considerations for pediatric patients

Before physically assessing an infant or a child, note the ear position. Ears that are set low or at an unusual angle may accompany urinary tract anomalies.

Throughout the abdominal assessment, the child's abdominal muscles must be relaxed. To promote relaxation, have the child flex the legs upward. If necessary, give an infant a bottle to prevent crying, which tenses the abdominal muscles.

After the child has been undressed (leaving on underclothes or diaper), ask the parent to help the child to a standing position to allow observation of the abdominal contour. Normally, the infant or child has a rounded or potbellied abdomen without masses. If an upper abdominal mass is present, *do not* physically assess it further. If the mass is a nephroblastoma (Wilms' tumor), palpation could increase tumor cell spread.

Developmental considerations for elderly patients

The kidneys of an elderly patient are easier to palpate because of reduced abdominal muscle tone and mass. However, reduced muscle tone can prevent the bladder from emptying completely, resulting in up to 100 ml of residual urine. This patient also may have little warning of the urge to void. Along with residual urine, this can lead to incontinence during the assessment.

Documentation

The following example shows how to document some normal physical assessment findings:

Weight: 157 lb

Vital signs: Temperature 98.6° F; pulse 72 and regular, respirations 18 and regular, blood pressure 130/70.

Oriented to person, place, and time. Skin color and integrity within normal limits, without lesions or bruising. Abdomen flat, no prominent veins, pulsations, or lesions. No bruits over renal arteries. Left kidney not palpable; right kidney palpable, smooth, firm, and nontender, size within normal limits. Bladder tympanic, nontender. No CVA tenderness. Urethral meatus centrally located on glans penis, no visible discharge.

The following example shows how to document some abnormal physical assessment findings:

Weight: 270 lb

Vital signs: Temperature 99.8° F, pulse 96 and regular, respirations 28 and regular, blood pressure 184/106.

Disoriented to person, place, and time. Dry oral mucous membranes with normal skin turgor. Skin: pallor, multiple 1- to 3-cm ecchymotic areas noted over extremities and trunk. Abdomen round, obese, with multiple well-healed scars. Bruits auscultated over renal arteries. Kidneys nonpalpable. Suprapubic and CVA tenderness noted. Urethral meatus centrally located on glans penis with scant amount of yellow discharge present. Ophthalmoscopic examination: disk margin blurred, retinal hemorrhages visible, arteries narrow and tortuous.

STUDY ACTIVITIES

Fill in the blank

1. In the adult, normal urinary output for 24 hours is _____ ml.

2. When fluid intake is high, urinary output _____. When fluid intake declines or when large amounts of fluid are lost, urinary output _____.

3. During physical assessment of the urinary system, the correct sequence of techniques is inspection, followed by _____, _____, and, finally, _____.

Matching related elements

Match the term on the left with the definition on the right.

4. ___ Dysuria   **A.** Difficulty starting the urinary stream

5. ___ Dyspareunia   **B.** Sensation of needing to void immediately

6. ___ Urinary urgency   **C.** Painful intercourse

7. ___ Urinary hesitancy   **D.** Painful urination

8. ___ Phimosis   **E.** Foreskin constriction

Short answer

9. Regina Farentino, age 68, is an obese patient hospitalized with congestive heart failure and chronic renal failure. The nurse formulates a care plan that includes daily weight measurement. What is the purpose of measuring daily weight in this patient?

_____

10. What guidelines should the nurse follow when measuring Ms. Farentino's daily weight?

_____

Multiple choice

11. Which of the following is a sign of dehydration that the nurse may detect during a physical assessment?

     A. Pitting edema
     B. Poor skin turgor
     C. Uremic frost
     D. Petechiae

12. Which of the following is an abnormal finding during physical assessment of the urinary system?

    A. Nonpalpable left kidney

    B. Absence of vascular sounds over the renal arteries

    C. Suprapubic tenderness

    D. Tympany upon percussion of an empty bladder

ANSWERS

Fill in the blank

  1. 720 to 2,400

  2. increases, decreases

  3. auscultation, percussion, palpation

Matching related elements

  4. D

  5. C

  6. B

  7. A

  8. E

Short answer

  9. Daily weight measurement assesses fluid loss or gain over a 24-hour period.

10. To ensure accuracy, the nurse should measure the patient's weight at the same time each day, use the same scale, and have the patient wear the same amount of clothing for each weigh-in.

Multiple choice

11. B. When testing skin turgor, the nurse should suspect dehydration if the skin does not return to its normal position immediately after gently pinching it.

12. C. Suprapubic tenderness upon palpation may indicate bladder infection.

CHAPTER 14

Female reproductive system

OBJECTIVES
After studying this chapter, the reader should be able to:
1. Locate the female reproductive organs.
2. Develop interview questions that will elicit pertinent information about the female patient's reproductive system.
3. Describe a physical assessment of the female reproductive organs and external genitalia.
4. Describe developmental considerations related to assessment of the female reproductive system.
5. Differentiate normal from abnormal findings during physical assessment of the female reproductive system.
6. Document reproductive assessment findings for the female patient.

OVERVIEW OF CONCEPTS
Women's health care issues have emerged as important discussion topics. Concerns, such as contraception, infertility, premenstrual syndrome (PMS), hormone replacement therapy (HRT), human sexuality, and sexually transmitted diseases (STDs) are frequently addressed in hospitals, clinics, and physician's offices. Because of their knowledge, nurses are particularly qualified to provide care and instructions related to these reproductive concerns.

The female reproductive system consists of external and internal genitalia. External genitalia include the mons pubis, clitoris, labia majora, labia minora, and adjacent structures (Bartholin's glands, Skene's glands, and urethral meatus). Internal genitalia include the vagina, uterus, ovaries, and fallopian tubes. (For illustrations of the external and internal genitalia, see *Female genitalia,* page 234.) Before menarche (the onset of menstruation) and after childbearing, the uterus changes in size and shape.

The hypothalamus, pituitary gland, and ovaries secrete hormones cyclically that affect the buildup and shedding of the uterine lining during the menstrual cycle. Ovulation is controlled by a network of positive and negative feedback loops from the hypothalamus to the pituitary gland to the ovaries and then back to the hypothalamus and pituitary gland.

Female genitalia

External and internal structures comprise the female genitalia.

View of external genitalia in lithotomy position

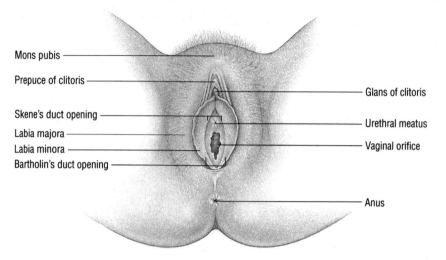

Mons pubis

Prepuce of clitoris

Skene's duct opening

Labia majora

Labia minora

Bartholin's duct opening

Glans of clitoris

Urethral meatus

Vaginal orifice

Anus

Lateral view of internal genitalia

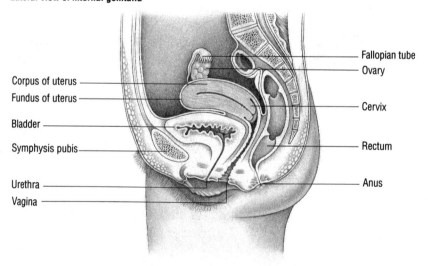

Corpus of uterus

Fundus of uterus

Bladder

Symphysis pubis

Urethra

Vagina

Fallopian tube

Ovary

Cervix

Rectum

Anus

Health history   During the reproductive health history interview, obtain health history data in a comfortable environment that provides privacy. In the outpatient clinic setting, always ask health history questions with the patient fully clothed. Also, use terms the patient understands, explaining technical language and avoiding jargon. Focus questions on the reproductive system, but maintain a holistic approach by inquiring about the status of other body systems and psychosocial concerns as well. Use the following questions to assess the female patient's reproductive system.

Health and illness patterns

Ask about the patient's current, past, and family health status and the patient's developmental status.

Current health status

Because current health status is foremost in the patient's mind, start here. Document the patient's own words, using the PQRST method to help the patient describe the chief complaint and any others completely. (For a detailed explanation of this method, see *Symptom analysis,* page 15.)

When was the first day of your last normal menstrual period?
(RATIONALE: Knowing when the last true menses occurred is necessary for evaluating the usual menstrual pattern and such conditions as pregnancy or dysfunctional uterine bleeding.)

How often do your periods occur?
(RATIONALE: The menstrual cycle length, from day 1 of one menses to day 1 of the next menses, should be more than 21 days and less than 35 days. Spotting may indicate an ectopic pregnancy, cervical infection, or inadequate hormonal support of the endometrium.)

How long do your periods normally last?
(RATIONALE: The usual flow duration is 3 to 7 days, and can vary for each woman from cycle to cycle. Extremely long or short periods that constitute a change from the patient's baseline may signal an abnormality, such as anovulation or anorexia nervosa.)

How would you describe your menstrual flow? How many pads or tampons do you use on the heaviest day of your period?
(RATIONALE: The number of heavy flow days, the flow on the heaviest day, and whether blood clots larger than a dime are expelled help reveal the patient's normal pattern. Heavy flow and clots that constitute a new pattern for the patient could indicate uterine fibroids or another uterine or ovarian abnormality. Menstrual flow greater than one pad or tampon per hour is considered very heavy. The usual flow ranges from 30 to 80 ml per cycle.)

Do you ever bleed between periods? If so, how much and for how long?
(RATIONALE: Bleeding between menstrual periods can indicate a problem, such as hormonal imbalance or cancer in the postmenopausal patient.)

Do you ever have vaginal bleeding or spotting after vaginal penetration?
(RATIONALE: Postcoital bleeding can indicate cervicitis, an endocervical polyp, or hypoestrogenic vaginal epithelialization in a postmenopausal patient or in one who has had bilateral surgical oophorectomy.)

Are you sexually active? If so, when was the last time you had intercourse?
(RATIONALE: Sexual functioning is an important part of the assessment. Avoid making assumptions regarding the patient's sexual activity. Not all women are sexually active with a male partner or some may abstain from sexual activity. If the patient has never had intercourse, begin the physical assessment with a small speculum. For optimal microscopic evaluation, the patient should not have had intercourse for at least 48 hours before the examination.)

Are you satisfied with communication between you and your partner about your sexual needs? Are your needs for affection and intimacy being met?
(RATIONALE: If the patient shows dissatisfaction with her sexuality or sexual relations, some self-help educational materials or counseling may be helpful. If the patient wants help with problems related to a specific sexual dysfunction, such as primary anorgasmia or vaginismus, refer her to a specialist.)

Do you have a need for birth control? Are you satisfied with your current method of birth control?
(RATIONALE: A patient who is satisfied with a contraceptive method is more likely to use it routinely. Discussion of contraceptive methods and their correct use may reveal that the patient lacks knowledge of the full range of contraceptive options available. A patient who reports troublesome adverse reactions to any contraceptive method requires further evaluation. [An elderly patient need not be questioned about current contraceptive use. However, a climacteric patient should be questioned because conception is possible for up to 12 months after menses ceases.])

Do you currently take any prescription or over-the-counter medications?
(RATIONALE: Some medications interfere with the action of oral contraceptives. Drugs that alter gastrointestinal absorption or liver function, such as rifampin, phenytoin, carbamazepine, ampicillin, and tetracycline, may reduce the effectiveness of oral contraceptives. Inform the patient of this possible effect and discuss the use of an alternative contraceptive method, such as condoms.)

Are you using any recreational drugs or alcohol? If so, what do you use? How much do you use?
(RATIONALE: Alcohol or drug use can impair judgment and may lead to high-risk sexual behavior, which can result in STDs. When taken during pregnancy, cocaine and other drugs can cause severe withdrawal symptoms and long-term adverse neurologic effects in neonates. Fetal alcohol exposure can cause serious birth defects.)

Do you smoke cigarettes?
(RATIONALE: Smoking is a health hazard for both pregnant and nonpregnant women. Lung cancer is the most prevalent form cancer in

women. Smoking significantly increases the risk of cardiovascular disease and thrombi [blood clots] in women over age 35 who use oral contraceptives. Smoking during pregnancy is associated with low neonatal birth weight, intrauterine growth retardation, and fetal and infant morbidity and mortality.)

Do you have any unusual signs or symptoms of infection, such as discharge, itching, painful intercourse, sores or lesions, fever, or chills?
(RATIONALE: Such signs and symptoms could result from an STD, vaginitis, or toxic shock syndrome. Urge a patient seeking a reproductive system health assessment not to douche or use vaginal creams or jellies for at least 48 hours before the assessment. Douching, unless medically indicated, is not recommended as a routine activity; it may wash away healthy, normal vaginal flora, upsetting the normal pH balance of the vagina [3.8 to 4.2] and predisposing the patient to infection.)

Does your sexual partner have any signs or symptoms of infection, such as genital sores or penile discharge?
(RATIONALE: Such symptoms may result from an STD. If the patient's partner has symptoms of an infection and is untreated, instruct the patient to insist her partner undergo diagnostic testing to treat the STD and prevent further spread.)

Past health status
Ask the following questions related to the female reproductive system:

Have you ever been pregnant? If so, how many times? What was the outcome of each pregnancy?
(RATIONALE: Information about the antepartal period, labor and delivery, the postpartal period, complications, and neonatal weight are important in assessing a patient of childbearing age.)

Have you ever had problems conceiving?
(RATIONALE: Inability to become pregnant after more than 1 year of regular coitus may indicate a fertility problem and the need for referral to a gynecologist or a fertility specialist if the couple desires children. The couple trying unsuccessfully to conceive may be experiencing significant stress and anxiety and may welcome a counseling referral.)

Have you had any uncomfortable signs and symptoms before or during your periods?
(RATIONALE: PMS can involve a wide variety of signs and symptoms, which occur cyclically during the premenstrual [luteal] phase of the cycle. Common symptoms include dysphoria [depression, irritability, anxiety, tension, and nervousness], breast tenderness, fluid retention [bloating, edema], headache, and food cravings. Primary dysmenorrhea [discomfort or pain during menstruation] or "normal" menstrual cramping commonly begins in adolescence when a normal ovulatory cyclic pattern is established. Pain that is not limited strictly to the men-

strual phase, that begins after adolescence, or that becomes more severe over time warrants a thorough investigation.)

Have you ever had an STD or other genital or reproductive system infection?
(RATIONALE: Repeated infections may indicate several problems. For example, a woman who continues to have candidal infections may have diabetes mellitus. Constant STD reinfections may reflect inadequate treatment or follow-up or an untreated partner. STDs require prompt evaluation and treatment. Some STDs, such as pelvic inflammatory disease [caused by such organisms as *Chlamydia trachomatis* and *Neisseria gonorrhea,* can lead to infertility.)

Have you had reproductive system surgery?
(RATIONALE: Tubal ligation, therapeutic abortion, dilatation and curettage, and hysterectomy are common gynecologic surgical procedures.)

Family health status
Ask about family reproductive history because several reproductive problems have familial tendencies. The following questions relate to family health status of the reproductive system:

Has anyone in your family ever had a reproductive health problem?
(RATIONALE: Ovarian cancer, breast cancer, cervical cancer, spontaneous abortion, menstrual problems, multiple births, congenital anomalies, and difficult pregnancies can have a familial tendency.)

Has anyone in your family had hypertension, coronary artery disease, diabetes mellitus, gestational diabetes (diabetes occurring only during pregnancy), obesity, or cancer?
(RATIONALE: Such conditions tend to be familial and can affect the health of both the nonpregnant and the pregnant patient and her fetus.)

Developmental considerations for adolescent patients
Bodily changes occurring as sexual maturity approaches may trigger fears and questions in the adolescent female, who may be reluctant to express them. The nurse should anticipate these concerns and offer opportunities for questions and explanations to help the patient understand her body and its functions.

Adolescents need simple, clear explanations. To introduce a topic in a comfortable and nonjudgmental manner, use open-ended questions with prefaces, such as "A lot of girls have questions about their bodies and their development. Maybe you have some questions about . . . (your periods or birth control)." Also touch on these topics:

At what age did you first notice hair on your pubic area? When did you first notice your breasts growing?
(RATIONALE: In females, the appearance of secondary sex characteristics is the most accurate indicator of physical maturity. Pubic hair growth usually begins between ages 8 and 14. For information about breast development, see Chapter 11, Female and male breasts.)

How do you feel you are developing compared with your friends?
(RATIONALE: Adolescent females need assurance that they are normal when their development seems to lag behind that of their peers. Unless no maturational changes occur by age 14, most girls can be reassured that they will menstruate normally when their bodies are ready.)

Have you noticed any moistness on your underwear?
(RATIONALE: Infection as well as increasing estrogen and androgen production from the ovaries cause increased vaginal secretions. To deal with body changes, the adolescent patient must understand them. Any signs of infection should be evaluated and frank, open explanations provided. Anatomic models and clear pictorials can aid the history taking and teaching.)

Have you experienced any new feelings or emotions? If so, would you like to talk about them?
(RATIONALE: During this time of rapid body change the patient may experience confusion and receive misinformation. Routine physical assessments for school or camp, during which evolving sexual changes can be evaluated, are ideal opportunities for the patient to ask questions and for the nurse to provide information in a supportive context. Assess the patient's knowledge and understanding of sexuality and provide anticipatory, preventive health information.)

When did you start having menstrual periods?
(RATIONALE: The mean onset of menarche is age 12.8; the normal age range, 9.1 to 17.7. The patient requires medical evaluation if she has not begun menses by age 14 and no growth and development or secondary sex characteristics appear, if she has not begun menses by age 16 despite normal growth and development or secondary sex characteristics, or if her menstrual periods are absent for more than three cycles. Also consider the possibility of pregnancy in a patient with amenorrhea.)

How old were you when you first had sex? Do you ever have pain with sex? Do you protect yourself from STDs and unintended pregnancy?
(RATIONALE: Many adolescents are sexually active. Ask these questions in a matter-of-fact manner. Protection from STDS and protection from pregnancy are separate issues, both of which the nurse should address.)

Developmental considerations for climacteric patients
During the reproductive health history interview, the following questions are appropriate for the climacteric patient:

Do you experience hot flushes or flashes? If so, how bothersome are they?
(RATIONALE: Hot flashes or flushes may bother one woman and not another. They may be associated with sleep disturbances, night sweats, mood changes, headaches, libido changes, and nervousness. If the pa-

tient rejects HRT or is not a candidate for HRT, reassure her that hot flashes and night sweats will resolve on their own within a few years.)

Do you experience vaginal dryness, pain, or itching during sexual intercourse?
(RATIONALE: These symptoms result from reduced estrogen levels that lead to decreased vaginal secretions. Although vaginal dryness may worsen, it responds well to hormonal treatment [vaginal, oral, or transdermal]. Patient teaching should include information on such nonpharmacologic treatments as water-soluble lubricants. Mention that increased frequency of coitus also improves lubrication.)

Are you experiencing any menstrual irregularities?
(RATIONALE: Reassure the patient that climacteric menstrual irregularities are common. However, refer the patient to a physician or nurse practitioner if she has excessive bleeding during menses [menorrhagia], bleeding at any time other than the menstrual period [metrorrhagia], or both [menometrorrhagia].)

Do you practice contraception?
(RATIONALE: Fertility declines with menopause but may be erratic. A woman can safely stop using contraception when she has had no menses for 12 months and when her follicle-stimulating hormone level is elevated in the menopausal range [above 50 IU/ml]).

How do you feel about approaching menopause (or about menopause, if it has occurred)?
(RATIONALE: Menopausal experiences are subjective and highly individual. Feelings associated with menopause can range from delight to decreased self-worth related to loss of reproductive function. Asking this question allows the patient to vent feelings about menopause and the life changes occurring during that time. Listen actively.)

Are you receiving hormone therapy for menopause?
(RATIONALE: HRT includes a combination of estrogen and a progestin. Regardless of the patient's age, estrogen prevents bone loss by inhibiting calcium absorption from bone. Estrogen also has a cardioprotective effect, increasing the level of high-density lipoproteins [the "good" cholesterol] and decreasing the level of low-density lipoproteins [the "bad" cholesterol]. Also, estrogen may alter vasomotor tone and have a direct vasodilatory effect on arterial walls. Progesterone may lessen the cardioprotective effects of estrogen but probably does not eliminate them entirely. Progesterone is used to reduce the risk of endometrial cancer in a patient with an intact uterus. The known and potential benefits and risks of HRT must be weighed carefully for each patient, taking into account risk factors, past history, and family history.)

If you have completed menopause, have you had any vaginal bleeding?
(RATIONALE: Any bleeding in a postmenopausal woman, except when associated with estrogen-progesterone replacement therapy, is abnor-

mal and a possible sign of endometrial cancer. The patient requires further medical evaluation.)

Health promotion and protection patterns

Continue with assessment of the patient's nutrition, sleep and waking patterns, and health behaviors. Ask the following questions:

When was your last Pap test? Do you know the results?
(RATIONALE: A Pap test can detect precancerous and cancerous cell changes in the cervix. It also may detect human papillomavirus [which causes venereal warts] and herpes simplex, which may not produce symptoms but may cause abnormal cellular changes. Remind the patient that she needs an annual Pap test even if the uterus has been removed surgically.)

Are you currently having any problems that you feel are related to your reproductive system, or any other problems that we have not covered?
(RATIONALE: These questions give the patient a chance to air any concerns.)

Role and relationship patterns

To assess the effect of a reproductive system disorder on role and relationship patterns, ask the following questions:

Have you noticed any changes in your sexual interest, frequency of intercourse, or sexual functioning?
(RATIONALE: Changes in libido [psychic energy or instinctual drive associated with sexual desire or pleasure] or sexual function could indicate pain, infection, hormonal changes, disease [for example, diabetes mellitus], changes in mental status [for example, depression], or altered role and relationship patterns.)

Are you experiencing any sexual problems?
(RATIONALE: Physical problems in the reproductive system can alter sexual relationships. The patient's answer may lead not only to exploring possible changes in sexual relations but also to assessing whether a physical problem is contributing to the changes.)

Physical assessment

In many health care facilities, a nurse may assist a physician or nurse practitioner with a gynecologic assessment. In some health care facilities, the nurse performs the assessment. This section describes how to prepare for a female reproductive system assessment and how to inspect the external genitalia. (Because the complete gynecologic assessment is an advanced assessment skill, it is discussed only briefly.)

Preparing for the assessment

Before beginning the assessment, gather the necessary equipment and supplies. (For detailed information, see *Gynecologic assessment equipment,* page 242.) Keep in mind that many women feel anxious when undergoing a gynecologic assessment. To allay the patient's anxiety and help her to relax, use the guidelines that follow.

Gynecologic assessment equipment

When assisting with a gynecologic assessment, the nurse assembles the equipment before helping the patient into position and draping her. Below is a description of necessary equipment and guidelines for use.

Gloves
Proper-fitting and medically clean examination gloves protect both the examiner and the patient from infection.

Specula
Several sizes and types of sterilized specula should be available, such as the Graves and the Pederson. Disposable plastic specula also may be obtained; some make loud clicking noises when the blades are opened. Warn the patient about this before the assessment begins.

Lubricant
The examiner applies a water-soluble lubricant to the fingers for the manual assessment. The lubricant should not be used during the speculum assessment.

Cytobrush, swabs, and endocervical brush
A cytobrush is used to obtain cells from the endocervix (internal cervix); a spatula, to obtain cells from the external cervix for the Pap test.

Glass slides and cover slides
Glass slides are used for wet mounts to diagnose such vaginal infections as *Trichomonas vaginalis,* bacterial vaginosis, or *Candida albicans.* Normal saline solution or 10% potassium hydroxide may be added to the specimen on the slide to create a wet mount.

Cytologic fixative
Cytologic fixative must be available for immediate fixation of Pap test samples. The fixative preserves tissue cells to allow accurate interpretation. Spray within 5 seconds.

Culture bottles or plates
Many examiners routinely test for *Neisseria gonorrhoeae* and *Chlamydia trachomatis.*

Sponge forceps
Sponge forceps are used for such procedures as applying pressure or medication with a gauze sponge or for cleaning. Keep at least one pair sterilized.

Mirror
A hand mirror is useful for the patient who wishes to watch the assessment and view her cervix. Because this provides an opportunity to teach the patient about her body, offer her the mirror.

Light source
Good lighting is essential. If a goosenecked lamp is used, the examiner must remember not to touch the lamp with the contaminated gloved hand.

Ask if this is the patient's first gynecologic assessment. If it is, explain the procedure beforehand so the patient knows exactly what to expect. If possible, use a model of the pelvis to demonstrate how the speculum works, and reassure the patient that it will not cause pain. If this is not the patient's first gynecologic examination, ask about previous experiences, which may help her express feelings.

Because a full bladder causes discomfort and interferes with accurate palpation, instruct the patient to empty her bladder before the pelvic examination.

Help the patient into the proper position, usually the dorsal lithotomy position. Secure the patient's heels in stirrups (preferably, padded ones.) Adjust the foot supports so the legs are equally and comfortably separated and symmetrically balanced. (With unpadded stirrups, the patient's shoes or socks can remain on for comfort.) The hips and knees will be flexed and thighs abducted. The patient places her feet in the stirrups and "inches" down to the proper position. (Use the palm of the hand as a guide so she feels secure when she reaches the end of the examination table.) A pillow placed beneath her head may increase her comfort and relax the abdominal muscles. Her arms should rest comfortably at her sides. The examiner sits on a movable swivel stool an arm's length away from and between the patient's abducted legs. In this way, equipment can be reached readily and the genitalia can be seen and palpated easily.

An alternative position for the patient who cannot assume the lithotomy position because of age, arthritis, back pain, or other reasons is Sims' (left lateral) position. To assume this position, the patient lies on her left side almost prone, with her buttocks close to the edge of the table, her left leg straight, and her right leg slightly bent in front of her left leg.

Privacy and adequate draping give the patient a sense of security, although some patients prefer no draping. Positioning the drape low on the patient's abdomen allows her to see the examiner. If the patient wishes to watch the assessment, supply a hand mirror for her to hold.

When assisting with the gynecologic assessment, stand beside the examination table, offer your hand for the patient to hold (if she wishes), and explain what is occurring and what will happen next. To help the patient relax as the assessment begins, describe what she will feel. Also, show the patient how to relax by inhaling slowly and deeply through the nose, exhaling through the mouth, and concentrating on breathing regularly to relax the muscle. If the patient begins to tense up and hold her breath, remind her to breathe and relax.

Inspection and palpation

Wash the hands thoroughly, then position the patient supine with the pubic area uncovered. Begin the inspection by determining sexual maturity, observing pubic hair for amount and pattern. Normally, pubic hair is thick and appears on the mons pubis as well as the inner aspects of the upper thighs. Then, using a gloved index finger and thumb, gently spread the labia majora and look for the following: labia majora and labia minora, which should be pink and moist with no lesions; and normal vaginal discharge, which varies in color and consistency, being clear and stretchy before ovulation, white and opaque after ovulation, and usually odorless and nonirritating to the mucosa. Check the vaginal Ph with a small strip of Ph paper; normally, it should be 3.8 to 4.2.

Next, palpate the Skene's and Bartholin's glands, noting any swelling, tenderness, or discharge. Specimens of all discharges should be examined with a microscope. Obtain gonorrhea cultures and a Chlamydia test if the patient is at risk for STDs.

Abnormal findings

Clitoromegaly (an enlarged clitoris) accompanied by other signs of androgen excess or masculinization, such as facial hair and voice changes, may warrant referral to a gynecologic endocrinologist. Pediculosis pubis (crab lice) or nits (louse eggs) may be attached to the hair shaft and cause intense pruritus. Note any wartlike lesions (condyloma acuminata or condylomata lata); malodorous vaginal discharge that is yellow, green, or gray; or ulcerations (such as from herpes simplex, chancroid, or syphilitic chancre) in the labial, vaginal, urethral, cervical, or anal areas. Also note any redness or erythema in these regions.

Developmental considerations for pediatric patients

The labia majora of an infant or a young child are soft and somewhat resilient compared with the firmer labia of a mature woman. In a child of any age, an inflamed vulva with open, irritated areas could indicate sexual abuse. If sexual abuse is suspected, follow the health care facility protocol for reporting such cases.

Pubic hair growth begins in early puberty and is sparse, long, and fine and found along the labia. In adolescents, the hair texture is similar to an adult's but not as thick and is limited to the mons pubis. As the adolescent becomes an adult, hair quantity increases, thickens, and extends to the inner aspects of the thighs.

Developmental considerations for elderly patients

The elderly patient's external genitalia show thinning and atrophy of the labia majora, with a smaller clitoris than in a younger woman. The pubic hair becomes sparse, thin, brittle, gray, and straight.

Advanced assessment skills

With experience, some nurses may choose to practice in facilities specializing in women's health care where, with appropriate preparation, they may perform complete gynecologic assessments independently.

As part of the complete gynecologic assessment, a Pap test (a routine cancer screening test) is performed after examining the cervix. Other specimens also are taken if an abnormal cervical or vaginal discharge is present. The nurse plays a key role in assisting the physician or nurse practitioner with this part of the assessment.

Documentation The following example shows how to document normal findings related to a basic assessment of the female reproductive system:
External genitalia: no lesions, inflammation, edema, varicosities, or other abnormalities. Labia majora, labia minora, clitoris intact, without clitoromegaly. Hair pattern distribution of mature female. No discharge from urethra and Skene's and Bartholin's glands. Vagina: pink.

The following example shows how to document abnormal findings:
External genitalia: Three tender ulcerations, each less than 1 mm, on right labia minora. Clear fluid from lesions. No other external abnormalities.

STUDY ACTIVITIES

Matching related elements

Match the female reproductive assessment finding on the left with its possible cause on the right.

1. ___ Bleeding between periods   **A.** Aging

2. ___ Vaginal sores   **B.** Hormonal imbalance

3. ___ Postcoital bleeding   **C.** Uterine fibroids

4. ___ Thin labia majora   **D.** STD

5. ___ Heavy menstrual flow with clots   **E.** Cervicitis

Fill in the blank

6. The menstrual cycle length normally ranges from more than

_____ days to less than _____ days.

7. Although variable, the average duration of menstrual flow is

_____ to _____ days.

8. The usual menstrual flow ranges from _____ to _____ ml per cycle.

Multiple choice

9. Pat Dwyer, age 25, comes to the clinic for her yearly gynecologic examination. During the health history, the nurse learns that Ms. Dwyer uses oral contraceptives. Which factor increases the risk of cardiovascular disease in women using oral contraceptives?

A. Smoking
B. Barbiturate use
C. Phenothiazine use
D. High-protein diet

10. To perform physical assessment of Ms. Dwyer's reproductive system, the nurse should place her in which position?

A. Sims'
B. Semi-Fowler's
C. Dorsal lithotomy
D. Lateral recumbent

11. Helen McCloskey, age 75, seeks care for irregular menopausal bleeding. Because of her age, she cannot assume the usual position for physical assessment of the reproductive system. The nurse should assist her into which alternate position?

A. Supine
B. Left lateral
C. Fowler's
D. Trendelenburg's

12. On inspection, Ms. McCloskey's external genitalia may display which normal age-related changes?

    A. Hypertrophy of the labia majora
    B. Sparse, thin pubic hair
    C. Thick, coarse pubic hair
    D. Cystocele

ANSWERS

Matching related elements

    1. B
    2. D
    3. E
    4. A
    5. C

Fill in the blank

    6. 21, 35
    7. 3, 7
    8. 30, 80

Multiple choice

    9. A. Smoking increases the risk of cardiovascular disease and thrombi in women who use oral contraceptives.

10. C. Usually, the patient is placed in the dorsal lithotomy position for physical assessment of the reproductive system.

11. B. The left lateral (Sims') position is an alternate position for the patient who cannot assume the dorsal lithotomy position.

12. B. In the elderly patient, pubic hair appears sparse, thin, brittle, gray, and straight.

CHAPTER 15

Male reproductive system

OBJECTIVES   After studying this chapter, the reader should be able to:

1. Locate the normal male reproductive organs and structures.
2. Discuss health history questions that elicit information about a male patient's reproductive system.
3. Inspect and palpate the penis and scrotum.
4. Describe normal and abnormal findings detected during physical assessment of the male reproductive system.
5. Document male reproductive system assessment findings properly.

OVERVIEW OF CONCEPTS   Assessing the male reproductive system, although potentially uncomfortable for the nurse and patient, is an essential part of a complete health assessment. Careful assessment may uncover actual or potential problems or concerns that the patient probably would not volunteer willingly. Such information may be crucial. Many common disorders of the male reproductive system have potentially serious physical or psychological consequences. For example, sexually transmitted diseases (STDs)—the most common communicable diseases in the United States—can produce devastating complications unless detected and treated early.

The male reproductive system consists of two major organs—the penis and the testes (testicles)—and associated structures, including the transport ducts, prostate gland, and inguinal structures. (For an illustration, see *The male reproductive system,* page 248.) This system is involved in three basic functions: sexual reproduction (including sexual function and spermatogenesis), male sex hormone secretion, and urine elimination.

Male sex hormones (androgens) are produced in the testes and the adrenal glands. Testosterone, the most significant male sex hormone, is secreted by Leydig cells located in the testes between the seminiferous tubules. (These cells become numerous during puberty and remain in large numbers throughout life.) Testosterone, which is responsible for developing and maintaining male sex organs and secondary sex characteristics, is required for spermatogenesis.

The male reproductive system

The male reproductive system consists of the penis, the scrotum and its contents, the prostate gland, and the inguinal structures.

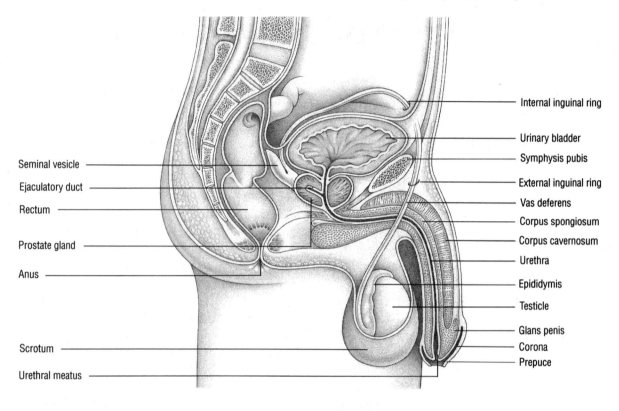

Seminal vesicle

Ejaculatory duct

Rectum

Prostate gland

Anus

Scrotum

Urethral meatus

Internal inguinal ring

Urinary bladder

Symphysis pubis

External inguinal ring

Vas deferens

Corpus spongiosum

Corpus cavernosum

Urethra

Epididymis

Testicle

Glans penis

Corona

Prepuce

Health history   Interviewing a male patient about his reproductive system requires sensitivity, tact, and a professional approach. The initial goal should be to establish a rapport with the patient so he will relax and confide in the nurse. An uncomfortable patient may withhold valuable information.

A patient having a problem with sexual function may be uncomfortable discussing it. Ask questions in a sensitive manner and assure the patient that his replies will be kept strictly confidential. To put such a patient at ease, begin the interview with general questions regarding his reproductive health. Then proceed to more sensitive areas, reserving questions about sexual function for last.

During the interview, take the patient's cultural, religious, and personal views on sexuality and reproduction into account and remain nonjudgmental and supportive. Use terms the patient can understand.

Health and illness patterns

Begin the health assessment by obtaining information about the patient's current, past, and family health status as well as developmental considerations.

Current health status

Because current health status is the patient's most pressing concern, begin the health history by exploring this area. Using the PQRST method, ask the patient to describe his chief complaint and any other complaints. (For a detailed explanation of this method, see *Symptom analysis*, page 15.) Be sure to document the patient's description in his own words. To investigate the patient's current health status further, ask the following questions about the male reproductive system:

Have you noticed any changes in the color of the skin on your penis or scrotum? Have you noticed the appearance of a sore, lump, or ulcer on your penis?
(RATIONALE: Such findings may point to an STD, an inflammatory disorder, or cancer.)

If you are uncircumcised, can you retract and replace the foreskin easily?
(RATIONALE: Inability to retract the prepuce [foreskin] from the glans penis [a condition called phimosis] sometimes occurs in uncircumcised men. If untreated, the inability of the retracted prepuce to return to its normal position over the glans penis [paraphimosis] could impair local circulation and lead to edema and, possibly, gangrene.)

Have you noticed any discharge or bleeding from the opening where urine comes out?
(RATIONALE: Copious amounts of thick, yellowish discharge may indicate gonorrhea. Thin, watery discharge may point to nonspecific urethritis or prostatitis. Bloody discharge may indicate infection or cancer in the urinary or reproductive tract.)

Have you noticed any bulging or swelling in your scrotum?
(RATIONALE: Scrotal bulging or swelling may indicate an inguinal hernia, hematocele, epididymitis, or a testicular tumor.)

Are you experiencing any pain in the penis, testes, or scrotal sac? If so, where? Does the pain radiate? If so, to where? What measures aggravate or relieve the pain? When does it occur?
(RATIONALE: Dull, aching pain in the scrotal sac may indicate inguinal hernia. Sudden onset of extremely sharp pain may point to testicular torsion. Sharp pain of more gradual onset usually indicates infection, such as orchitis or epididymitis.)

Have you felt a lump, a painful sore, or tenderness in the groin?
(RATIONALE: These findings may point to a tumor or an infection.)

Do you get up during the night to urinate? Do you have urinary frequency, hesitancy, or dribbling? Do you have pain in the area between your rectum and penis, hips, or lower back?
(RATIONALE: These signs and symptoms are especially significant in men over age 50; they may point to a prostate problem, such as benign prostatic hypertrophy or prostate cancer.)

Do you have any trouble achieving and maintaining an erection during sexual activity? If so, do you have erections at other times, such as on awakening? Do you have any difficulty with ejaculation?
(RATIONALE: The ability to achieve an erection is an important diagnostic clue in evaluating the cause of impotence.)

Do you ever experience pain from erection or ejaculation?
(RATIONALE: Painful erection or ejaculation suggests inflammation in the genitourinary tract.)

What medications (prescribed and over-the-counter) or illegal drugs do you take? At what dosage and for what reason?
(RATIONALE: Certain medications can interfere with reproductive system function.)

Past health status

Next, ask the patient about past health problems because other body system dysfunctions or past reproductive problems may affect the current condition of the reproductive system. Include these questions in this part of the assessment:

Have you fathered any children? If so, how many and what are their ages? Have you ever had a problem with infertility? Is it a current concern?
(RATIONALE: If infertility is a problem, further exploration is required— preferably by a professional who specializes in this field.)

Have you ever had surgery on the genitourinary tract or for a hernia? If so, where, when, and why? Did you have any complications after surgery? Have you ever experienced trauma to the genitourinary tract? If so, what happened, when did it occur, and what symptoms, if any, have developed as a result of the trauma?
(RATIONALE: A history of surgery may predispose the patient to adhesions or may alter reproductive structure and function. Trauma to the genitourinary tract may alter normal physiologic processes and affect sexual and reproductive function.)

Have you ever been diagnosed with a sexually transmitted disease or any other infection in the genitourinary tract? If so, what was the specific problem? How long did it last? What treatment was provided? Did any complications develop?
(RATIONALE: Depending on its nature and course, infection can cause infertility and other reproductive system abnormalities.)

Do you have diabetes mellitus, cardiovascular disease (such as arteriosclerosis), neurologic disease (such as multiple sclerosis or amyotrophic lateral sclerosis), or malignancy in the genitourinary tract?
(RATIONALE: These conditions can affect sexual and reproductive function, causing impotence, infertility, or both.)

Do you have a history of undescended testes (cryptorchidism) or an endocrine disorder (such as hypogonadism)?
(RATIONALE: These conditions may cause infertility.)

Family health status
Determine the patient's family history as it relates to the patient's reproductive system, looking for disorders with known familial tendencies. Include these questions:

Has anyone in your family had infertility problems?
(RATIONALE: Infertility often has a familial tendency.)

Has anyone in your family had a hernia?
(RATIONALE: Hernias also tend to occur in families.)

Developmental considerations for pediatric patients
Try to involve the child and the parent or guardian in the interview. Obviously, the parent or guardian will answer for an infant or a very young child. Questions to ask include:

Did the mother use any hormones during pregnancy?
(RATIONALE: Some hormones taken during pregnancy can adversely affect the development of a male child's reproductive system.)

If the child is uncircumcised, what hygienic measures are used?
(RATIONALE: Poor hygiene increases the risk of infection under the prepuce.)

Do you notice any scrotal swelling when the child cries or has a bowel movement?
(RATIONALE: This finding may point to an inguinal hernia.)

Did the child exhibit any genitourinary abnormalities at birth? If so, what treatment, if any, did he receive?
(RATIONALE: If uncorrected, such congenital defects as hypospadias and epispadias can lead to further problems.)

Developmental considerations for adolescent patients
When interviewing an adolescent, determine his knowledge of sexual and reproductive function and his level of sexual development by asking the following questions:

Do you have pubic hair? If so, at what age did it appear?
(RATIONALE: Pubic hair typically appears between ages 12 and 14, usually indicating normal sexual development.)

How would you describe your sexual activity?
(RATIONALE: This question gives the adolescent patient the opportunity to ask questions and express concerns about sexual function. It also al-

lows the nurse to share information and clear up any misconceptions the patient may have.)

If you are sexually active, do you use condoms?
(RATIONALE: This question elicits information about the adolescent's knowledge of contraception and STD prevention. It also gives the nurse a chance to teach the patient about the proper use of condoms.)

Developmental considerations for elderly patients
When interviewing an elderly patient, ask questions that elicit information about changes in sexual patterns.

Have you experienced any change in your frequency of or desire for sex?
(RATIONALE: Depression, loss a partner, or physical illness may cause these changes.)

Have you noticed any changes in your sexual performance?
(RATIONALE: Such physiologic changes as slower and softer erections, a longer time required to reach orgasm, and decreased ejaculatory volume normally occur with age or may result from physical illness or use of certain drugs.)

Health promotion and protection patterns
Continue the health history by eliciting information about the patient's lifestyle to determine his risk of reproductive system trauma or disease. Ask the following questions:

Do you examine your testes periodically? Have you been taught the proper procedure?
(RATIONALE: Testicular cancer, the most common form of cancer in males between ages 15 and 35, is treated most successfully after early detection. For information on testicular self-examination to detect, see *Testicular self-examination*.)

If you are sexually active, do you have more than one partner?
(RATIONALE: Having multiple partners increases the risk of contracting STDs.)

Do you take any precautions to prevent contracting STDs or acquired immunodeficiency syndrome (AIDS)? If so, what do you do?
(RATIONALE: Take this opportunity to discuss ways to prevent these diseases, such as using condoms during intercourse and avoiding exchange of body fluids during any sexual activity.)

What is your job?
(RATIONALE: Certain occupations—for example, construction or assembly-line work with heavy machinery—put a patient at increased risk for genital injury.)

Are you now or have you ever been exposed to radiation or toxic chemicals?
(RATIONALE: Such exposure may increase the patient's risk for infertility or testicular cancer.)

Testicular self-examination

To help detect abnormalities early, every male should examine his testes once a month. Instruct the patient to follow this procedure:

1 If possible, take a warm bath or shower before beginning. The scrotum tends to contract when cold; a warm bath or shower will relax the scrotum, making the testes easier to examine.

2 With one hand, lift the penis and check the scrotum (the sac containing the testes) for any change in shape, size, or color. The left side of the scrotum normally hangs slightly lower than the right.

3 Next, check the testes for lumps and masses. Locate the crescent-shaped structure at the back of each testis. This is the epididymis, which should feel soft.

4 Using the thumb and first two fingers of your left hand, squeeze the spermatic cord gently; it extends upward from the

epididymis, above the left testis. Then repeat on the right side, using your right hand. Check for lumps and masses by palpating along the entire length of the cord.

5 Next, examine each testis. To do so, place your index and middle fingers on its underside and the thumb on top, then gently roll the testis between your thumb and fingers. A normal testis is egg-shaped, rubbery, firm, and movable within the scrotum; it should feel smooth, with no lumps. Both testes should be the same size.

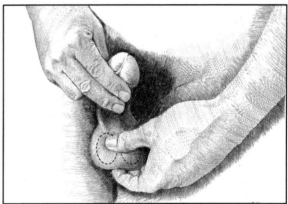

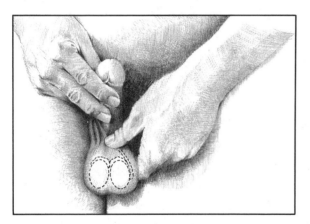

6 Promptly report any lumps, masses, or changes to your health care provider.

Do you engage in sports or any activity that requires heavy lifting or straining? If so, do you wear protective or supportive devices, such as a jock strap, protective cup, or truss?
(RATIONALE: Any activity involving heavy lifting or abdominal straining can increase the risk of hernia formation. Certain sports activities—for example, playing the catcher's position in a baseball or softball game—can predispose the patient to genital trauma.)

Would you describe yourself as being under a lot of stress?
(RATIONALE: Stress can adversely affect sexual and reproductive function.)

Role and relationship patterns

Obtain information about the patient's role and relationship patterns by asking these questions:

What is your self-image? Do you consider yourself attractive to others?
(RATIONALE: A poor self-image and lack of self-confidence can predispose a patient to sexual dysfunction.)

What is your cultural and religious background? Do any cultural or religious factors affect your beliefs or practices regarding sexuality and reproduction?
(RATIONALE: Knowledge of the patient's cultural and religious beliefs may help explain normal variants and identify potential risk factors. For example, if the patient's religion or culture prohibits condom use, he may be at increased risk for contracting AIDS and STDs.)

Do you have a supportive relationship with another person?
(RATIONALE: Problems with family or other relationships can produce stress, which in turn can cause sexual dysfunction.)

Are your sexual partners male, female, or both?
(RATIONALE: The answer to this question provides information about the patient's possible risk for certain STDs and about certain sexual practices that can injure the anal sphincter.)

If you are experiencing sexual difficulty, is it affecting your emotional and social relationships?
(RATIONALE: Feelings of emotional or social isolation can increase stress, which in turn can exacerbate sexual dysfunction.)

Physical assessment

A complete physical assessment of the patient's reproductive system should include general inspection of the groin; inspection and palpation of the penis and scrotum; and inspection and palpation of the groin to detect hernias. (Prostate gland palpation in men over age 50 and in others with prostate problems is an advanced skill not discussed here.)

Before beginning the physical assessment, wash the hands and gather gloves and a flashlight. Then instruct the patient to urinate (to reduce discomfort from a full bladder) and to undress to expose the groin area. If the patient wishes, he may wear a gown to prevent unnecessary exposure.

Because reproductive system assessment involves genital exposure and touching, the patient may feel anxious and embarrassed. To minimize such discomfort, explain each assessment step beforehand and expose only the necessary areas. If the patient objects to being examined by a female, a female nurse might defer to a male nurse or physician. If the patient relieves his embarrassment by using language that a female nurse finds offensive, continue the assessment in a professional manner; if the situation becomes threatening, defer the assessment to a male nurse or physician.

When assessing patients who are at high risk for AIDS, such as men who have sex with men or who inject drugs intravenously, make an extra effort to maintain a professional, nonjudgmental demeanor. Such patients are entitled to the same assessment and nursing care as other patients.

Inspection

Physical assessment of the male reproductive system begins with inspection of the genitals and inguinal area. Be sure to put on gloves before starting.

Penis

Start by evaluating the color and integrity of the penile skin. Over the shaft, the skin should appear loose and wrinkled; over the glans penis, taut and smooth. The skin should be pink to light brown in Caucasians and light to dark brown in Blacks, and should be free of scars, lesions, ulcers, or breaks of any kind.

If the patient is uncircumcised, ask him to retract his prepuce to allow inspection of the glans penis. Normally, the patient should be able to retract the prepuce with ease, revealing a glans with no ulcers or lesions, and then easily replace it over the glans after inspection. A white substance (smegma) may be present.

The urethral meatus, a slit-like opening, should be located at the tip of the glans. Inspection of the urethral meatus should reveal no discharge.

Scrotum

Begin with evaluation of the amount, distribution, color, and texture of pubic hair. Pubic hair should cover the symphysis pubis and scrotum.

Next, inspect the scrotal skin for obvious lesions, ulcerations, induration, or reddened areas, and evaluate the sac for size and symmetry. The scrotal skin should be coarse and more deeply pigmented than the body skin. The left testicle usually hangs slightly lower than the right; both should hang freely in the scrotum.

Inguinal area

Inspect the inguinal area for obvious bulges—a sign of hernias. Then ask the patient to bear down as if passing a stool, and repeat the inspection. (Bearing down or coughing momentarily increases intra-abdominal pressure, which pushes any herniation downward and makes it more easily visible.)

Abnormal findings

Inspection of the penis may reveal lesions or similar problems. If so, document the location, size, and color of any lesions as well as the presence of any exudate. Lesions may indicate an STD. In an uncircumcised patient, inspection of the prepuce may reveal phimosis (abnormal tightness of the prepuce that prevents its retraction from the glans penis) or paraphimosis (strangulation of the glans penis caused by a prepuce that will not return over the glans).

Inspection of the urethral meatus may detect epispadias (a congenital defect involving opening of the urethral meatus on the dorsal surface of the penis), hypospadias (a congenital defect involving opening of the urethral meatus on the ventral surface of the penis), or discharge. If discharge is present, obtain a smear to send to a laboratory for culture and sensitivity testing. Discharge indicates infection and may signal an STD, such as gonorrhea.

On the scrotum, absence of pubic hair or the presence of bald spots is abnormal. Absence of pubic hair may indicate a vascular or hormonal problem. Other abnormal findings include lesions, ulcers, induration, and reddened areas, which may indicate infection or inflammation. Scrotal bulging may indicate a hernia.

Inspection of the inguinal area may reveal obvious bulging, suggesting a hernia.

Palpation

After inspection, palpate the penis and scrotum for structural abnormalities; then palpate the inguinal area for hernias.

Penis

Gently grasp the shaft of the penis between the thumb and first two fingers; palpate along its entire length, noting any indurated, tender, or lumpy areas. The nonerect penis should feel soft and free of nodules.

Scrotum

Like the penis, the scrotum can be palpated using the thumb and first two fingers. Start by examining the scrotal skin, palpating its rough, wrinkled surface for nodules, lesions, or ulcers.

Normally, the right and left halves of the scrotal sac are identical in content and feel the same. The testes are felt as separate, freely movable, oval masses low in the scrotal sac. Their surface should feel smooth and be even in contour. Slight compression should elicit a dull, aching sensation that radiates to the patient's lower abdomen. This pressure-pain sensation should not occur when the other structures are compressed. No other pain or tenderness should be present.

Absence of a testis may reflect cryptorchidism (failure of one or both testes to descend into the scrotal sac) or may result from temporary migration. The cremasteric muscle surrounding the testicles contracts in response to such stimuli as cold air, cold water, or touching the inner thigh. This contraction raises the contents of the scrotum toward the inguinal canal. When the muscle relaxes, the scrotal contents resume their normal position. This temporary migration is normal and may occur throughout the course of the assessment.

The epididymis is palpated on the posterolateral surface by grasping each testicle between the thumb and forefinger and palpating up from the epididymis along the spermatic cord or vas deferens to the inguinal ring. The epididymis should feel like a ridge of tissue lying vertically on the testicular surface. The vas deferens should feel like a smooth cord and be freely movable. Arteries, veins, lymph vessels, and nerves, which are located next to the vas deferens, may be felt as indefinite threads.

Any lumps, nodular regions, or areas of swelling should be transilluminated. To perform this technique, darken the room, then hold a flashlight behind the scrotum and direct its beam through the mass. If the swollen area contains serous fluid, it will transilluminate, marked by an orange-red glow; if the area contains blood or tissue, it will not transilluminate. Describe a lump or mass anywhere in the scrotal sac according to its placement, size, shape, consistency, tenderness, and response to transillumination.

Inguinal area

After assessing the penis and scrotum, palpate the patient's inguinal area for hernias—protrusions of the bowel through the abdominal wall into the inguinal or femoral canal or, in some cases, into the scrotum. (For more information, see *Palpating for hernias in the inguinal area,* page 258.)

Abnormal findings

Indurated, tender, or lumpy areas of the penis may indicate Peyronie's disease, characterized by a fibrous band in the corpus cavernosum.

Surface nodules on the scrotum may be sebaceous cysts. Abnormal testicular pain or tenderness may result from an inflammation, such as orchitis or epididymitis. Absence of a testis may stem from congenital maldescent, or cryptorchidism. In this condition, one or both testes fail to descend from the abdomen into the scrotal sac. Fixed or tender areas in the scrotum may indicate a testicular tumor.

In men of any age, palpation of the inguinal area may reveal three major types of hernias. An *indirect inguinal hernia* occurs when the herniation enters the internal inguinal canal, possibly descending into the scrotum. A *direct inguinal hernia* develops when the herniation penetrates the inguinal canal through an abnormal opening in the abdominal wall. A *femoral hernia* occurs in the femoral canal, a space below the inguinal ligament lateral to the pubic tubercle.

Developmental considerations for pediatric patients

In an infant, the scrotum is pink, small, and wrinkled, with a well-defined median raphe (seam of union of the two halves). Both testes should be easily palpated in the scrotal sac at birth. The penis should appear pink and smooth. In neonates, small white cysts on the distal prepuce are considered a normal finding. In an uncircumcised infant, the prepuce usually is tight for 2 to 3 months after birth. It does not retract easily but should retract enough to allow urine to flow freely from the urinary meatus.

When assessing an uncircumcised infant, retract the prepuce only enough to expose the urethral meatus. Forced retraction may cause tearing of the prepuce from the glans. (By age 3 or 4, the child's pre-

Palpating for hernias in the inguinal area

When assessing the male reproductive system, palpate the inguinal area for inguinal and femoral hernias.

Palpating for inguinal hernias

First, place the index and middle finger of each hand over each external inguinal ring, and ask the patient to bear down or cough to increase intra-abdominal pressure momentarily. Then, with the patient relaxed, proceed as follows: Gently insert the middle or index finger (if the patient is an adult) or the little finger (if the patient is a young child) into the scrotal sac and follow the spermatic cord upward to the external inguinal ring, to an opening just above and lateral to the pubic tubercle known as Hesselbach's triangle. Holding the finger at this spot, ask the patient to bear down or cough again. A hernia is felt as a mass or bulge.

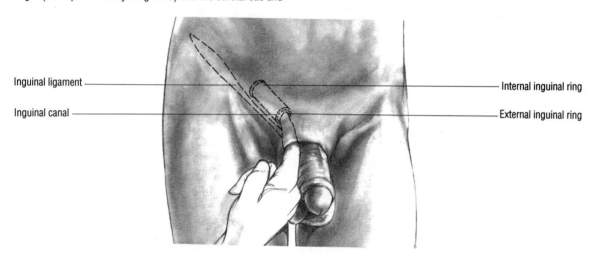

Inguinal ligament — — Internal inguinal ring

Inguinal canal — — External inguinal ring

Palpating for femoral hernias

Place the right hand on the patient's thigh, with the index finger over the femoral artery. The femoral canal is then under the ring finger with an adult patient and between the index and ring finger with a child. A hernia here is felt as a soft bulge or mass.

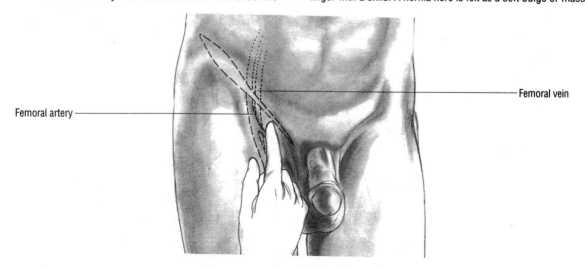

Femoral vein

Femoral artery —

puce should be completely retractable.) If an infant has been circumcised, the penis may appear reddened.

During infancy, any congenital malformations, such as epispadias, hypospadias, or cryptorchidism, should be detected.

Throughout childhood, the scrotum and penis remain hairless and pink. The genitals grow in proportion to the child, but usually remain small. During puberty, the genitals enlarge and develop and secondary sex characteristics appear, including pubic hair and typical male facial and body hair distribution. By the end of puberty, the male reaches full adult sexual appearance and functional capability.

Pubic hair on a preschooler and extremely small genitals in an adult male are abnormal. Absence of secondary sex characteristics after puberty also is abnormal, as are secondary sex characteristics before puberty.

Developmental considerations for elderly patients

After full maturity is reached, the genitals remain fairly constant in appearance until about age 50. At this point, pubic hair turns gray or white and scrotal skin becomes less taut over the testes, giving the scrotum a more pendulous appearance.

Documentation   The following example shows how to document some normal physical assessment findings:

Normal male pubic hair distribution. Penis circumcised; no lesions, inflammation, or structural alterations; urethral opening patent. Testes descended and symmetrical without redness, masses, or tenderness.

The following example shows how to document some abnormal physical assessment findings:

Normal male pubic hair distribution. One testicle undescended; no scrotal masses. Circumcised penis with two small raised vesicles on lip of circumcised fold; no penile discharge.

STUDY ACTIVITIES   **Multiple choice**

1. Testicular cancer is the most common form of cancer for which age group?
  A. Age 15 and under
  B. Ages 15 to 35
  C. Ages 30 to 45
  D. Age 45 and over

2. When inspecting a patient's scrotum, the nurse should consider which finding normal?
  A. The testes hang evenly and freely.
  B. The left testicle is larger than the right testicle.
  C. The right testicle hangs lower than the left testicle.
  D. The left testicle hangs lower than the right testicle.

3. How should the testicles feel upon palpation?
  A. Rough and hard
  B. Rubbery and smooth
  C. Nodular and soft
  D. Granular and firm

4. The prepuce of an uncircumcised male should be completely retractable by what age?
  A. At birth
  B. Age 1 or 2
  C. Age 3 or 4
  D. Age 5 or 6

5. To accentuate the presence of an inguinal hernia during assessment, the nurse should ask the patient to perform which action?
  A. Bend to the side.
  B. Flex the knees.
  C. Bear down.
  D. Stretch.

6. When inspecting the external genitalia of an elderly male patient, the nurse may note which normal age-related change?
  A. Pendulous scrotum
  B. Testicular atrophy
  C. Testicular hypertrophy
  D. Taut scrotal skin

Short answer

7. What is the significance of an inability to retract and replace the prepuce in an uncircumcised adult male?

_____

8. Which hormone is required for spermatogenesis?

_____

9. During physical assessment of a patient with a testicular mass, how should the nurse proceed?

_____

Fill in the blank

10. Copious amounts of thick, yellowish penile discharge suggests

_____; thin, watery discharge suggests _____.

11. _____ refers to failure of one or both testes to descend into the scrotal sac.

ANSWERS   **Multiple choice**

1. B. Testicular cancer is the most common form of cancer in males between ages 15 and 35.

2. D. The left testicle usually hangs slightly lower than the right.

3. B. Normally, the testicles feel smooth, rubbery, firm, and movable within the scrotum.

4. C. The prepuce should be completely retractable by age 3 or 4.

5. C. Bearing down or coughing momentarily increases intra-abdominal pressure, causing the hernia to become more palpable as a mass or bulge.

6. A. At about age 50, the male patient may display a more pendulous scrotum and gray or white pubic hair.

Short answer

7. The inability to retract the prepuce (phimosis) sometimes occurs in uncircumcised men. If untreated, the inability of the retracted prepuce to return to its normal position (paraphimosis) could impair local circulation and lead to edema and, possibly, gangrene of the glans penis.

8. Testosterone is required for spermatogenesis.

9. The nurse should inspect the scrotum, comparing the testes for symmetry and noting any obvious bulges, lesions, ulcerations, induration or reddened areas. Next the nurse should palpate and transilluminate the scrotum. Describe any lump or mass according to its placement, size, shape, consistency, tenderness, and response to transillumination.

Fill in the blank

10. gonorrhea, nonspecific urethritis or prostatitis

11. Cryptorchidism

CHAPTER 16

The nervous system

OBJECTIVES

After studying this chapter, the reader should be able to:

1. Identify the major components of the nervous system.
2. Describe the neuron and explain how it conducts an impulse.
3. Identify the function of each of the 12 cranial nerves and describe one assessment technique for each.
4. Formulate interview questions that elicit information about the status of the patient's nervous system.
5. Explain the differences among a neurologic screening assessment, a complete neurologic assessment, and a neuro check.
6. Describe how to assess a patient's level of consciousness.
7. Differentiate between normal and abnormal neurologic findings in pediatric, adult, and elderly patients.
8. Document a neurologic assessment accurately.

OVERVIEW OF CONCEPTS

The nurse may encounter signs and symptoms of neurologic disorders in patients of any age. Neurologic dysfunction may manifest as a change in the level of consciousness (LOC), inability to understand or use language, slurred speech, vision changes, headache, dizziness, numbness or tingling, paralysis, or weakness. Any of these warning signs warrants a nervous system assessment.

The patient's age and health status determine the depth of a neurologic assessment. Usually, a simple neurologic screening is adequate for children and healthy adults; most of the information needed for this screening can be obtained during a routine interview and physical examination. An elderly patient or one with signs or symptoms of neurologic dysfunction requires a more comprehensive assessment, including evaluation of mental status, cranial nerves, motor and cerebellar function, sensory function, and reflexes.

The nervous system consists of the central nervous system (CNS)—the brain and spinal cord—and the peripheral nervous system (PNS)—the cranial nerves, spinal nerves, and autonomic nervous system (ANS). (For illustrations of central nervous system structures, see *Central nervous system*.)

Central nervous system

The central nervous system consists of the brain and spinal cord.

Brain

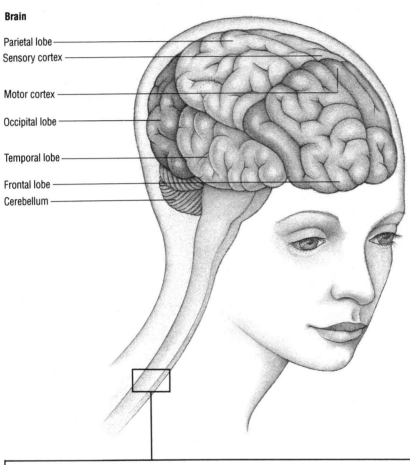

Parietal lobe
Sensory cortex
Motor cortex
Occipital lobe
Temporal lobe
Frontal lobe
Cerebellum

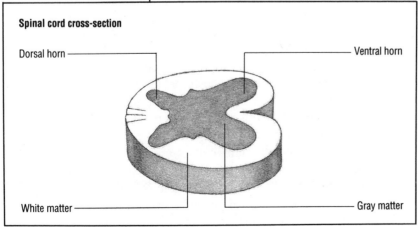

Spinal cord cross-section

Dorsal horn
Ventral horn
White matter
Gray matter

Twelve pairs of cranial nerves transmit motor or sensory messages, or both, primarily between the brain or brain stem and the head and neck. All cranial nerves except the olfactory and optic nerves exit from the midbrain, pons, or medulla oblongata.

Thirty one pairs of spinal nerves are each named according to the vertebra immediately below its point of exit from the spinal cord. Each spinal nerve consists of afferent (sensory) and efferent (motor) neurons, which carry messages to and from particular body regions, called dermatomes.

The vast ANS innervates all internal organs. The nerves of the ANS, sometimes called visceral efferent nerves, carry messages to the viscera from the brain stem and neuroendocrine systems. The ANS has two major divisions: the sympathetic (thoracolumbar) nervous system and the parasympathetic (craniosacral) nervous system.

Two major cell types, neurons and neuroglia, make up the nervous system. Neurons (nerve cells) are the conducting cells of the CNS. They detect and transmit stimuli by electrochemical messages. Neuroglia (glial cells) are the supportive cells of the CNS. They nourish neurons, remove their waste products, and produce cerebrospinal fluid and myelin (a fatlike substance that coats nerve fibers).

Neurons detect and transmit stimuli in the form of electrochemical impulses. *Sensory impulses* travel by two major pathways to the sensory cortex in the parietal lobe of the brain. Pain and temperature sensations enter the spinal cord through the dorsal horn, then immediately cross over to the opposite side of the cord and travel to the thalamus via the spinothalamic tract. Tactile, pressure, and vibration sensations enter the cord via the dorsal root ganglia. After traveling up the cord in the dorsal column to the medulla, these stimuli cross to the opposite side and enter the thalamus. The thalamus relays all incoming sensory impulses, except olfactory ones, to the sensory cortex in the parietal lobe for interpretation.

Motor impulses originating in the motor cortex of the frontal lobe reach the lower motor neurons of the peripheral nervous system via upper motor neurons of the pyramidal or extrapyramidal tract. In the pyramidal tract, impulses travel from the motor cortex, through the internal capsule, to the medulla, where they cross to the opposite side and continue down the cord. In the anterior horn of the cord, impulses are relayed to lower motor neurons, which carry them to the muscles via spinal and peripheral nerves, producing a motor response.

Motor impulses regulating involuntary muscle tone and control travel along the extrapyramidal tract from the premotor area of the frontal lobe to the pons of the brain stem, where they cross to the opposite side. The impulses then travel down the cord to the anterior horn, where they are relayed to lower motor neurons, which carry the impulses to the muscles.

Health history   A complete and accurate neurologic assessment begins with the health history. Although the history presented here focuses on the nervous system, the nurse also should inquire about the patient's general well-being and overall functional ability. Remember that the nervous system is not always the primary source of a neurologic disorder. Also, nervous system disorders can cause problems in other body systems. No matter what their source, neurologic signs and symptoms can disrupt a patient's vocational, social, and family life and interfere with the ability to perform activities of daily living. The questions in this section are designed to help evaluate the patient's nervous system.

Health and illness patterns

Investigate the current, past, and family health status as well as any pertinent developmental considerations.

Current health status

Begin by obtaining information about the patient's current health status. Use the following questions as a guide:

Do you get headaches? If so, how would you describe them?
(RATIONALE: The pattern and characteristics of a headache can help identify its etiology.)

Have you noticed a change in your ability to concentrate or remember things?
(RATIONALE: Such a change may be an early sign of cerebral degeneration. High stress levels and fatigue also can impair memory.)

Do you ever feel dizzy? If so, how would you describe the dizziness?
(RATIONALE: Simple dizziness is a sensation of unsteadiness, light-headedness, or faintness without movement. Vertigo is a sensation that the patient or the environment is spinning. Dizziness evoked by position changes suggests a middle ear problem.)

Have you ever fainted? If so, please describe what happened.
(RATIONALE: Syncope may indicate a temporary decrease in blood supply to the brain [transient ischemic attack].)

Do you have any vision problems, such as double vision, blurred vision, or blind spots? Do you wear glasses?
(RATIONALE: Blurred or double vision may indicate a disorder of cranial nerves II, IV, and VI. Blind spots suggest localized damage to optic tracts in the brain caused by trauma, a cerebrovascular accident [CVA], or a tumor. Uncorrected vision contributes to disorientation in the elderly. Expect some loss of visual acuity with age.)

Do you have any difficulty hearing? If you wear a hearing aid, does it help?
(RATIONALE: A hearing problem may indicate a disorder of cranial nerve VIII. Expect some loss of auditory acuity with age.)

Have you noticed any change in your sense of smell or taste?
(RATIONALE: Such a change may signal a brain tumor or lesion. A decreased sense of taste always accompanies an impaired sense of smell. Expect some loss of these sensations with age.)

Do you have any difficulty swallowing?
(RATIONALE: This symptom may indicate a disorder of cranial nerve IX, X, or XII. Poor neuromuscular control, caused by such disorders as a CVA or Parkinson's disease, also can impair swallowing.)

Do you have difficulty speaking or expressing yourself?
(RATIONALE: Difficulty using or understanding language [aphasia] indicates injury to the cerebral cortex. As needed, provide appropriate tools to assist communication.)

Have you noticed any numbness, tingling, weakness, or inability to move a part of your body (paralysis)?
(RATIONALE: Degenerative neurologic disorders produce progressive bilateral symptoms. CVA or peripheral nerve damage produces sudden localized or unilateral symptoms. Spinal nerve or cord compression can cause unilateral or bilateral symptoms below the lesion level.)

Do you have problems with balance or coordination? Do you ever have trouble walking? Have you ever fallen?
(RATIONALE: Poor balance suggests a cerebellar disorder or impairment of the vestibular portion of cranial nerve VIII. Disturbed coordination suggests disease of the cerebellum, basal ganglia, or extrapyramidal tracts. Ataxia is the first sign of cerebellar dysfunction. A shuffling gait suggests disease of the basal ganglia or extrapyramidal tracts, such as Parkinson's disease.)

Do you experience uncontrollable twitches, tremors, or body movements?
(RATIONALE: These symptoms may indicate a disorder of the cerebellum or basal ganglia.)

Are you taking any prescription or over-the-counter medications?
(RATIONALE: Some medications can affect nervous system functioning.)

Do you smoke cigarettes or drink alcohol? Do you use recreational drugs? If so, which ones, how much, how often, and for how long?
(RATIONALE: These substances affect nervous system functioning.)

Past health status

Next, ask about any previous neurologic disorders.

Have you ever had a head injury? If so, when? Can you describe what happened? Have you experienced any symptoms since the injury?
(RATIONALE: Even minor head injuries can produce long-term effects.)

Have you ever been treated by a neurologist or neurosurgeon? If so, when and why?
(RATIONALE: The answer to this question helps identify existing or potentially recurring neurologic problems.)

Have you ever had a seizure? If so, can you describe what happened? When was your last seizure? Have you ever taken medications for seizures?
(RATIONALE: Seizures may be hereditary or acquired; they sometimes stem from metabolic causes, such as fever. Partial seizures do not impair consciousness and produce focal seizure activity [which helps to localize the structural lesion in the cerebral cortex]. Generalized seizures involve loss of consciousness and bilateral body movements; they suggest a larger area of cortical disturbance. Urge the patient to wear a Medi-alert bracelet or carry other medical identification. Review first aid with the patient's family or caregiver.)

Have you ever had a stroke? If so, can you describe what happened? Have you experienced any symptoms or changes since the stroke?
(RATIONALE: A previous CVA predisposes a patient to another one. Residual deficits may be minimal and hard to detect without specific questioning.)

Family health status
Then ask the patient about the neurologic health status of relatives, such as parents and siblings. Ask the following questions:

Have any family members ever had a neurologic problem?
(RATIONALE: Many neurologic diseases and disorders, including certain types of brain tumors, Alzheimer's disease, and epilepsy, have a familial tendency. Some degenerative neurologic disorders, such as Huntington's disease, are genetic.)

Have any family members ever had high blood pressure or a stroke?
(RATIONALE: Hypertension has a familial tendency and can predispose the patient to a CVA.)

Developmental considerations for pediatric patients
For a young child, gather information about prenatal, perinatal, and developmental history from the parent or guardian. For an older child, gather information from the child as well as the parent. Examples of developmental questions include:

During the pregnancy with this child, was the mother exposed to a TORCH virus (toxoplasmosis, other rubella viruses, cytomegalovirus, herpes simplex)? Did she lose weight, gain too little weight, become ill, suffer an injury, smoke cigarettes, or use alcohol or recreational drugs?
(RATIONALE: Such factors can increase the risk of congenital neurologic defects.)

Was the baby full term at birth or premature? If premature, how early was the baby born?
(RATIONALE: The nervous system of a premature neonate is not fully developed at birth; therefore, age-related developmental milestones will not be accurate.)

Was the child delivered vaginally or by cesarean delivery? If by vaginal delivery, was it assisted? If by cesarean delivery, was the procedure planned or an emergency, and why?
(RATIONALE: Difficult labor and delivery can cause neurologic birth injuries, leading to cerebral palsy and peripheral neuropathies.)

Did the mother receive medications during delivery?
(RATIONALE: Analgesics or anesthetics may decrease the neonate's responsiveness immediately after birth and contribute to insufficient oxygenation and cerebral ischemia.)

During the first month after birth, did the baby have any problems?
(RATIONALE: Sucking or swallowing problems may indicate a neurologic disorder. Metabolic disorders, such as phenylketonuria [PKU], can affect neurologic functioning.)

Are the child's immunizations up to date? Has the child had any major illnesses or injuries?
(RATIONALE: Many childhood illnesses, such as mumps, measles, meningitis, and chicken pox, can produce neurologic symptoms. A head injury, even if minor, can cause subtle behavioral changes up to 1 year later [as in postconcussional syndrome].)

At what age did the child reach the following developmental milestones: hold the head up while prone, roll over, sit without support, walk without support, talk, dress without assistance, and tie the shoes? Has the child lost any skills previously mastered?
(RATIONALE: Delayed neuromuscular development in a full-term infant or loss of previously mastered skills suggests an underlying neurologic disorder.)

Is the child in school? How is the child's progress?
(RATIONALE: Poor school performance may indicate a visual or auditory deficit and warrants immediate screening. Learning disabilities, such as dyslexia and attention deficit disorder, may have a neurologic basis.)

Developmental considerations for elderly patients

Because visual and auditory acuity normally diminish with age, make sure the elderly patient wears glasses or a hearing aid for the interview, if necessary. Be alert for complaints of transient neurologic signs and symptoms (such as vision disturbance, extremity weakness, clumsiness, sudden falls, dizziness, or language impairment). These problems could reflect cerebrovascular disease and impending CVA. Ask about a family history of neurologic disorders or degenerative diseases occurring later in life, such as CVA, senile dementia, blindness, and neuromuscular disorders. Use the following questions as a guide:

Are you less agile than you used to be? Do you trip or fall more frequently?
(RATIONALE: These changes are common effects of aging; however, an extreme change suggests a cerebellar or brain stem disorder.)

How would you describe your walking pattern? Has it changed? Have you developed tremors?
(RATIONALE: Gait changes or tremors could signify Parkinson's disease or another degenerative neurologic disorder.)

Have you noticed a change in your memory, thinking ability, vision, hearing, or sense of smell or taste?
(RATIONALE: A change in any of these functions may indicate cerebral or cranial nerve changes, which may jeopardize the patient's lifestyle, health maintenance, and safety.)

Health promotion and protection patterns

Continue the health history by asking the patient about nutrition, daily activities, recreational patterns, stress and coping patterns, sleep, and personal habits. Also assess for occupational and environmental health patterns that might affect the nervous system.

Please describe your typical daily food intake, including the number of meals and types of foods.
(RATIONALE: An inadequate diet may lead to vitamin B_{12}, folic acid, and niacin deficiencies, which can result in peripheral neuropathy.)

Do you usually feel ready for activities or do you need to rest during the day?
(RATIONALE: Symptoms of certain degenerative neurologic disorders may vary with activity. For example, symptoms of myasthenia gravis, such as muscle weakness, tend to worsen with activity and improve after rest.)

Have you ever been exposed to toxic chemicals, such as insecticides, solvents, or lead, at home or on the job?
(RATIONALE: Exposure to toxins can cause neurologic signs and symptoms. As indicated, plan for poison prevention education.)

Do you perform heavy lifting or repetitive activities on the job?
(RATIONALE: Repetitive motions, such as those used on an assembly line, can cause peripheral nerve injury from overuse. Heavy lifting increases the risk of intervertebral disc injuries. To help prevent such injuries, review body mechanics.)

Do you use seat belts? Do you use recommended protective equipment for recreational and occupational activities?
(RATIONALE: Failure to use seat belts and protective equipment may indicate a potential problem and a need for education.)

Do you have difficulty concentrating on activities you once found enjoyable, such as reading, listening to music, or watching television?
(RATIONALE: Such difficulty may be an early sign of auditory, visual, or cognitive impairment; as indicated, arrange for screening. Depression also can cause loss of interest in previous pastimes.)

How do you know when you are under stress? How do you deal with stress?
(RATIONALE: Some neurologic disorders produce emotional lability, causing the patient to respond inappropriately or excessively.)

Role and relationship patterns

Nervous system disorders can affect the patient's self-concept and impair the ability to perform self-care, fulfill role expectations, and function sexually. Ask the following questions:

In general, how do you feel about yourself?
(RATIONALE: Nervous system disorders that cause obvious deficits, such as paralysis, can adversely affect the patient's self-image.)

Can you do the things for yourself that you would like to do?
(RATIONALE: Neurologic disorders may prevent the patient from attaining personal goals or pursuing satisfying activities.)

Can you fulfill your usual family responsibilities? If not, who assumes them?
(RATIONALE: Neurologic impairment may prevent the patient from fulfilling certain roles, which then must be assumed by another family member.)

Has your illness or disability affected family members? If so, how?
(RATIONALE: Nervous system disorders can devastate the family emotionally. Chronic or degenerative diseases commonly require prolonged treatment, hospitalization, or special equipment, which can drain family finances.)

Do you have any sexual concerns?
(RATIONALE: Injury or damage to the nervous system, especially to the lumbosacral spinal cord, may impede sexual functioning. Brain injuries also can alter libido and sexual functioning.)

Physical assessment   A complete neurologic assessment provides information about five broad categories of neurologic function—cerebral function (including LOC, mental status, and language), cranial nerves, motor system and cerebellar function, sensory system, and reflexes.

Typically, the nurse performs a neurologic screening assessment. This simple, brief assessment quickly evaluates the key indicators of neurologic status to help identify any areas of dysfunction. The neurologic screening assessment includes:
• brief evaluation of mental status (including LOC and verbal responsiveness)
• selected cranial nerve assessment (usually cranial nerves II, III, IV, and VI)
• motor screening (strength, movement, and gait)
• sensory screening (tactile and pain sensations in extremities).

If the screening assessment identifies areas of neurologic dysfunction, the nurse must perform a complete neurologic assessment to evaluate those areas in greater detail.

Finally, the nurse should be able to perform a very brief neurologic assessment, called a neuro check or neuro vital signs. This assessment is used to make rapid, repeated evaluations of several key indicators of neurologic status: vital signs, LOC, verbal responsiveness, pupil size and reaction, and muscle strength and movement.

Preparing for the assessment

Gather a penlight, cotton, and a sterile needle or sharp object. For a complete neurologic assessment, also gather an ophthalmoscope, reflex hammer, tuning fork, tongue depressor, hot and cold test tubes, and substances for testing the patient's sense of smell and taste.

Always start by assessing the patient's cerebral function, including mental status. Changes in mental status usually are the earliest signs of a developing CNS disorder; if they are present, further neurologic evaluation is difficult, if not impossible. Keep in mind that an elderly patient or one with a neurologic disorder affecting balance and coordination may be unable to perform certain maneuvers.

Cerebral function

Basic assessment of cerebral function includes vital signs, general appearance, mood, behavior, LOC, and communication. Advanced assessment of cerebral function includes a more formal evaluation of speech and language, thought processes, and cognitive function. It usually is conducted by a physician or nurse practitioner.

A brief screening examination may be used to help identify the patient with a mental status disorder. A typical screening examination consists of 10 questions, each addressing one area of the complete mental status examination. Conduct a mental status screening when the patient's responses seem unreliable or indicate a possible impairment of memory or cognitive processes. (For details, see *Mental status screening questions,* page 272.) Such a screening may help identify the need for additional testing of cerebral function.

Vital signs

The CNS controls heart rate and rhythm; respiratory rate, depth, and pattern; blood pressure; and body temperature. However, because the control centers for these vital functions lie deep within the cerebral hemispheres and brain stem, vital sign changes usually are late signs of CNS deterioration. (For details on assessing vital signs, see Chapter 3, Physical assessment skills.)

General appearance, mood, and behavior

Observe the patient's posture and body movements. Note any unusual postures, involuntary movements, or immobility. Are movements smooth, controlled, symmetrical, and appropriate? Is the patient calm and relaxed, or restless and fidgety?

Mental status screening questions

As part of a neurologic screening assessment, the nurse can ask specific questions to help identify patients with disordered thought processes. An incorrect answer to any of the questions below indicates the need for a complete mental status examination.

QUESTION	FUNCTION SCREENED
What is your name?	Orientation to person
What is today's date?	Orientation to time
What year is it?	Orientation to time
Where are you now?	Orientation to place
How old are you?	Memory
Where were you born?	Remote memory
What did you have for breakfast?	Recent memory
Who is the U.S. president?	General knowledge
Can you count backwards from 20 to 1?	Attention and calculation skills
Why are you here?	Judgment

Next, observe the patient's prevailing mood and affect. Do facial expressions vary with conversation? Are they appropriate? Does the patient appear happy, anxious, angry, or depressed? To verify your conclusions, ask about the patient's moods and feelings.

Finally, note the patient's dress, grooming, and personal hygiene. Are they appropriate for the weather and the patient's age, health, and socioeconomic status?

Level of consciousness

To evaluate LOC, assess the patient's level of arousal and orientation.

Level of arousal. Arousal—the degree of wakefulness—varies from full consciousness to coma. Decreased arousal often precedes disorientation.

To evaluate arousal, observe the patient's behavior. If the patient is dozing or sleeping, attempt arousal by providing an appropriate auditory, tactile, or painful stimulus, in that sequence. Always start with a minimal stimulus, increase the intensity as necessary, and note the type and intensity of stimulus required to elicit a response. Use painful stimuli only to assess the patient who does not respond to other stimuli. Never use an unsterile pin, apply supraorbital pressure, pinch a nipple, or rub the sternum; these actions can spread infection and cause bruising or other injury.

After assessing the patient's arousal level, compare the findings with those of previous assessments, noting any trends. Because most terms used to describe level of arousal are subjective, be sure to include a description of the patient's action or response when documenting. A *fully conscious* patient quickly responds to an appropriate auditory stimulus (such as calling the patient's name). A *lethargic* patient requires a tactile stimulus (such as a touch or gentle shake) to respond. A *stuporous* patient responds only to painful stimuli, such as pressure applied over a nail bed with a pen. A *comatose* patient remains unresponsive despite painful stimuli.

Orientation. Assess orientation to person, place, and time by asking questions that require the patient to provide information rather than a simple yes or no answer.

Person. Is the patient aware of personal identity? Ask for the patient's name and note the response. Self-identity usually remains intact until late in decreasing LOC, making disorientation to person an ominous sign.

Place. Can the patient state the location correctly? For example, can the patient interpret the environment and sensations and conclude that this is a health care facility? Or does the patient think this is home?

Time. Does the patient know the year or month, or the day's date? Disorientation to time is one of the first signs of decreasing LOC. A patient who is oriented to time usually can state the correct year, provide the correct month or date, and, if in an appropriate environment, differentiate day from night.

Many health care facilities use assessment scales to evaluate LOC according to three objective behaviors: eye opening, verbal responsiveness (which includes orientation), and motor response.

Communication

Language skills, which reflect the brain's ability to comprehend communication, are essential to most mental functions. When language is impaired, a reliable history cannot be obtained and mental status evaluation is difficult, if not impossible.

Verbal responsiveness. Most information regarding the quantity and quality of the patient's verbal responsiveness can be obtained during the health history and physical examination. When asking a question, note the patient's verbal responses.

Note the quantity of the patient's speech. Does the patient speak in complete sentences? In phrases? In single words? Is communication spontaneous? Or does the patient rarely speak?

Note the quality of the patient's speech. Is it unusually loud or soft? Does the patient articulate clearly, or are words hard to understand? What is the rate and rhythm of speech? What language does the patient speak?

Are the patient's verbal responses appropriate? Does the patient choose the correct words to express thoughts, or seem to have problems finding or articulating words? Does the patient use nonsense or made-up words (neologisms)?

Can the patient understand and follow commands? When given a multistep command, does the patient forget what follows the first step?

If communication is difficult, is the patient aware of the difficulty? Does the patient appear frustrated or angry when attempts at communication fail? Or does the patient continue to try to talk, unaware that the nurse does not comprehend?

If observations of and interactions with the patient suggest a language difficulty, show the patient a common object, such as a cup or a book, and ask for its name. Or ask the patient to repeat a word, such as *dog, running,* or *breakfast.*

If the patient seems to have trouble understanding spoken language, ask the patient to follow a simple instruction, such as "Touch your nose." If the patient can do that, try a two-step command, such as "Touch your right knee, then touch your nose."

Keep in mind that language performance tends to fluctuate with the time of day and the patient's physical condition. Even a healthy person may have language problems when ill or fatigued. However, marked or increasing language problems may signal neurologic deterioration, warranting further evaluation and physician notification. Impaired language function results in aphasia (inability to use or understand language, or both). Speech disorders include articulation problems and slurred speech, which may result from facial muscle paralysis. Neuromuscular speech impairment is called dysarthria; voice impairment, dysphonia.

Developmental considerations for pediatric patients

To assess LOC in an infant or young child, observe the child's behavior, noting activity, curiosity, shyness, or sleepiness. To assess orientation, observe the child's response to parents or other familiar people. The parents can be a valuable resource because they may detect subtle changes in the child's behavior before any overt change in LOC. Also note the child's speech. If unable to speak yet, does the child try to imitate speech or "coo" in response to the parent's voice? Or does the child use single words or short sentences? Are they appropriate to the situation?

Developmental considerations for elderly patients

Decreased visual and auditory acuity related to aging can prevent the elderly patient from properly recognizing or interpreting environmental stimuli. Also, keep in mind that an elderly patient may process information more slowly. Before concluding that the patient is disoriented, repeat the question and allow adequate response time.

Cultural considerations

A language barrier can lead to inaccurate assessment of the patient's mental status. Cultural differences cause misinterpretation of the patient's appearance, behavior, and orientation. Ask a family member or friend about the patient's behavior and orientation. Arrange for an interpreter, as needed, to complete the assessment.

Cranial nerves

Cranial nerve assessment provides valuable information about the condition of the CNS, particularly the brain stem. As with other assessment techniques, adjust this evaluation to the patient's age. (For specific information on assessing cranial nerves, see *Cranial nerve assessment,* pages 276 to 278.)

Motor system and cerebellar function

The neurologic screening assessment of the motor system includes assessment of the patient's muscle strength (such as muscle size and symmetry), arm and leg movement, and gait. Gait reflects the integrated activity of muscle strength and tone, extremity movement and coordination, balance, proprioception (sense of position), and ability of the cerebral cortex to plan and sequence movements.

A complete neurologic assessment of the motor system includes evaluation of motor functions (muscle size, tone, strength, and movement), cerebellar functions (balance and coordination), and gait. When performing a complete assessment, proceed from head to toe (for example, moving from the neck to the shoulders, arms, trunk, hips, and finally to the legs), assessing all muscles of the major joints. Then assess the patient's gait and cerebellar function. Usually, the complete motor system assessment (muscle tone and cerebellar function) is reserved for patients who display a motor deficit during the screening assessment or who need a complete neurologic examination. Muscle tone and cerebellar function evaluations are advanced assessment skills.

Motor function

Evaluate muscle strength of the patient's arms and legs, movement of the arms and legs, and gait. When evaluating arm strength, never assess hand grasps. The primitive grasp reflex may return with brain dysfunction (especially with frontal lobe involvement), making the hand grasp an unreliable indicator of strength and voluntary movement. Instead, assess arm strength by applying resistance to the patient's forearms and asking the patient to push the nurse away. Then grade muscle strength and movement on a scale of 0 to 5. (See *Grading muscle strength,* page 299, for details.)

Expect some mild bilateral loss of muscle mass and strength with age. If unilateral weakness is present, confirm suspicions by evaluating for downward drift and pronation of the arm. Ask the patient to close both eyes, extend both arms with palms up, and maintain this position for 20 to 30 seconds. Observe for downward drift and pronation (palms-down movement) of the arm. Pronator drift occurs with a motor deficit because the patient cannot rely on visual cues to keep the arm raised. A sideways or upward drift suggests loss of proprioception.

(Text continues on page 278.)

Cranial nerve assessment

The techniques for cranial nerve (CN) assessment vary with the nerve being tested. The chart below lists the type and function of the cranial nerves and describes related assessment techniques and normal findings.

CRANIAL NERVE	ASSESSMENT TECHNIQUE	NORMAL FINDINGS
Olfactory (CN I) Type: Sensory Function: Smell	After checking patency of patient's nostrils, have patient close both eyes. Then occlude one nostril and hold a familiar, pungent-smelling substance (such as coffee, tobacco, soap, or peppermint) under patient's nose and ask its identity. Repeat this technique with other nostril.	Patient should be able to detect and identify smell correctly. If patient reports detecting the smell but cannot name it, offer a choice, such as, "Do you smell lemon, coffee, or peppermint?"
Optic (CN II) and oculomotor (CN III) Type: Sensory Function: Vision	*Optic nerve:* Check visual acuity, visual fields, and retinal structures. *Oculomotor nerve:* Check pupil size, pupil shape, and pupillary response to light. (For a description of how to perform these assessments, see Chapter 8, Eyes and ears.)	Pupils should be equal, round, and reactive to light. When assessing pupil size, be especially alert for any trends. For example, watch for a gradual increase in the size of one pupil or appearance of unequal pupils in patient whose pupils previously were equal.
Oculomotor (CN III) Type: Motor Function: Extraocular eye movement; pupil constriction; upper eyelid elevation **Trochlear (CN IV)** Type: Motor Function: Extraocular eye movement **Abducens (CN VI)** Type: Motor Function: Extraocular eye movement	To test coordinated function of these three nerves, assess them simultaneously by evaluating patient's extraocular eye movement. (For a description of how to perform these assessments, see Chapter 8, Eyes and ears.)	Eyes should move smoothly and in a coordinated manner through all six directions of eye movement. Observe each eye for rapid oscillation (nystagmus), movement not in unison with that of other eye (dysconjugate movement), or inability to move in certain directions (ophthalmoplegia). Also note any complaint of double vision (diplopia).
Trigeminal (CN V) Type: Sensory and motor Function: Transmitting stimuli from face and head; corneal reflex; chewing, biting, and lateral jaw movement	*Sensory portion:* Gently touch right side, then left side, of patient's forehead with cotton ball while patient's eyes are closed. Instruct patient to state the moment the cotton touches area. Compare patient's responses on both sides. Repeat technique on right and left cheek and on right and left jaw. Next, repeat entire procedure using sharp object. Cap of disposable ballpoint pen can be used to test light touch (dull end) and sharp stimuli (sharp end). (If abnormality appears, also test for temperature sensation by touching patient's skin with test tubes filled with hot and cold water and asking patient to differentiate between them.)	Patient with normal trigeminal nerve should report feeling both light touch and sharp stimuli in all three areas (forehead, check, and jaw) on both sides of face.

Cranial nerve assessment *(continued)*

CRANIAL NERVE	ASSESSMENT TECHNIQUE	NORMAL FINDINGS
Trigeminal (CN V) *(continued)*	*Motor portion:* Ask patient to clench jaws. Palpate temporal and masseter muscles bilaterally, checking for symmetry. Try to open patient's clenched jaws. Next, watch opening and closing of patient's mouth to for asymmetry.	Jaws should clench symmetrically and remain closed against resistance.
	Corneal reflex: Ask the patient to look straight ahead. Lightly touch the patient's cornea with a wisp of cotton.	Lids of both eyes should close when wisp of cotton is lightly stroked across cornea.
Facial (CN VII) Type: Sensory and motor Function: Taste receptors (anterior two-thirds of tongue); facial muscle movement, including muscles of expression (those in the forehead and around the eyes and mouth)	*Motor portion:* Ask patient to wrinkle forehead, raise and lower eyebrows, smile to show teeth, and puff out cheeks. Also, with patient's eyes tightly closed, attempt to open eyelids. With each movement, observe closely for symmetry.	Normal facial movements are symmetrical.
	Sensory portion: First prepare four marked, closed containers — one containing salt, another sugar, a third, vinegar (or lemon), and a fourth, quinine (or bitters). Then, with patient's eyes closed, place salt on anterior two-thirds of tongue using cotton swab or dropper. Ask patient to identify taste as sweet, salty, sour, or bitter. Rinse patient's mouth with water. Repeat procedure, alternating flavors and sides of tongue until all four flavors have been tested on both sides. Taste sensations to posterior third of tongue are supplied by the glossopharyngeal nerve (CN IX) and usually are tested at the same time.	Normal taste sensations are symmetrical.
Acoustic (CN VIII) Type: Sensory Function: Hearing and balance	*Acoustic portion:* Test patient's hearing acuity. (For a description of how to perform these tests, see Chapter 8, Eyes and ears.)	Patient should be able to hear a whispered voice or watch tick.
	Vestibular portion: Observe for nystagmus and lack of balance, and note reports of dizziness or the room spinning.	Patient should display normal eye movement and balance and have no dizziness or vertigo.
Glossopharyngeal (CN IX) Type: Sensory and motor Function: Taste receptors (posterior third of tongue); sensations of the throat **Vagus (CN X)** Type: Sensory and motor Functions: Sensations of the throat; taste receptors (posterior third of the tongue); swallowing movements	First, assess patient's voice for hoarse or nasal quality. Then watch patient's soft palate as patient says "ah." Next, test gag reflex (after warning patient). To evoke this reflex, touch posterior wall of pharynx with cotton swab or tongue depressor.	Patient's voice should sound strong and clear. Soft palate and uvula should rise when patient says "ah," and uvula should remain midline. Palatine arches should remain symmetrical during movement and at rest. Gag reflex should be intact. If gag reflex is decreased or pharynx moves asymmetrically, evaluate each side of posterior wall of pharynx to confirm integrity of both cranial nerves.

(continued)

Cranial nerve assessment (continued)

CRANIAL NERVE	ASSESSMENT TECHNIQUE	NORMAL FINDINGS
Accessory (CN XI) Type: Motor Function: Shoulder movement; head rotation	Press down on patient's shoulders while patient tries to shrug against this resistance. Note shoulder strength and symmetry while inspecting and palpating trapezius muscle. Then apply resistance to patient's turned head while patient attempts to return to midline position. Note neck strength while inspecting and palpating sternocleidomastoid muscle. Repeat for opposite side.	Normally, both shoulders should overcome resistance equally well. Neck should overcome resistance in both directions.
Hypoglossal (CN XII) Type: Motor Function: Tongue movement	Observe patient's protruded tongue for deviation from midline, atrophy, or fasciculations (very fine muscle flickerings indicating lower motor neuron disease). Next, ask patient to move tongue rapidly from side to side with mouth open, curl tongue up toward nose, then curl tongue down toward chin. Then use tongue depressor or folded gauze pad to apply resistance to patient's protruded tongue, and ask patient to try to push depressor to one side. Repeat on other side and note tongue strength. Listen to patient's speech for *d, l, n,* and *t* sounds, which require use of tongue. If general speech suggests a problem, have patient repeat phrase or series of words containing these sounds.	Normally, tongue should be midline and patient should be able to move it right to left equally. Patient should be able to move tongue up and down. Pressure exerted by tongue on tongue depressor should be equal on either side. Speech should be clear.

Assess the patient's movement in response to a command. Instruct the patient who is very weak to open and close each fist or to move each arm without raising it off the bed or examination table. If the patient fails to respond, observe for spontaneous arm movements.

If no spontaneous movements occur, test for movement in response to tactile stimuli. Begin with a gentle touch or tickle on the arm. If the patient does not move the arm, use a stronger stimulus, such as firm pressure applied over the nail bed with a blunt object—for example, the side of a pen. Describe the patient's response. Does the patient attempt to withdraw the arm or try to push the stimulus away (a purposeful response)? Or does the patient extend or flex the arm in an abnormal or unusual position (a nonpurposeful response)?

Assess leg movement in the same manner. Throughout the assessment, stay alert for involuntary movement of the limbs, trunk, or face.

Abnormal findings

Motor dysfunction can indicate several types of neurologic disorders. Muscle atrophy can signal absent nerve stimulation (denervation) caused by a peripheral nerve disorder (lower motor neuron disease), or it may indicate disuse secondary to a lesion on the corticospinal tracts.

Unilateral weakness or paralysis of the arm and leg on the same side of the body (hemiparesis) suggests a lesion in the corticospinal tracts or in the motor cortex on the opposite side of the weakness or paralysis. Spasticity in the affected extremities can indicate an upper motor neuron lesion, such as from trauma, CVA, or brain tumor.

Bilateral weakness or paralysis suggests a spinal cord lesion or a disease affecting overall neuromuscular function. Involuntary movements suggest a disorder of the basal ganglia, extrapyramidal tracts, or cerebellum. Nonpurposeful flexion or extension in response to stimuli usually indicates a severe cerebral or brain stem lesion.

Disorders of the motor cortex or corticospinal tracts produce spastic hemiparesis and a characteristic gait. If the disorder involves both corticospinal tracts, as in spinal cord disease, expect bilateral spastic paresis of the legs, causing a scissors gait (the legs tend to cross each other). If the disorder affects peripheral nerves or muscles, foot drop and flaccidity result (one leg seems to drag as the toes fail to lift with each step).

Developmental considerations for pediatric patients

Until age 2 months, fine tremors and occasional involuntary movements are normal. To assess motor function in the pediatric patient, note balance, coordination, and muscle strength as the child rolls over, sits, crawls, stands, or walks. Observe an older infant's or a toddler's ability to grasp and manipulate objects. Carefully watch for indications of hand preference, which normally develops after age 2.

Observe the child's gait. A wide-based gait after age 6 could indicate a neuromuscular or cerebellar disorder.

Developmental considerations for elderly patients

Aging normally causes some loss of muscle mass and strength and also may cause fine tremors. The elderly patient's gait commonly is slower and may be less certain and steady. Observe for mild unilateral weakness, which may indicate a small CVA, or a shuffling, accelerating gait, which could signal Parkinson's disease.

Sensory system

The basic neurologic screening examination consists of evaluating light-touch sensation in all extremities and comparing for symmetry. Some experts also recommend assessing the patient's sense of pain and vibration in the hands and feet as part of this examination. To assess sensory function further requires advanced assessment skills, including a complete assessment of the patient's sensory system to test such functions as the sense of touch, vibration, and position and discriminative sensations.

Because the sensory system becomes fatigued with repeated stimulation, complete sensory system testing in all dermatomes tends to produce unreliable results. Instead, a few screening procedures usually can reveal any dysfunctions. If a localized deficit appears or if the patient complains of localized numbness or an unpleasant sensation (dysesthesia), perform a complete sensory assessment. Expect to conduct a complete neurologic assessment on a patient with motor or reflex abnormalities or trophic skin changes, such as ulceration or atrophy. For a pediatric patient, expect variable and unreliable results until language skills are well developed.

Before beginning the sensory function screening, ask the patient about any areas of numbness or unusual sensations. These areas require special attention.

To perform the assessment, have the patient sit with both eyes closed. Ask the patient to say "now" when the nurse lightly touches the patient's forearm with a cotton wisp. Allow time for the patient's response, then lightly touch the same area on the other arm.

Compare sensations bilaterally on the patient's upper arm, back of the hand, thigh, lower leg, and top of the foot. Occasionally skip an area to test the reliability of the patient's responses. However, be sure to check the skipped area for sensory response before concluding the assessment.

Stay alert for complaints of numbness, tingling, or unusual sensations accompanying the tactile stimulus. Also note the degree of stimulation required to evoke a response. A light, brief touch should be sufficient.

Abnormal findings

The need for repeated, prolonged, or excessive contact to evoke a response indicates reduced sensory acuity. Suspect a sensory deficit if the patient repeatedly fails to detect tactile stimuli in one body area or if sensory acuity in one extremity appears to differ from that on the opposite side of the body.

Reflexes

Evaluation of reflexes usually is reserved for a complete neurologic assessment. Reflexes fall into one of two groups: deep tendon reflexes and superficial reflexes. Commonly tested deep tendon reflexes include the biceps, triceps, quadriceps, patellar (knee jerk), brachioradialis (elbow jerk), and Achilles tendon (ankle jerk) reflexes. Superficial reflexes include the gag, abdominal, cremasteric, and plantar reflexes. Pathologic reflexes, including the grasp, sucking, snout, and Babinski reflexes, may be tested if the patient has suspected CNS damage. (For information on assessment techniques, see *Assessing selected reflexes.*)

Use a grading scale to rate each reflex. Commonly, a scale of 0 to +4 is used. In this scale, 0 denotes an absent reflex, +1 denotes a diminished reflex, +2 signifies a normal reflex, +3 reflects an increased (but not necessarily pathologic) reflex, and +4 denotes a hyperactive reflex. Document the rating for each reflex at the appropriate site on a stick figure.

Assessing selected reflexes

This chart describes the assessment techniques and normal responses for some commonly tested deep tendon and superficial reflexes.

REFLEX	ASSESSMENT TECHNIQUE	NORMAL RESPONSES
Deep tendon reflexes		
Biceps	Have patient partially flex one arm at elbow, with palm facing down. Place thumb or finger over biceps tendon. Tap lightly over thumb or finger with reflex hammer.	Visible and palpable flexion.
Triceps	Have patient partially flex one arm at elbow, with palm facing body. Support arm and pull it slightly across patient's chest. Tap triceps tendon with direct blow of reflex hammer at tendon insertion site.	Brisk elbow extension with visible and palpable contraction of triceps muscle.
Brachioradialis (elbow jerk)	Have patient rest hand on abdomen or lap with forearm partly pronated. Strike radius 1″ to 2″ above wrist.	Flexion and supination of forearm.
Patellar (knee jerk)	Seat patient with one knee flexed and lower leg dangling. Tap patellar tendon with reflex hammer.	Knee extension and quadriceps contraction.
Achilles (ankle jerk)	Place patient with knee bent and ankle dorsiflexed. Tap the Achilles tendon.	Plantar flexion followed by muscle relaxation.
Superficial reflexes		
Cremasteric	Scratch inner aspect of each of patient's thighs with tongue depressor.	Elevation of testicles.
Abdominal	Using fingernail or tip of reflex hammer, stroke one side, then opposite side, of patient's abdomen above umbilicus. Repeat on lower abdomen.	Abdominal muscle contraction; deviation of umbilicus to stimulated side.
Plantar response	Stroke lateral aspect of sole from heel to ball of foot, curving medially across ball.	Flexion of toes. Note presence of fanning (abnormal Babinski response).

Abnormal findings

Increased (hyperactive) reflexes occur with upper motor neuron disorders. Damaged CNS neurons in the cerebral cortex or corticospinal tracts prevent the brain from exerting its usual inhibitory control over peripheral reflex activity. This allows any small stimulus to trigger reflexes, which then tend to overrespond. Examples of hyperactive peripheral reflexes include spasticity associated with spinal cord injuries or other upper motor neuron disorders, such as multiple sclerosis.

Reflexes typically diminish with normal aging. However, markedly decreased or absent reflexes may indicate a disorder of the lower motor neurons or the anterior horn of the spinal cord, where peripheral nerves originates. Lower motor neuron disorders characterized by hyporeflexia (or areflexia) include Guillain-Barré syndrome and amyotrophic lateral sclerosis.

A compressed spinal nerve root can diminish the reflex associated with the affected cord level. For example, a herniated intervertebral disc at lumbar nerve 3 or 4 may diminish the knee jerk reflex.

Documentation

The following sample illustrates the correct way to document normal findings of the nervous system assessment:

Vital signs: Temperature 98.2° F; pulse 76 and regular; respirations 20 and unlabored; blood pressure 124/72.

Cerebral function: Awake, alert, and oriented to person, place, and time. Recent and remote memory intact. Thought processes coherent. Cooperative and relaxed. Language comprehension and expression intact. Well groomed and appropriately dressed. (Complete mental assessment not performed.)

Cranial nerves: CN II through XII intact. (CN I not tested.)

Motor system and cerebellar function: Moves all extremities on command without difficulty. Upper extremities (UE) strong and equal bilaterally. Lower extremities (LE) strong and equal bilaterally. Muscle tone normal. No evidence of muscular atrophy or hypertrophy. No involuntary movements noted. Gait stable. Good balance and coordination. Right-handed.

Sensory system: Light touch and pain intact.

Reflexes: Deep tendon and superficial reflexes intact.

The following sample illustrates the correct way to document abnormal findings of the nervous system assessment:

Vital signs: Temperature 98.4° F; pulse 82 and irregular; respirations 22 and unlabored, Cheyne-Stokes pattern with 15-second periods of apnea occurring approximately once a minute; blood pressure 162/50.

Cerebral function: Lethargic, falls asleep when left alone. Opens eyes when name called loudly. Oriented to person, but can give only first name. Disoriented to place ("my house") and time ("1967"). Responses to many questions inappropriate or unintelligible. Speech slurred and garbled.

Cranial nerves:

CN I: Unable to identify peppermint, coffee, or orange odors. Pungent odor (acetone) does not produce facial grimacing, withdrawal, or other signs of detection.

CN II: Visual acuity corrected with glasses OS, legally blind OD.

CN III, IV, and VI: Right pupil 3 mm, round, reacts sluggishly. Left pupil 7 mm, round, nonreactive. Extraocular movements: upward, lateral, and nasal gazes intact (III, VI). Unable to direct eye downward and nasally (IV). Reports diplopia in lower, medial portion of both visual fields.

CN V: Unable to detect light touch on right side of forehead or right cheek. Touch sensation intact over right jaw and on left side of face.

Jaw clench weak on right, strong on left. Mouth deviates to left with jaw opening and closing. Corneal reflex absent.

CN VII: Facial movement decreased on right side: unable to puff right cheek, wrinkle forehead on right, or close eyelid tightly. Smile droops on right. Left-sided facial movement intact. Unable to differentiate sweet from salt on left anterior two-thirds of tongue; sense of taste intact on right side.

CN VIII: Auditory acuity decreased in right ear; intact in left ear. Complains of vertigo and nausea. Balance poor; falls to left side when sitting without support.

CN IX and X: Taste sensation absent in posterior one-third of tongue bilaterally. Left side of soft palate does not rise, uvula deviates to the right. Voice sounds nasal. Gag reflex absent.

CN XI: Decreased strength in left sternocleidomastoid; right intact.

CN XII: Tongue deviates to left. Fasciculations noted.

Motor system and cerebellar function: Muscle atrophy noted in bilateral UE, most pronounced in hand. Moves all extremities on command. Decreased UE strength, more pronounced on right: overcomes gravity with difficulty. LE strong bilaterally. Gait shuffling and unsteady, leans forward while walking.

Sensory system: Light touch absent in left arm, left leg, and left side of face. Reports dysesthesia characterized by intense burning sensation in response to light touch on right forearm. Paresthesia in feet and lower legs.

Reflexes: Upper extremity deep tendon reflexes intact. Achilles and patellar reflexes absent. Superficial reflexes absent. Babinski's reflex present.

STUDY ACTIVITIES Fill in the blank

1. The CNS consists of the _____ and the _____.

2. _____ are the conducting cells of the CNS.

3. A disorder of cranial nerve _____ is associated with hearing problems.

Short answer

4. What are the three functions of neuroglial cells?

_____

_____

5. What five broad categories are evaluated during a complete neurologic assessment?

_____

_____

6. A neuro check assesses which key indicators of neurologic status?

_____

_____

Multiple choice

7. To help assess a patient's cerebral function, the nurse should ask which health history question?
   A. "How would you describe your eyesight?"
   B. "Have you noticed a change in your ability to remember?"
   C. "Have you noticed a change in your muscle strength?"
   D. "Have you noticed a change in your coordination?"

8. To evaluate the trigeminal nerve (cranial nerve V), the nurse should assess which reflex?
   A. Corneal reflex
   B. Corneal light reflex
   C. Gag reflex
   D. Cough reflex

9. When assessing a patient's level of consciousness, the nurse should use which type of stimulus first?
   A. Painful
   B. Tactile
   C. Auditory
   D. Olfactory

10. What is a normal response to eliciting the Achilles reflex?
   A. Plantar flexion
   B. Dorsiflexion
   C. Foot eversion
   D. Toe fanning

ANSWERS   ### Fill in the blank
   1. brain, spinal cord
   2. Neurons
   3. VIII

Short answer
   4. Neuroglial cells nourish the neurons, remove neuron waste, and produce cerebrospinal fluid and myelin.
   5. The five broad categories evaluated during a complete neurologic assessment include cerebral function, cranial nerves, motor system and cerebellar function, sensory system, and reflexes.
   6. A neuro check (neuro vital signs) assesses these key indicators of neurologic status: vital signs, LOC, verbal responsiveness, pupil size and reaction, and muscle strength and movement.

Multiple choice

7. B. A change in the ability to concentrate or remember things may be an early sign of cerebral degeneration.

8. A. As part of assessing the motor function of the trigeminal nerve, the nurse should test the corneal reflex by stroking a wisp of cotton lightly across the cornea.

9. C. When assessing LOC, the nurse should attempt arousal by providing an appropriate, minimal auditory stimulus, followed by tactile or painful stimulus, if necessary.

10. A. Eliciting the Achilles reflex normally causes plantar flexion followed by muscle relaxation.

CHAPTER 17

Musculoskeletal system

OBJECTIVES
After studying this chapter, the reader should be able to:

1. Identify the structures of the musculoskeletal system.

2. Discuss health history questions useful in eliciting information about musculoskeletal complaints.

3. Identify appropriate modifications of a musculoskeletal physical assessment for a pediatric and an elderly patient.

4. Explain the key elements to be evaluated during the assessment of body symmetry, posture, and gait.

5. Describe techniques used to inspect and palpate musculoskeletal structures, test range of motion, evaluate muscle strength, and estimate muscle mass.

6. Document musculoskeletal assessment findings appropriately.

OVERVIEW OF CONCEPTS
Assessment of the musculoskeletal system involves examination of muscles, bones, and joints. Because the central nervous system (CNS) coordinates muscle and bone function, the examiner must understand how it interrelates with the musculoskeletal system. (For information about the CNS, see Chapter 16, Nervous system.)

Typically, the musculoskeletal assessment is only a small portion of the complete physical assessment. However, if the patient's chief complaint and symptom analysis reveal musculoskeletal involvement, comprehensive assessment of this system is necessary.

Structurally, the musculoskeletal system consists of muscles, bones, and connecting structures (tendons, ligaments, cartilage, joints, and bursae). These structures act together to produce skeletal movement. (For illustrations, see *Musculoskeletal system*.)

The body contains three major muscle types: visceral (involuntary, smooth), skeletal (voluntary, striated), and cardiac (striated). This chapter discusses only skeletal muscle, which is attached primarily to bone. Under voluntary control, skeletal muscle contraction is initiated by impulses from motor neurons to the motor unit of the muscle. Such contraction is responsible for supporting and moving the skeleton—the primary purposes of skeletal muscle.

Musculoskeletal system

The musculoskeletal system is composed of the muscular system and the skeletal system.

MUSCULAR SYSTEM

Anterior view

Posterior view

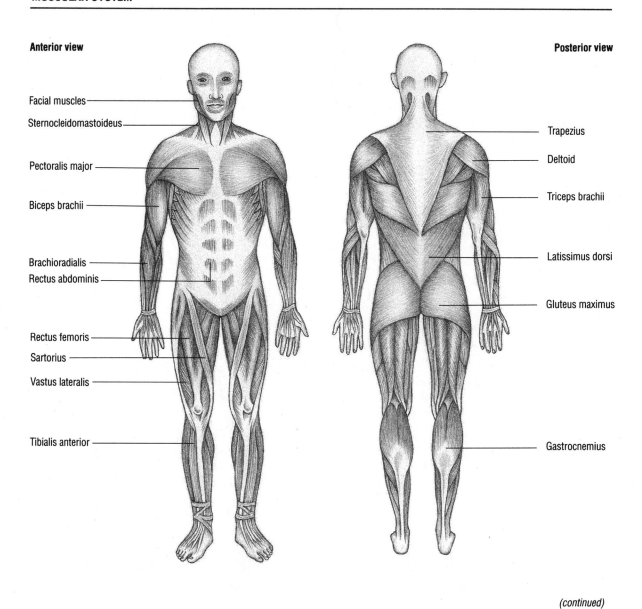

Facial muscles

Sternocleidomastoideus

Pectoralis major

Biceps brachii

Brachioradialis

Rectus abdominis

Rectus femoris

Sartorius

Vastus lateralis

Tibialis anterior

Trapezius

Deltoid

Triceps brachii

Latissimus dorsi

Gluteus maximus

Gastrocnemius

(continued)

Musculoskeletal system *(continued)*

SKELETAL SYSTEM

Anterior view

Posterior view

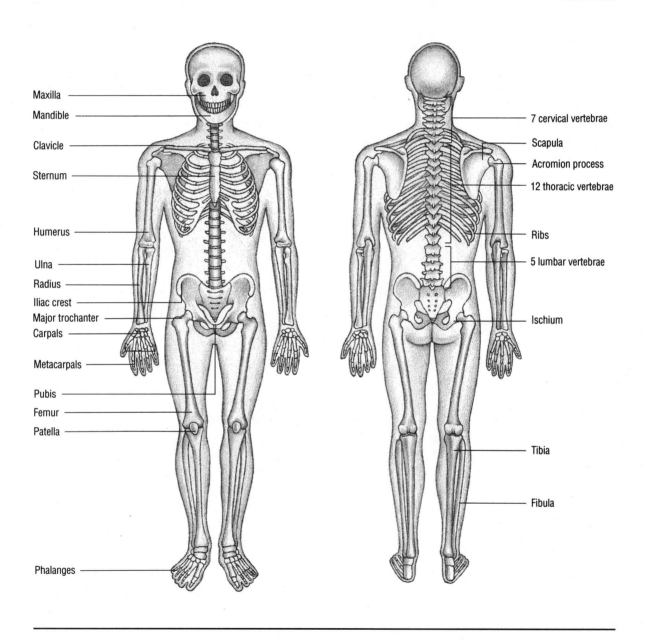

Maxilla

Mandible

Clavicle

Sternum

Humerus

Ulna

Radius

Iliac crest

Major trochanter

Carpals

Metacarpals

Pubis

Femur

Patella

Phalanges

7 cervical vertebrae

Scapula

Acromion process

12 thoracic vertebrae

Ribs

5 lumbar vertebrae

Ischium

Tibia

Fibula

Bones are classified by location (axial or appendicular skeleton) and by shape. The axial skeleton includes the bones of the skull, face, auditory ossicles, ribs, vertebrae, sternum, and hyoid bone. The appendicular skeleton includes the bones of the extremities, shoulders, and pelvis.

When classified by shape, a bone may be long (such as the humerus), short (such as the carpals), flat (such as the scapula), irregular (such as the vertebrae), or sesamoid (such as the patella).

The 206 bones of the human skeleton have various mechanical and physiologic functions. They protect internal organs; stabilize and support the body, thereby allowing erect posture; provide a surface for muscle, ligament, and tendon attachment; and move through "lever" action when contracted. Bones also produce red blood cells in the bone marrow and store minerals (primarily calcium and phosphorus).

Health history The nurse should conduct a complete symptom analysis for each patient complaint. With a musculoskeletal complaint, however, the patient's activity-exercise pattern and health promotion pattern may require in-depth questioning.

Health and illness patterns

Explore the patient's current, past, and family health status as well as developmental considerations.

Current health status

Begin the health history interview with questions that explore current health status. Using the PQRST method, ask the patient to describe completely the current musculoskeletal complaint and any others. (For a detailed explanation of the PQRST method, see *Symptom analysis*, page 15.) Use the following questions to explore the patient's complaint thoroughly:

When did you first notice your symptom? Did it start gradually or suddenly?
(RATIONALE: These questions establish whether onset was gradual or sudden and whether the symptom is acute or chronic. Acute symptoms typically arise over 24 hours; subacute symptoms, over several days to weeks; and slowly progressive symptoms, over weeks to months.)

Are you having any pain? If so, can you point to the area where you feel the pain?
(RATIONALE: The answer helps determine whether the pain is diffuse or localized. For instance, arthritis tends to cause localized pain, whereas tendinitis causes more diffuse pain. Many patients have trouble localizing their pain with words, so asking the patient to point to the painful area may be helpful. Patients with fibromyalgia [psychogenic component of muscular pain] typically present with diffuse pain.)

Does the pain also occur in other locations?
RATIONALE: Pain may be felt in a location other than the one of origin. For example, pain in the leg associated with lower back pain may signify lumbosacral nerve root irritation. A hip problem may present as groin pain.)

What activities increase the pain?
(RATIONALE: Movements and weight-bearing activities typically aggravate pain resulting from osteoarthritis, especially if it affects the hips, knees, or spine. Trauma may precipitate gout.)

What makes the pain feel better? Rest? Exercise?
(RATIONALE: Rest of affected parts typically reduces symptoms of osteoarthritis. Symptoms of rheumatoid arthritis usually decrease with mild exercise or 30 minutes after awakening.)

How would you describe the pain? Is it mild, moderate, severe, or unbearable? Is it aching, burning, stabbing, throbbing, dull, sharp, constrictive, sharp, diffuse, or intense?
(RATIONALE: These terms may help the patient clarify and classify the pain. Trauma, gout, and septic arthritis usually cause severe pain. Neoplasms tend to cause throbbing pain; aching suggests a muscle or joint problem.)

How often does the pain occur? Is it episodic? Recurrent? Constant? Intermittent? Does it worsen as the day progresses? Does it vary from day to day?
(RATIONALE: Intermittent and recurrent pain may indicate gout. Pain lasting more than 6 weeks suggests rheumatoid arthritis or osteoarthritis.)

Are you taking any prescription or nonprescription drugs or using home remedies to treat the problem? If so, which ones, at which strengths, for how long, and with what results? Do you use heat or ice applications? Have you ever had a steroid injection? Have you undergone physical or occupational therapy to reduce the pain or improve your functional ability?
(RATIONALE: The answers to these questions may help identify remedies that can be continued, or may uncover inappropriate patient actions. Also, many prescription drugs can adversely affect musculoskeletal function; for instance, thiazide diuretics can trigger gout. The patient's responses also may reveal which nonprescription agents have been effective for musculoskeletal symptoms. Long-term oral steroid use can lead to osteoporosis.)

Do you have any associated symptoms, such as tingling, weakness, loss of sensation in the limbs, urinary incontinence, or inability to void?
(RATIONALE: Tingling may indicate paresthesia, which can accompany nerve compression. The other symptoms listed could indicate a vertebral fracture or spinal cord lesion.)

Do you have any swelling? If so, when did you first notice it? Have you ever injured this area? Is the area tender? Does the overlying skin look red or feel hot?
(RATIONALE: This finding could indicate infection or recent trauma. Swelling with pain could signal rheumatoid arthritis or bursitis. Swelling months after the onset of pain could indicate osteoarthritis.)

Do you have any stiffness? Do you feel stiff all the time or only on awakening?
(RATIONALE: Remission and periods of exacerbation occur with some diseases. With rheumatoid arthritis, stiffness typically is present on awakening and decreases with activity.)

Is pain associated with the stiffness? Do you sometimes hear a grating sound or feel a grating sensation, as if your bones are scraping together?
(RATIONALE: Pain, stiffness, and a crackling noise [crepitus] indicate rough, irregular articular cartilage, as in osteoarthritis. With some diseases, such as osteoarthritis, stiffness typically subsides 15 minutes after awakening. Stiffness associated with rheumatoid arthritis may last more than 30 minutes.)

Is your movement limited?
(RATIONALE: Impaired movement can result from pain, tumors, rheumatic disorders, inflamed joints, contractures, or deformities.)

Do you have a sore throat, fever, joint pain, rash, weight loss, or diarrhea?
(RATIONALE: Certain musculoskeletal diseases may produce multiple symptoms. For example, acute rheumatic fever, gout, and systemic lupus erythematosus can cause fever and joint pain. A female with back pain and vaginal discharge may have a gynecologic disease, such as pelvic inflammatory disease. Lower back pain and weight loss suggest tuberculosis of the spine. Bowel and bladder dysfunction may indicate a herniated disk.)

Do you engage in social activities? Are you confined to your bed? Are you able to work? Can you sleep through the night?
(RATIONALE: The answers to these questions help reveal the severity of the symptoms.)

Past health status
Use the following questions to gather additional information related to the musculoskeletal system.

Have you ever had an injury or trauma to the limbs or to a bone, muscle, ligament, cartilage, joint, or tendon? If so, what was the injury? How and when did it occur? How was it treated? Have you had any aftereffects?
(RATIONALE: The patient's answers help guide the physical assessment, particularly evaluation of muscle strength and joint range of motion.)

Do you have a history of low back pain?
(RATIONALE: Anyone with a history of low back pain may be experiencing an escalation of a preexisting condition. Previous history may

give insight to the presenting problem, such as trauma or mechanical stress causes by heavy lifting.)

Have you had X-rays or a magnetic resonance imaging (MRI) scan of your bones? What was X-rayed or scanned, and when? What were the results?
(RATIONALE: X-ray studies reveal bone and joint integrity as well as previous injuries. MRI scans help diagnose soft-tissue injuries as well as those of bone structure.)

Have you had blood or urine tests because of a muscle or bone problem? If so, when? What were the results?
(RATIONALE: Certain test results may point to specific musculoskeletal problems; for example, hypercalciuria and urine positive for Bence Jones protein may indicate multiple myeloma [malignant neoplasm of the bone marrow] that has infiltrated bone.)

Have you ever had joint fluid removed or a biopsy performed?
(RATIONALE: Synovial fluid analysis and tissue biopsy usually provide important diagnostic information.)

Have you ever had polio with resultant neuromuscular involvement? Rubella with subsequent arthralgias?
(RATIONALE: The answers to these questions can help guide the physical assessment.)

Have you had surgery or other treatment involving a bone, muscle, joint, ligament, tendon, or cartilage? If so, what was the outcome?
(RATIONALE: The answers to these questions provide useful guides to physical assessment. Previous surgical procedures, such as total joint replacement, can give insight to potential present or future surgical evaluation.)

What immunizations have you had, and when?
(RATIONALE: Tetanus and polio can cause musculoskeletal signs and symptoms. Especially in elderly patients, tetanus may be misdiagnosed as arthritis because of joint stiffening).

The following questions complete this portion of a female patient's musculoskeletal health history:

At what age did you start menstruating? If you have undergone menopause, at what age did it occur? Are you taking estrogen? Have you ever had pelvic inflammatory disease?
(RATIONALE: Late menarche and early menopause allow fewer years for exposure to the estrogen levels that promote bone mass, thus placing a woman at risk for osteoporosis. A female patient with pelvic inflammatory disease may have referred back pain.)

Family health status
Investigate possible familial tendencies regarding musculoskeletal problems by asking the following question:

Has anyone in your family had osteoporosis, gout, arthritis, psoriasis, or tuberculosis?
(RATIONALE: A family history of certain diseases or a history of infectious tuberculosis increases the patient's risk for these conditions. Approximately 30% of patients with psoriatic arthritis have a family history of this disease.)

Developmental considerations for pediatric patients

When assessing a child, try to involve the child as well as the parent in the interview. A complete musculoskeletal assessment of a child should include the following questions (directed to the parent or guardian):

Was labor and delivery difficult?
(RATIONALE: Birth injuries may include fractures or nerve damage. Difficulty breathing at birth may cause neonatal hypoxia, leading to decreased muscle tone.)

At what age did the child first hold up the head, sit, crawl, and walk?
(RATIONALE: This information helps determine whether the child is achieving appropriate developmental milestones or if a musculoskeletal problem is impeding normal development.)

Have you noticed any lack of coordination in your child? Can the child move about normally? Would you describe your child's strength as normal for his or her age?
(RATIONALE: Poor coordination may point to a serious musculoskeletal problem, such as cerebral palsy, or may indicate something less serious, such as a vision problem. Muscle weakness may signify muscular dystrophy.)

Has your child ever broken a bone? If so, which one and when? Did any complications occur during the healing?
(RATIONALE: The answers to these questions help guide subsequent physical assessment.)

Developmental considerations for elderly patients

Ask the following questions of an elderly patient:

Have you broken any bones recently? If so, how?
(RATIONALE: Bones lose density with age. The vertebrae, hips, and wrists are particularly susceptible to fractures in an elderly patient. Some fractures result from trauma; others, from a pathologic [nontraumatic] cause.)

Have you noticed any change in your agility, in the speed at which you can move, or in your endurance?
(RATIONALE: Decreased agility, reaction time, and endurance are normal effects of aging.)

Health promotion and protection patterns

Next, explore the patient's personal habits, sleep and waking patterns, and daily activities. Functional health status, as reflected by activities of daily living, may be the best indicator of how well a patient is managing with a musculoskeletal problem. Ask the following questions:

Do you engage in an exercise routine? If so, please describe it. How has your current problem affected your usual exercise routine?
(RATIONALE: The answer reflects the patient's functional ability. Routine exercise helps maintain strength, muscle tone, bone density, and flexibility.)

What is your typical food and fluid intake over 24 hours?
(RATIONALE: Intake of calories, calcium, protein, and vitamins A, C, and D affects the musculoskeletal system. Excessive consumption of purine-rich foods, such as liver, kidney, fish roe, and alcohol, can precipitate gouty arthritis.)

What is your current weight? Is this your normal weight?
(RATIONALE: A marked weight gain may add stress to weight-bearing joints, such as the knees, placing the patient at greater risk for such musculoskeletal disorders as osteoarthritis. Weight loss may indicate rheumatoid arthritis, tuberculosis of the spine, or neoplasm.)

How much coffee, tea, or other beverages containing caffeine do you consume? How much alcohol do you drink daily? Do you smoke cigarettes? Do you use recreational drugs?
(RATIONALE: Excessive alcohol intake could lead to gouty arthritis. Excessive caffeine intake and smoking may contribute to osteoporosis, especially in postmenopausal women. Intravenous drug abuse is a risk factor for septic arthritis.)

Does your current problem affect your ability to prepare food or to eat? For instance, do you have difficulty opening cans or cutting meat? Do you have trouble holding a cup or utensils?
(RATIONALE: The finger stiffness that accompanies osteoarthritis or rheumatoid arthritis can interfere with such tasks, possibly compromising the patient's nutritional status.)

Are you now using or do you think you would be helped by an assistive device, such as a cane, walker, or brace?
(RATIONALE: The answer shows how the patient feels about an assistive device and its effects on daily life.)

Does your current problem prevent you from falling asleep? Does it cause you to wake up during the night?
(RATIONALE: A patient with osteoarthritis may have difficulty getting comfortable. Tendinitis or bursitis may cause the patient to wake up in the middle of the night.)

Has this problem adversely affected your hobbies, leisure pursuits, and social life?
(RATIONALE: An affirmative answer indicates the need to help identify new activities within the patient's capabilities.)

Do you have problems with personal hygiene because of limited mobility?
(RATIONALE: This question gives the patient an opportunity to detail physical concerns and limitations.)

Are you having any problems with written communication?
(RATIONALE: The patient with severe rheumatoid arthritis may have great difficulty using writing implements.)

Have any of your usual activities, such as dressing, grooming, climbing stairs, or rising from a chair, become difficult or impossible for you to do?
(RATIONALE: The patient's response helps establish the degree of weakness and assesses its impact on daily living.)

Role and relationship patterns
Because musculoskeletal problems can profoundly affect role and relationship patterns, explore this area by asking the following questions:

What is your occupation? Does it involve heavy lifting?
(RATIONALE: Certain occupations, such as truck driving and nursing, increase the risk for lower back injury by straining the lumbar vertebrae.)

Have you experienced significant changes in your life over the past 1 or 2 years? Do you feel any stress because of your current problem?
(RATIONALE: Such stressors as financial problems, marital problems, divorce, and job insecurity can strain the patient's coping abilities, thereby exacerbating pain.)

In general, how do you feel about yourself?
(RATIONALE: Certain musculoskeletal problems can interfere with lifestyle and self-image. For example, finger flexion associated with Dupuytren's contracture [progressive thickening and tightening of subcutaneous tissue of the palm] severely limits dexterity. Pronounced scoliosis [lateral curvature of the spine] can cause self-consciousness and low self-esteem in a child or adolescent.)

Status of other body systems
While assessing health and illness patterns, use these questions to address body system functions that are particularly important to a musculoskeletal complaint:

Have you had fever, chills, fatigue, anorexia, weight loss, or weakness?
(RATIONALE: Rheumatoid arthritis and systemic lupus erythematosus commonly cause these generalized symptoms in the early stages.)

Do you have a history of rashes or skin eruption?
(RATIONALE: Inflammatory diseases, such as rheumatoid or psoriatic arthritis, initially may manifest as a rash or skin eruption.)

Are you having any problems with bowel or bladder function?
(RATIONALE: Lack of exercise because of a musculoskeletal complaint can lead to constipation. Loss of bowel, bladder, or sexual function could indicate a herniated disk—a medical emergency that requires immediate referral. Unilateral back pain associated with fever and chills could indicate a urinary tract infection.)

Have you been through menopause?
(RATIONALE: Vertebral compressions are more common in postmenopausal women.)

Do you take steroids? If so, how long have you been taking them?
(RATIONALE: Long-term steroid therapy and a history of diabetes mellitus are known risk factors for osteoporosis.)

Do you frequently engage in unsafe sex?
(RATIONALE: Sexually transmitted or sexually related diseases that affect the musculoskeletal system include gonorrhea, which may result in tenosynovitis of wrists, fingers, ankles, and toes as well as inflammation of the knees; hepatitis B, which may exhibit rheumatic symptoms or articular symptoms, including symmetric involvement of such small joints as the hands, feet, knees, wrists, and ankles; and acquired immunodeficiency syndrome, which can cause neuralgia.)

Physical assessment

Physical assessment of the musculoskeletal system is divided into two main parts: observing posture, gait, and coordination; and inspecting and palpating the muscles, joints, and bones.

When examining the musculoskeletal system, direct attention to function as well as structure and keep the patient's history in mind—for example, the ability to perform activities of daily living. Move slowly through the assessment, allowing the patient to show how he or she functions.

To prepare, provide the patient with warmth, privacy, and respect. Allow the patient to wear underwear or a swimsuit, removing it only when necessary. Gather a tape measure and a goniometer for measuring angles.

During the assessment, compare both sides of the body for such characteristics as size, strength, movement, and tenderness. As the assessment proceeds, ask additional health history questions, as needed. For example, if inspection reveals a scar over a joint, ask about surgery or injury to that joint.

Because a complete musculoskeletal assessment may exhaust a patient with limited strength, provide adequate rest periods during the assessment. To enhance the patient's comprehension of musculoskeletal tests, demonstrate the activity to the patient while giving instructions.

Observing posture, gait, and coordination

Physical assessment begins as the patient enters the examining room. Observe the patient for approximate muscle strength, symmetry of facial muscle movements, and physical or functional deformities. As the patient assumes different postures and makes diverse movements, assess overall body symmetry.

Posture

Evaluation of posture—the position body parts assume in relation to other body parts and to the external environment—involves inspection of spinal curvature. To assess spinal curvature, instruct the patient to stand as straight as possible. Standing to the patient's side, back, and front, respectively, inspect the spine for alignment and inspect the shoulders, iliac crests, and scapulae for symmetry of position and height. Then have the patient bend forward from the waist with arms relaxed and dangling. Standing behind the patient, inspect the straightness of the spine, noting the position and symmetry of the flank and thorax.

Normally, convex curvature prevails in the thoracic spine, whereas concave curvature is normal in the cervical and lumbar spine when the patient is standing. Normal findings also include a midline spine without lateral curvatures; a concave lumbar curvature that changes to a convex curvature in the flexed position; and iliac crests, shoulders, and scapulae at the same horizontal level.

Gait

Gait consists of two main phases: stance and swing. To assess gait, ask the patient to walk away, turn around, and walk back. Observe and evaluate the patient's posture, movement, foot position, coordination, and balance. (*Note:* Stay close to an elderly or infirm patient and be prepared to help.)

Normal findings include smooth, coordinated movements, the head leading the body when turning, and erect posture with approximately 2″ to 4″ (5 to 10 cm) of space between the feet.

Coordination

Assessing coordination involves evaluating how well a patient's muscles produce movement. Coordination results from neuromuscular integrity. Assess gross motor skills with such tests as lifting the arm to the side or other range-of-motion exercises (any body action involving the muscles and joints in natural directional movements). To evaluate fine motor coordination, have the patient unbutton the shirt or rapidly touch alternating index fingers to the nose, first with eyes open, then closed.

Abnormal findings. Abnormal gait may result from joint stiffness and pain, muscle weakness, and deformities. Other abnormal findings may include an excessively wide support base (which may indicate CNS dysfunction in an adult), toes pointed inward or outward, arms held out to the side or in front, jerky or shuffling motions, and the ball of the foot striking the floor instead of the heel.

Examples of coordination problems associated with voluntary movement include ataxia (impaired movement coordination characterized by unusual or erratic muscular activity); spasticity (awkward, jerky, and stiff movements); and tremor (muscular quivering). (For more information, see Chapter 16, Nervous system.)

Developmental considerations for pediatric patients

For an infant or a small child, the parent's lap can serve as an examination surface. If the child cannot follow directions well, observe active and passive motions to assess strength. Palpate any affected part last to promote the child's cooperation with the rest of the assessment.

The neonate has a generalized convexity (C-shape) of the spine. When the infant begins to hold up the head, a concave cervical curve develops. When the infant begins to walk, a lumbar concavity (lordosis) develops and may appear exaggerated. The school-age child usually stands with the normal adult spinal curvature, which should continue until old age.

A toddler's gait normally involves a wide support base—that is, with feet wide apart. Common knee deviations in children include knock-knee (genu valgum) and bowlegs (genu varum). In a child with genu valgum, the knees touch and the medial malleoli are $3/4''$ to $1\frac{1}{8}''$ (2 to 3 cm) or more apart when the child stands. (This is common during the first year the child walks.) In a child with genu varum, the knees are more than $1''$ (2.5 cm) apart and the medial malleoli touch when the child stands. This is normal in children from ages 2 to $3\frac{1}{2}$ and may persist until age 6.

Lateral curvature (scoliosis) may become apparent during adolescence, with a higher incidence among girls. The spine does not grow straight and the shoulders and iliac crests are not the same height. To assess the difference between functional scoliosis (related to posture) and true scoliosis, ask the patient to flex the spine by bending over. Functional scoliosis will disappear but true scoliosis will remain, its appearance emphasized by a thoracic hump.

Developmental considerations for elderly patients

Kyphosis (exaggerated convexity of the thoracic curvature) typically accompanies aging. An elderly patient may have an abnormal gait with an uneven rhythm, a wide support base, and short steps. Contributing factors include loss of muscle strength and coordination and painful arthritic joints.

Inspecting and palpating muscles

Inspection and palpation are performed simultaneously during the musculoskeletal assessment. Muscle assessment includes evaluating muscle tone, mass, and strength. Palpate the muscles gently, never forcing movement if the patient reports pain or if resistance is felt. Observe the patient's face and body language for signs of discomfort.

Grading muscle strength

Grade muscle strength on a scale from 0 to 5, using the following definitions:
0: No muscle contraction
1: Slight muscle contraction; no joint movement
2: Movement of the body part without gravity
3: Movement against gravity
4: Movement against gravity and light resistance
5: Movement against gravity and full resistance (normal muscle strength)

Tone

Assess muscle tone—consistency or tension in the resting muscle—by palpating a muscle at rest and during passive range of motion. Palpate a muscle at rest from the muscle attachment at the bone to the edge of the muscle. Normally, a relaxed muscle feels soft, pliable, and nontender; a contracted muscle feels firm.

Mass

Muscle mass is the actual size of a muscle. Assessment of muscle mass usually involves measuring the circumference of the thigh, calf, and upper arm. When measuring, establish landmarks to ensure measurement at the same location on each area.

When measuring midarm circumferences to assess muscle size, be sure to ask the patient which side is dominant. Expect symmetry of size; a ½″ (1 cm) or more difference in circumference between opposite thighs, calves, and upper arms is considered abnormal unless increased muscle size results from specific physical activities.

Abnormal findings. Abnormalities include decreased muscle size (atrophy), excessive muscle size (hypertrophy) without a history of muscle-building exercises, flaccidity (atony), weakness (hypotonicity), spasticity (hypertonicity), and fasciculation (involuntary twitching of muscle fibers).

Strength

To evaluate muscle strength, apply resistance as the patient performs active range-of-motion movements. Note the strength the patient exerts against resistance. If the muscle group is weak, lessen the resistance to permit a more accurate assessment. Record findings according to a five-point scale. (For information, see *Grading muscle strength.*)

Inspecting and palpating joints and bones

Assessment of joints and bones includes measuring the patient's height and the length of extremities, evaluating joint and bone characteristics, and assessing joint range of motion.

Measure the patient's height as well as the length of extremities for comparison. (For a description of how to measure height, see Chapter 3, Physical assessment skills.)

To measure extremities, place the patient in the supine position on a flat surface, with arms and legs fully extended and shoulders and hips abducted. Measure each arm from the acromion process to the tip of the middle finger. Measure each leg from the anterior superior iliac spine to the medial malleolus, with the tape crossing at the medial side of the knee. More than $\frac{3}{8}$" (1 cm) disparity in the length of limbs on either side is abnormal.

Examine one extremity at a time, always comparing it to the opposite limb. During joint assessment, never force joint movement if resistance occurs or the patient complains of pain.

Head and neck

The temporomandibular joint is assessed by palpation and range of motion. Place the fingers on the tragus in front of each ear, and ask the patient to open the mouth widely. Range of motion should not be limited. Palpate for swelling, crepitus, and tenderness. Abnormal findings include crepitation, tenderness, swelling, and limited range of motion.

Inspect the cervical spine from three viewpoints: from behind, from the side, and facing the patient. The patient may sit or stand. Observe the neck for deformities and abnormal posture. Inspect the alignment of the head with the body. The nose should be in line with the midsternum and extend beyond the shoulders when viewed from the side. The head should align with the shoulders. Palpate the cervical spinous process and surrounding soft tissues, such as the trapezius muscles, the muscles between the scapulae, and the sternocleidomastoid muscles. Normally, the seventh cervical and first thoracic vertebrae are more prominent than the others.

Abnormal findings include arthritis (which commonly affects cervical joints, causing audible crepitus on movement, tenderness, stiffness, or sensory changes in the arm and hand); loss of a normal cervical curve; and abnormally protruding vertebrae.

Shoulders

Inspect the skin covering the shoulder joints for deformities, erythema, nodules, lesions, or edema. Palpate moving joints for crepitus.

Palpate the acromioclavicular joint and the area over the greater humeral tuberosity. Shoulder joint palpation begins with the patient's arm at the side. Ask the patient to move the arm across the chest (adduction). Then, place the thumb on the anterior portion of the patient's shoulder joint and the fingers on the posterior portion of the joint. Ask the patient to move the arm backward, to externally rotate and abduct the arm; palpate the shoulder joint as the patient's arm moves.

Next, stand behind the patient. With the fingertips placed over the greater humeral tuberosity, instruct the patient to rotate the shoulder internally by moving the arm behind the back. A portion of the musculo-tendinous rotator cuff also can be palpated in this way.

Abnormal findings include pain or crepitus resulting from movement or palpation, less than normal range of motion, asymmetrical movements or contours, edema, nodularities, and erythema.

Suspect a rotator-cuff tear if the patient has difficulty abducting the arm and, during palpation, complains of pain in the deltoid muscle or over the supraspinatus tendon insertion site.

Elbows

Inspect joint contour and the skin over each elbow. Palpate the joint at rest and during movement. Abnormal findings include tenderness with range of motion or palpation, decreased range of motion, erythema, nodules, edema, and crepitus.

Wrists

Inspect the wrists for masses, erythema, skeletal deformities, and edema. Palpate the wrist at rest and during movement by gently grasping it between the thumb and fingers. Abnormal findings include pain from movement or palpation, reduced range of motion, erythema, edema, crepitus, nodules, and asymmetry of movement.

A positive Tinel's sign (tingling sensations in the thumb, index, and middle fingers), elicited by briskly tapping the patient's wrist over the median nerve, may indicate carpal tunnel syndrome (a painful disorder of the wrist and hand caused by median nerve compression between the carpal ligament and other structures within the carpal tunnel). Similar tingling sensations in response to Phalen's sign, in which the patient holds the wrists in acute flexion for 60 seconds, also suggest this disorder.

Fingers and thumbs

Inspect the fingers and thumb of each hand for nodules, erythema, or deformities. Palpate the fingers and thumb at rest and during movement for crepitus, erythema, and tenderness.

Abnormal findings include pain during movement or rest, decreased range of motion, asymmetry of movement, crepitus, edema, erythema, nodules (for example, Heberden's nodes of osteoarthritis), and deformities (for example, extra digits, ulnar deviation of chronic rheumatoid arthritis, or contracture).

Thoracic and lumbar spine

Besides evaluating thoracic and lumbar spinal curvatures during the postural assessment, palpate the length of the spine for tenderness and vertebral alignment. To check for tenderness, lightly percuss each spinous process with the ulnar side of the fist. Normal spinal assessment findings include ability of the patient to perform movements with a full range of motion while maintaining balance and coordination.

Abnormal findings include scoliosis, kyphosis, or lordosis. With the patient in the upright position, scoliosis appears as a lateral curvature of the spine; in the flexed position, as one shoulder more prominent than the other. Kyphosis is an exaggerated dorsal convexity of the spine. Other abnormal findings include horizontal misalignment of the shoulders and iliac crests; decreased range of motion; and tenderness during movement, palpation, or percussion.

Hips and pelvis

Inspect and palpate over the bony prominences—the iliac crests, ischial tuberosities, and greater trochanter. Palpate the hip at rest and during movement.

Abnormal findings include decreased range of motion, pain or crepitus during movement (common in elderly patients with osteoarthritis of the hip), pain during palpation of bony prominences, and flexion of the opposite hip when flexion is tested (flexion deformity).

Knees

Inspect the knees for symmetry with the patient seated. Palpate the knees at rest and during movement. Inspect and palpate the popliteal spaces (behind the knee joint). Knee movements should be smooth.

Abnormal findings include decreased range of motion, pain during palpation or movement, erythema, Baker's cysts, edema, effusions, asymmetrical movement, crepitus, nodules in the popliteal space, genu valgum, or genu varum.

Ankles and feet

Inspect and palpate the ankles and feet at rest and during movement.

Abnormal findings include decreased range of motion, pain, crepitus, edema, nodules, erythema, ulcerations, calluses, and such deformities as pes varus (inverted foot), pes valgus (everted foot), pes planus (flatfoot with low, longitudinal arch), and pes cavus (exaggerated arch, or high instep).

Toes

With the patient sitting or lying supine, inspect all toe surfaces. Palpate the toes at rest and during movement.

Abnormal findings include decreased range of motion; pain with movement or palpation; crepitus; erythema; edema; calluses; bunions; such deformities as hallux malleus, or hammer toe (hyperextension of metatarsophalangeal joint with flexion of the proximal toe joint) and hallux valgus (lateral deviation of the great toe, possibly causing it to ride under the second toe).

Developmental considerations

In a child with rheumatic fever, the wrist is a common site for migratory arthritis, characterized by tenderness, pain, and inflammation. A toddler normally has lumbar lordosis when learning how to walk.

In elderly patients, the normal convexity of the thoracic spine increases, thrusting the head and cervical spine forward. The pronounced convex curvature may prevent an elderly patient from looking upward because the back of the head cannot tilt beyond the thoracic vertebrae.

Other common findings in elderly patients include a partially abducted and flexed hip joint with reduced range of motion during rotation and hyperextension; and arthritic changes of the knees and wrist, including crepitus, pain, stiffness, and joint enlargement.

Documentation

The following example shows how to document some normal physical assessment findings:

Weight: 185 lb

Height: 5′10″

Other findings: Posture erect, gait with normal stance and swing phases.

Left triceps, biceps, and deltoid: normal contour, tone, and strength; no pain or fasciculations.

Left elbow range of motion (ROM): extension, 0 degrees; flexion, 150 degrees; pronation, 90 degrees; supination, 90 degrees. Patient reports no pain with movement.

Right triceps, biceps, and deltoid: normal contour, tone, and strength; no pain or fasciculations.

Right elbow ROM: extension, 0 degrees; flexion, 150 degrees; pronation, 90 degrees; supination, 90 degrees. Patient reports no pain with movement.

No evidence of erythema of overlying skin and no swelling, nodules, or masses of joints or muscles in either arm.

The following example shows how to document some abnormal physical assessment findings:

Weight: 134 lb

Height: 6′3″

Other findings: Posture slumped, gait rolling with toes striking floor before heel in swing phase.

Left triceps, biceps, and deltoid: normal contour, tone, and strength; no pain or fasciculations.

Left elbow ROM: extension, 0 degrees; flexion, 150 degrees; pronation, 90 degrees; supination, 90 degrees. Patient reports no pain with movement.

Right biceps: normal contour, tone, and strength; no pain or fasciculations. Right triceps: normal contour and tone, slight weakness (4 rating; scale 1 to 10), no pain or fasciculations.

Right deltoid: flattened contour, reduced strength (3 rating), hypotonicity. Patient complains of pain during movement, although not during palpation.

Right elbow ROM: extension, 10 degrees; flexion, 120 degrees; pronation, 90 degrees; supination, 45 degrees. Patient complains of discomfort in right elbow during all ROM movements (pain rating, 4). Crepitus felt with extension and flexion but not with pronation or supination.

STUDY ACTIVITIES

Short answer

1. Barbara West is a nurse who works nights on a neurologic unit. Most of her patients require heavy lifting and repositioning. Also, she is a single mother of three toddlers and often lifts and bends when caring for them. Why is Ms. West at high risk for back injury?

_____

2. How should the nurse proceed when physically assessing a patient with lower back pain?

_____

3. For a patient with a musculoskeletal complaint, what is the most important part of the health history interview and why?

_____

Fill in the blank

4. Bones are classified by _____ and _____.

5. The two main phases of gait are the _____ and _____ phases.

6. The three primary techniques used in physical assessment of the musculoskeletal system are _____, _____, and _____.

Multiple choice

7. To assess for spinal curvature, the nurse should inspect the spine with the patient in which of the following positions?
- **A.** Sitting up and standing
- **B.** Supine and lateral recumbent
- **C.** Supine and standing straight
- **D.** Standing straight and bending forward from the waist

8. Which of the following is a normal gait variation in a toddler?
- **A.** Shuffling gait
- **B.** Increased stride length
- **C.** Wide support base
- **D.** Pointing toes inward

9. In an elderly patient, which joint commonly has a reduced range of motion?
- **A.** Hip
- **B.** Ankle
- **C.** Knee
- **D.** Finger

True or false

10. When grading muscle strength, a score of 4 reflects slight muscle contraction without joint movement.
☐ True   ☐ False

11. When the patient is standing, a concave curvature should prevail in the thoracic spine and a convex curvature should appear in the cervical and lumbar spine.
☐ True   ☐ False

12. A family history of osteoporosis or gout increases a patient's risk of developing these disorders.
☐ True   ☐ False

ANSWERS

Short answer

1. Ms. West is at high risk for back injury because she does extensive lifting and bending—both at work and at home. Heavy lifting can cause lower back injury by straining the lumbar vertebrae.

2. To ensure a thorough examination of a patient with lower back pain, the nurse should perform inspection and palpation, test range of motion, evaluate muscle strength, and estimate muscle mass.

3. The most important part of the health history for a patient with a musculoskeletal complaint is health promotion and protection patterns. This part of the history addresses the patient's functional ability (as reflected by activities of daily living), which is likely to be affected by a musculoskeletal complaint.

Fill in the blank

4. location, shape
5. stance, swing
6. observation, inspection, palpation

Multiple choice

7. D. The nurse should assess the spinal curvature with the patient standing straight and bending forward from the waist with arms relaxed and dangling.

8. C. A toddler's gait normally has a wide support base.

9. A. An elderly patient commonly has a partially abducted and flexed hip joint, with reduced range of motion during rotation and hyperextension.

True or false

10. False. A score of 4 reflects movement against gravity and light resistance.

11. False. Normally, a convex curvature prevails in the thoracic spine and a concave curvature prevails in the cervical and lumbar spine when the patient is standing.

12. True.

CHAPTER 18

Immune system and blood

OBJECTIVES

After studying this chapter, the reader should be able to:
1. Identify immune system structures and organs.
2. Name the elements that constitute blood.
3. Write interview questions that elicit information about the patient's immune system and blood.
4. Perform a physical assessment of the lymph nodes and spleen.
5. Document assessment findings for the immune system and blood.

OVERVIEW OF CONCEPTS

Unlike other body systems, the immune system and blood are not composed of simple organ groups. The immune system consists of specialized cells—lymphocytes and macrophages—and structures, including lymph nodes, spleen, thymus, bone marrow, tonsils, adenoids, and appendix. (For an illustration of immune system structures, see *Organs of the immune system.*) The immune system defends the body from assault by microorganisms. Through its lymphatic channels, it also performs a transport function.

The blood is composed of fluid (plasma) and formed elements—blood cells (erythrocytes, or red blood cells [RBCs], and leukocytes, or white blood cells [WBCs]), and thrombocytes (platelets)—that circulate throughout the body. As the body's major transportation fluid, blood maintains homeostasis (equilibrium of the body's internal environment). It transports gases, nutrients, metabolic wastes, blood cells, immune cells, and hormones throughout the body. To accomplish this task, the blood, which is confined to the vascular system, constantly interacts with extracellular fluid for exchange and transfer.

Although they are distinct entities, the immune system and the blood are closely related. For example, their cells share a common origin in the bone marrow, and the immune system uses the bloodstream to transport its components. The cells of the immune system and the blood develop from multipotential stem cells formed in the bone marrow by a process called hematopoiesis.

Because of their diffuse nature, the immune system and the blood can affect, and be affected by, every other body system. Assessing the immune system and blood is therefore complex.

Organs of the immune system

The immune system includes organs and tissues in which lymphocytes predominate, as well as cells that circulate in peripheral blood. Central lymphoid organs include the bone marrow and thymus, which play a role in developing B and T cells. Peripheral lymphoid organs include the lymph nodes (which help remove and destroy antigens circulating in blood and lymph); lymphatic vessels; and the spleen (which gathers and isolates worn-out red blood cells and filters and remove foreign material, worn-out cells, and cellular debris). Other lymphoid tissues include the tonsils, adenoids, appendix, and intestinal lymphoid tissue (Peyer's patches, which remove foreign debris).

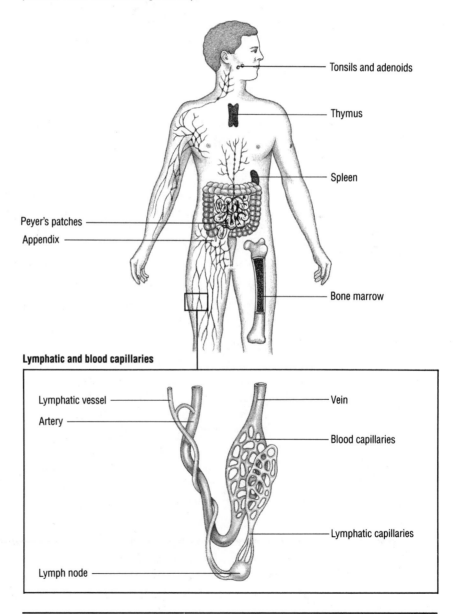

Tonsils and adenoids

Thymus

Spleen

Peyer's patches

Appendix

Bone marrow

Lymphatic and blood capillaries

Lymphatic vessel

Artery

Vein

Blood capillaries

Lymphatic capillaries

Lymph node

Once an antigen penetrates the skin or mucous membrane, the immune system launches nonspecific cellular responses in an attempt to identify and remove the invader.

Health history The nurse who is preparing to collect health history data about the patient's immune system and blood should review the following interview guidelines.

Establish a comfortable environment that ensures patient comfort and privacy. Allow enough time to conduct the interview at a comfortable, uninterrupted pace so that the patient and other participants do not feel rushed and omit important information.

Use familiar terms. For example, ask about bruises, not ecchymoses. If medical terms must be used, be sure to explain them and make sure the patient understands them.

Obtain full biographic data, including age, sex, race, and ethnic background, because some immune and blood disorders occur more frequently in certain groups of people.

Focus the health history on detecting the most common signs and symptoms of immune and blood disorders: abnormal bleeding, lymphadenopathy (hypertrophy of lymphoid tissue, often called swollen glands), fatigue, weakness, fever, and joint pain. While focusing on blood and immune system concerns, maintain a holistic approach by inquiring about the status of other systems and about health-related concerns. Blood and immune system disorders may result from problems in other systems, may cause problems in other systems, or may impair other aspects of the patient's life.

Health and illness patterns

Explore the patient's current and past health status, developmental status, and family health status.

Current health status

Because current health status usually is foremost in the patient's mind, begin the interview with this topic. Carefully document the chief complaint in the patient's own words. Then, using the PQRST method, obtain a complete description of this complaint and any others. (For a detailed explanation of this method, see *Symptom analysis*, page 15.)

The patient with an immune or blood disorder may report vague signs and symptoms. To avoid overlooking important clues, remember that any change from the patient's usual status could be significant and requires investigation. To assess the patient's current health status, ask the following questions:

How have you been feeling lately? Have you noticed any changes in your usual health? If so, please tell me more about them.
(RATIONALE: Because immune and blood disorder symptoms may be vague, open-ended questions usually elicit more information than a checklist. The patient may discuss seemingly insignificant health devia-

tions when comparing current and past health status. Ask the patient additional, detailed questions about vague, hard-to-pinpoint complaints. The more specific the information, the more readily the nurse can identify interrelationships among the patient's discomforts.)

Have you noticed any unusual bleeding—for example, frequent nosebleeds or bruises you don't remember getting?
(RATIONALE: In a patient with a low platelet count or clotting factor deficiencies, unusual bleeding or unexplained ecchymoses can occur secondary to minimal trauma. The extremities are most prone to such injuries, but no body part is exempt.)

Have you ever bled for a long time after accidentally cutting yourself?
(RATIONALE: Prolonged bleeding may indicate a platelet or clotting mechanism deficiency, which can occur with certain immune disorders. If it occurs regularly, it can lead to anemia.)

Have you noticed any bleeding from your gums?
(RATIONALE: Because oral mucosal tissues are highly vascular [and visible], the patient may notice bleeding from these tissues before noting abnormal bleeding in other areas. Gingivae may bleed after the patient chews coarse foods or roughage or after the patient performs daily oral hygiene; they may bleed vigorously after dental hygiene or repair.)

Have you noticed any rash or skin discolorations? If so, on which part of your body does it occur?
(RATIONALE: Petechiae, or pinpoint accumulations of blood in the skin or mucous membranes, may look to the patient like a rashlike discoloration. Petechiae occur when small vessels leak under pressure and too few platelets are present to stop the bleeding. They are most likely to arise where clothing constricts circulation, such as at the waist and wrists.)

Have you noticed any swelling in your neck, armpits, or groin? If so, are the swollen areas sore, hard, or red? Do they appear on one or both sides?
(RATIONALE: Lymphadenopathy may signal inflammation; infection, including human immunodeficiency virus [HIV]; or elevated lymphocyte production associated with certain leukemias. Primary lymphatic tumors rarely cause pain; nontender, swollen lymph nodes may occur in Hodgkin's disease.)

Do you ever feel tired? If so, are you tired all the time or only after exertion? Do you need frequent naps, or do you sleep an unusually long time at night?
(RATIONALE: Fatigue is a prominent symptom of many hematologic disorders. The change may be subtle [the patient requires more sleep at night] or dramatic [the patient no longer can climb a flight of stairs comfortably or requires a longer time to do so]. The patient may complain of always feeling tired.)

Do you ever feel weak? If so, are you weak all the time or only at certain times? Does weakness ever interfere with your ability to perform your usual daily activities, such as cooking or driving a car?
(RATIONALE: Although weakness differs from fatigue, these symptoms commonly coexist in a patient with an immune or blood disorder. Exertional fatigue and weakness suggest moderate anemia; constant or extreme fatigue and weakness suggest severe anemia or neuropathy from an autoimmune disorder. *Note:* Instead of reporting weakness, the patient may complain of heavy extremities, "as if my ankles and wrists had weights around them.")

Have you had a fever recently? If so, how high was it? Was it constant or intermittent? Did it follow any particular pattern?
(RATIONALE: A fever that recurs every few days—for example, Pel-Ebstein fever—may indicate Hodgkin's disease; a temperature that rises and falls within 24 hours suggests an infection. Frequently recurring fevers may signal immune system impairment or rapid blood cell proliferation.)

Do you ever have joint pain? If so, which joints are affected? Do swelling, redness, or warmth accompany the pain? Do your bones ache?
(RATIONALE: Pain in the knees, wrists, or hands may indicate an autoimmune process or hemarthrosis [blood in a joint] resulting from a blood disorder. Pain accompanied by swelling, redness, or warmth typically suggests inflammation, which may be relieved by heat application or salicylate therapy. Aching bones may result from the pressure of expanding bone marrow [caused by blood cell proliferation and subsequent crowding].)

Have you noticed any change in your skin's texture, color, or other characteristics?
(RATIONALE: Hard, thickened skin may indicate scleroderma; dry skin, Hashimoto's disease; sallow skin, systemic lupus erythematosus [SLE].)

Have you noticed any sores that heal slowly?
(RATIONALE: A patient with too few WBCs to control infection and promote healing may have delayed wound healing resulting from compromised hematopoietic or immune functions.)

Have you recently experienced wheezing, a runny nose, or difficulty breathing?
(RATIONALE: Wheezing, rhinitis, and dyspnea may signify an allergy. Dyspnea may result from anemia, connective tissue disease, or infection.)

Do you have any allergies? If so, what causes them and which symptoms are most bothersome?
(RATIONALE: Multiple allergies to foods, drugs, insects, or environmental pollutants are common. A description of the allergic symptoms

helps distinguish a food intolerance or an adverse drug reaction from a true allergic reaction indicating an immune system dysfunction.)

Do you have an immune disorder, such as acquired immunodeficiency syndrome (AIDS)? Have you tested positive for HIV antibodies?
(RATIONALE: An immune disorder may predispose the patient to other diseases because the immune system does not function properly.)

Do you ever have heart palpitations?
(RATIONALE: Palpitations may indicate tachycardia, which can result from an infection in a patient with an immunodeficiency.)

Do you have a persistent or recurrent cough or cold? Do you cough up sputum? Do you feel chest pain when you cough, breathe deeply, or laugh?
(RATIONALE: Immunodeficiency increases the risk of persistent or recurrent respiratory infections, especially pneumonia. Pleuritic pain [a sharp, knifelike pain that worsens with coughing, deep breathing, or laughing] commonly accompanies pneumonia.)

Has your appetite changed recently? Do you experience nausea, flatulence, or diarrhea?
(RATIONALE: Such effects may result when anemia causes gastric hypoxia. The severity of these manifestations may reflect the severity of the hypoxia.)

Have you vomited recently? If so, how would you describe the vomitus?
(RATIONALE: Hematemesis [vomiting of blood] may produce bright-red, brown, or black vomitus of coffee-ground consistency. This sign may result from thrombocytopenia or a clotting factor disorder.)

Have you noticed any blood in your bowel movements, or have you had any black, tarry bowel movements? Do you experience discomfort when defecating?
(RATIONALE: Hematochezia [passage of bloody stools] can cause bright red, blood-streaked, or dark-colored stools. It may result from thrombocytopenia or a clotting factor deficiency; sometimes, it stems from a tear in the rectal mucosa caused by straining or hemorrhoidal irritation. In either case, the rectal mucosa is predisposed to infection in the patient with an immune or blood disorder because macrophages that normally inhabit the area are absent.)

Have you noticed any change in how your urine looks or in your urination pattern?
(RATIONALE: In a patient with a coagulation disorder, urine may appear pink or bloody as a result of bladder capillary hemorrhages. It may appear cloudy and malodorous in a patient with an external genital inflammation caused by a WBC deficiency, immunodeficiency, or a urinary tract infection. Such a patient also may experience changes in usual urinary patterns, such as nocturia [urination at night], dysuria

[painful urination], urinary frequency, urinary urgency, or urinary incontinence.)

Do you have any difficulty walking, or do you experience a pins-and-needles sensation?
(RATIONALE: These neurologic effects may result from pernicious anemia.)

Have you recently suffered from emotional instability, headaches, irritability, or depression?
(RATIONALE: These effects commonly occur with SLE and other chronic immune disorders.)

Ask a female patient the following questions:

Have your menstrual periods changed recently? For example, do they last longer or occur more frequently? Have your periods become irregular? Has your menstrual flow increased or changed in volume or nature?
(RATIONALE: A menstrual pattern change may be the first sign of a bleeding disorder stemming from inadequate platelet numbers or function or from deficient clotting factors.)

Do you experience any pain or discomfort during sexual intercourse?
(RATIONALE: In a patient with a WBC deficiency or an immunodeficiency, a genital infection may develop, causing dyspareunia [painful or difficult intercourse].)

Past health status
When compiling data on the patient's past health status, ask the following questions:

In the past, have you had any of the problems we've just discussed?
(RATIONALE: The patient may have experienced problems related to hematopoiesis, coagulation, or immune function in the past.)

Did you have sore throats frequently in the past?
(RATIONALE: Frequent sore throats suggest a poor immune response to infecting organisms.)

Do you recall being seriously ill as a child or having a long illness requiring frequent visits to a physician?
(RATIONALE: Information about childhood illnesses can provide clues to immune or blood disorders. For example, Hodgkin's disease, sarcoma, and acute lymphocytic leukemia, which usually arise in childhood and adolescence, require aggressive bone marrow suppression therapy with drugs or radiation. Certain chemotherapeutic agents, called alkylating agents, may induce bone marrow dysfunction or leukemia.)

Have you ever had asthma?
(RATIONALE: A history of asthma may indicate immunopathology.)

Have you had any other disorders or health problems?
(RATIONALE: Hepatitis and tuberculosis promote bone marrow failure. Liver failure or cirrhosis can disrupt normal production of prothrombin

and fibrinogen needed for blood coagulation. A history of peptic ulcer disease with excessive bleeding suggests anemia.)

Are you currently taking any prescription or over-the-counter medications? Have you taken any of these medications in the past few weeks? If so, which ones? How often do you take them?
(RATIONALE: Many drugs produce adverse reactions in the immune system and blood.)

Have you ever had surgery? If so, what kind and when? What follow-up care did you receive?

(RATIONALE: Surgery can adversely affect the immune system and blood. For example, gastric surgery can contribute to malabsorption of nutrients and vitamins needed for blood formation. A splenectomy places the patient at increased risk for disseminated infection.)

Have you had an organ transplant?
(RATIONALE: Organ transplants usually require prolonged treatment with immunosuppressant agents to prevent organ rejection. Such therapy compromises the immune system, predisposing the patient to numerous disorders, such as infections and lymphoreticular cancers.)

Have you ever had a blood transfusion? If so, when? How many units did you receive?
(RATIONALE: Blood products can transmit infectious agents, such as hepatitis virus [types B and C], cytomegalovirus, plasmodia that cause malaria, and Epstein-Barr virus. Donor blood is screened for hepatitis B and C, but early infection in the donor may be missed. Although donor blood now is screened for HIV [which causes AIDS], it was not tested routinely before March 1985 and could have transmitted this virus.)

Have you ever been rejected as a blood donor?
(RATIONALE: A blood donation rejection may stem from chronic anemia, a history of hepatitis or jaundice from an unknown cause, or participation in behaviors that put the patient at risk for HIV infection. A history of testing positive for hepatitis B, C, or D or for HIV antibodies would be grounds for rejection as a blood donor.)

Family health status
Investigate the immune system and blood status of the patient's family by asking the following questions:

How would you describe the health of your blood relatives? How old are your living relatives? How old were those who died? What caused their deaths? Do or did any of them have immune, blood, or other problems of the kinds we've discussed?
(RATIONALE: Several blood and immune disorders, including sickle cell anemia, hemophilia, and hemolytic anemia, are transmitted genetically. To determine the patient's risk for developing such disorders, trace the occurrence of these disorders on a family genogram.)

Developmental considerations for pediatric patients

Involve the child in the interview if the child is old enough. If not, direct your questions to the parent or guardian.

Is the infant breast-fed or bottle-fed? If the infant is bottle-fed, what type of formula do you use?
(RATIONALE: Breast-feeding introduces immunoglobulins into the infant's gastrointestinal (GI) tract, conferring some immunity. If the infant is bottle-fed, the formula should be fortified with iron to prevent anemia.)

Does your child ever seem pale or lethargic? Does the child sleep too much? Has the child been gaining weight at a normal rate?
(RATIONALE: Pallor, lethargy, fatigue, and failure to gain weight are common signs of anemia.)

Did the mother have any obstetric bleeding complications? Was the mother's blood Rh negative?
(RATIONALE: Obstetric bleeding complications or Rh incompatibility of the parents may lead to clotting disorders in the child.)

Does the child have frequent or continuous severe infections?
(RATIONALE: Such infections suggest thymic deficiency or bone marrow dysfunction.)

Does the child have any allergies? If so, to what? Does anyone else in the family have allergies?
(RATIONALE: Children are more susceptible to allergies than adults. A family history of infections and allergic or autoimmune disorders may indicate a pattern of immunodeficiencies.)

Which immunizations has the child received?
(RATIONALE: Immunizations can prevent many common communicable diseases. However, the timing of immunizations is important. Every effort should be made to follow the recommended immunization schedule.)

Developmental considerations for elderly patients

The elderly patient may have the same immune and blood disorder signs and symptoms as a younger adult. However, some effects, such as cerebral and cardiac changes, may be more pronounced. The following questions help elicit additional useful information from an elderly patient:

Do you take walks? If so, for how long?
(RATIONALE: Anemia and other disorders that impair the oxygen-carrying capacity of the blood can cause weakness, dyspnea, and light-headedness. These effects may become more pronounced with age, preventing the elderly patient from taking even short walks.)

Do you have any difficulty using your hands?
(RATIONALE: Weakness and numbness in the hands and impaired fine finger movement suggest a blood disorder, such as pernicious anemia.

Joint pain in the hands and other areas may indicate an autoimmune disorder, such as rheumatoid arthritis.)

Do you ever have headaches, faintness, vertigo, confusion, or ringing in the ears?
(RATIONALE: These symptoms are especially likely to occur in an elderly patient with anemia.)

Have you ever had arthritis, osteomyelitis, or tuberculosis?
(RATIONALE: These disorders may predispose the patient to anemia related to chronic illness.)

What do you eat during a typical day? Do you cook for yourself?
(RATIONALE: Because of limited income, resources, and mobility, an elderly patient may consume a diet deficient in protein, calcium, and iron—nutrients essential for hematopoiesis. Even with an adequate diet, nutrients may not be metabolized because an elderly patient has fewer digestive enzymes, which explains why about 40% of people over age 60 have iron deficiency anemia.)

Health promotion and protection patterns
Next, determine the patient's personal habits and activities that may affect the immune system and blood.

What is your typical daily diet? What types and amounts of food do you eat at each meal? What do you eat between meals?
(RATIONALE: Certain foods, such as beef, liver, milk, and kidney beans, contain iron, vitamin B_{12}, and folic acid, which are needed for RBC development. A diet lacking these foods may lead to anemia. Inadequate caloric and protein intake alter the immune response by compromising antibody formation, antigen recognition and processing, and phagocytosis. When this happens, the patient runs a higher risk of developing infections.)

Do you drink alcoholic beverages? If so, what kind, how much, and how often do you drink?
(RATIONALE: Alcohol, especially when combined with decreased food intake, may cause folic acid deficiency anemia.)

How would you rate your stress level? Have you recently experienced the death of a loved one, a job change, divorce, marriage, or other major changes?
(RATIONALE: Persistently high stress levels can reduce the patient's resistance to infection. Researchers are exploring the possible link between high stress levels and immune system suppression.)

Have you ever used injected drugs? If so, which ones and under what conditions?
(RATIONALE: All injected drugs compromise intact skin, one of the body's first defenses against invasion by microorganisms. Illegal injected drugs are more likely to be contaminated and thus promote transmission of infectious agents, such as HIV and hepatitis virus.)

Have you ever been in military service? If so, when and where did you serve?
(RATIONALE: A patient who served in Vietnam in the 1960s may have been exposed to such dioxin-containing defoliants as Agent Orange, which is linked to leukemia and lymphoma.)

What type of work do you do? In what kind of environment do you work?
(RATIONALE: On the job, many workers are exposed to substances that increase the risk of blood and immune disorders. For the patient in a hazardous occupational setting, emphasize safety regulations and investigate specific health-related problems.)

Role and relationship patterns

Ask the following questions to assess the patient's role and relationship patterns related to immune and blood disorders:

How supportive are your family members and friends? How do they perceive and cope with your illness?
(RATIONALE: Chronic autoimmune disorders, such as multiple sclerosis, and immunodeficiency diseases, such as AIDS, are devastating. If the patient receives little support from friends and family members or if these people have trouble coping with the patient's illness, plan to refer the patient to a supportive agency.)

Are you sexually active? If so, are you and your partner monogamous? Do you practice "safe sex"?
(RATIONALE: A patient with multiple sexual partners, or whose partner has multiple partners, may acquire or transmit infectious organisms, such as HIV. Condoms can help reduce this risk.)

Have you noticed any change in your usual pattern of sexual functioning? If so, can you describe this change?
(RATIONALE: Any chronic illness or pain can profoundly affect sexual performance and satisfaction. For example, anemia may cause such severe cellular hypoxia and fatigue that the patient loses sexual desire or has problems with erection or ejaculation.)

Physical assessment

To assess the patient's immune system and blood, the nurse evaluates factors that reflect changes in overall body function (for example, vital signs); the status of related body systems (for example, the skin and respiratory system); and the spleen and lymph nodes (the only accessible immune system structures). Initial patient complaints and physical findings commonly are nonspecific and may involve several body systems.

To prepare for the assessment, obtain the following equipment: flashlight (for transillumination), ruler, nonstretchable tape measure, and gown and drapes. Make sure the examination room is well-lit. Adjust the examination table to the proper height for supine and sitting positions. Have the patient void for comfort, undress, and put on a gown. Then drape the patient to provide adequate access while preventing unnecessary exposure.

Required physical assessment techniques include observation of general appearance, measurement of vital signs, assessment of related body structures, and inspection and palpation of superficial lymph nodes. Physical assessment of the immune system and blood typically is incorporated into the assessment of body systems where lymph nodes are located; for example, the cervical lymph nodes may be palpated during head and neck assessment.

General appearance and vital signs

Because signs and symptoms of immune and blood disorders typically are nonspecific, begin the assessment by observing the patient's general appearance. Look for signs of acute illness, such as grimacing or difficulty breathing, and of chronic illness, such as emaciation and listlessness. Determine whether the patient appears to be the stated age. Chronic disease and nutritional deficiencies related to immune and blood disorders may make a patient look older than the actual age.

Observe the patient's facial features. Note any edema, grimacing, or lack of expression. Next, measure the patient's height and weight, and compare the findings with normal values for the patient's structure. Weight loss may result from anorexia and other GI problems related to immune and blood disorders.

Finally, assess the patient's vital signs, noting especially whether they vary from normal baseline measurements. (For information about assessing vital signs, see Chapter 3, Physical assessment skills.) An elevated temperature, with or without a chill, suggests infection; a subnormal temperature usually accompanies gram-negative infections. Other signs of inflammation, such as redness, swelling, or tenderness, may accompany a fever. Caused by phagocytosis, these effects may be absent if the patient has a WBC deficiency, such as leukopenia (a decrease in total WBCs), granulocytopenia (a decrease in circulating granulocytes), or neutropenia (an absolute neutrophil count below $500/\text{mm}^3$).

Assess the patient's heart rate by checking the pulse. The heart pumps blood harder and faster to compensate for decreased oxygen-carrying capacity in anemia or for reduced volume from active or slow bleeding. Such compensation leads to tachycardia (a rapid but regular heart rate of 100 to 150 beats/minute) or other arrhythmias.

Check the rate and character of the patient's respirations. Particularly note tachypnea (an abnormally rapid respiratory rate) or labored breathing—especially with exertion. These abnormal findings may occur as the respiratory system tries to meet the body's oxygen needs when a disorder compromises the blood's oxygen-carrying capacity.

Measure blood pressure with the patient in the supine, seated, and standing positions. After the patient changes position, blood pressure usually rises or falls only slightly. A decrease of 20 mm Hg or more after a position change suggests orthostatic hypotension, which can result from hypovolemia (decreased circulating plasma volume).

Assessment of related body structures

Because immune and blood disorders affect several body systems, the assessment must include such areas as the skin, hair, and nails; head and neck; eyes; respiratory system; cardiovascular system; GI system; urinary system; nervous system; and musculoskeletal system. The following guidelines describe how to perform this assessment.

Skin, hair, and nails. Observe the color of the patient's skin. Normally, the skin has a slightly rosy undertone, even in dark-skinned patients. Note any pallor, cyanosis (bluish color), or jaundice. Pallor may indicate anemia or another blood disorder that disrupts oxygen delivery. Cyanosis suggests hypoxia in cutaneous blood vessels, which appears in some anemias. Pallor and jaundice may accompany hemolytic anemia. Also check for erythema (redness), which indicates local inflammation, and plethora (a red, florid complexion), which is a sign of polycythemia.

Because skin appearance may be the first sign of a bleeding disorder, such as thrombocytopenia, observe for petechiae or ecchymoses. Carefully check body areas prone to pressure, such as the elbow, wrist, waistline, or upper arm where a blood pressure cuff is applied. With a dark-skinned patient, check for petechiae or ecchymoses on the oral mucosa or conjunctivae.

Next, evaluate skin integrity. Look for signs of inflammation or infection—redness, swelling, heat, or tenderness. Also note other signs of infection, such as poor wound healing, wound drainage, induration (tissue hardening), or lesions. Assess for signs of wound healing at sites of recent invasive procedures, such as venipunctures, bone marrow biopsies, or surgery.

Also check for rashes, and note their distribution. For example, a butterfly-shaped rash over the nose and cheeks may indicate SLE; palpable, painless, purplish lesions on the lower extremities may be Kaposi's sarcoma, which occurs in AIDS.

Observe hair texture and distribution, noting any alopecia (hair loss) on the arms, legs, or head. Alopecia in these areas and broken hairs above the forehead (lupus hairs) occur in SLE.

Inspect the patient's nail color and texture, which should appear pink, smooth, and slightly convex. Pale nail beds may reflect compromised oxygen-carrying capacity (as in anemia). Longitudinal striations also indicate anemia. Koilonychia (spoon-shaped nails) suggests iron-deficiency anemia. Finger clubbing, characterized by a nail angle of 180 degrees or more, indicates chronic hypoxia, which sometimes accompanies an immune or blood disorder. (For more information about these findings, see Chapter 6, Skin, hair, and nails.)

Head and neck. An immune or blood disorder may affect the nose and mouth. Using a penlight, assess the nasal cavity. Position the patient's nose appropriately and look for mucous membrane ulceration, which may indicate SLE, and pale, boggy turbinates, which suggest chronic allergy.

Next, inspect the oral mucous membranes. They should be pink, moist, smooth, and free of lesions. Red mucous membranes suggest polycythemia; petechiae and ecchymoses suggest bleeding disorders. Fluffy white patches scattered throughout the mouth may be candidiasis, a fungal infection. Lacy white plaques on the buccal mucosa may result from hairy leukoplakia, which is associated with AIDS. Such lesions also may occur in a patient who has an immunosuppressive disorder or who receives chemotherapy.

Observe the gingivae (gums). They should be pink, moist, and slightly irregular with no spongy or edematous areas. Gingival swelling, redness, oozing, bleeding, or ulcerations can signal bleeding disorders. Also inspect the tongue. Pink and slightly rough, it should fit comfortably into the floor of the mouth. The tongue may appear smooth and beefy red in folic acid deficiency states or enlarged in Hashimoto's disease and multiple myeloma. In pernicious anemia, it may lack papillae. (For more information, see Chapter 7, Head and neck.)

Eyes. First, test the patient's eye muscle strength using the six cardinal positions of gaze and the convergence tests. The patient with myasthenia gravis may exhibit transient eye muscle weakness, especially when fatigued.

Next, inspect the color of the patient's conjunctivae (normally pink) and sclerae (normally white). Conjunctival pallor may accompany anemia or a bleeding disorder. Scleral icterus may occur with blood disorders that cause jaundice—such as hemolytic anemia—or with liver dysfunction, and may precede skin color changes. Observe the eyelids for drooping, which occurs in myasthenia gravis, and for signs of infection (lesions) or inflammation (swelling or redness).

Respiratory system. Besides observing the patient's respiratory rate and rhythm and energy expenditure related to respiratory effort, note the position the patient assumes to ease breathing. During an asthma attack, the patient may sit up to use accessory respiratory muscle. Chest expansion may be limited in a patient with scleroderma. Exertional dyspnea, tachypnea, and orthopnea (difficulty breathing except in an upright position) commonly accompany the cardiac effort needed to supply oxygen to hypoxic tissues.

Percuss the patient's anterior, lateral, and posterior thorax, comparing one side with the other. A dull sound indicates consolidation, which may occur in pneumonia; hyperresonance may result from trapped air, which occurs in bronchial asthma.

Auscultate over the lungs for adventitious (abnormal) sounds. Wheezing suggests asthma or an allergic response. Crackles can denote a respiratory infection, such as pneumonia, which commonly is seen in immunodeficient patients. (For more information about these assessment procedures, see Chapter 9, Respiratory system.)

Cardiovascular system. Besides assessing the pulse rate and rhythm for anemia-related tachycardia or other arrhythmias, palpate and auscultate the heart and vessels for other signs of immune system or blood disorders.

Auscultate for heart sounds over the precordium. Normally, auscultation reveals only the first and second heart sounds ("lub-dub"). An apical systolic murmur may signify severe anemia; a pericardial friction rub suggests endocarditis or pericardial effusion (which occurs in about 50% of patients with SLE).

Finally, assess the patient's peripheral circulation. Begin by inspecting for Raynaud's phenomenon (intermittent arteriolar vasospasm of the fingers or toes and sometimes of the ears and nose). This phenomenon, which may be caused by SLE or scleroderma, produces blanching in the affected area, followed by cyanosis, pallor, and reddening. Next, palpate the peripheral pulses, which should be symmetrical and regular. Weak, irregular pulses may indicate anemia. (For more information about these procedures, see Chapter 10, Cardiovascular system.)

Gastrointestinal system. Use auscultation, percussion, palpation, and inspection to assess the GI system for signs and symptoms of blood and immune disorders.

First, auscultate the abdomen for bowel sounds. These sounds increase in autoimmune disorders that cause diarrhea, such as ulcerative colitis, and decrease in scleroderma and autoimmune disorders that cause constipation.

Next, percuss the patient's liver. Normally, the liver produces a dull sound over a span of $2\frac{1}{2}''$ to $4\frac{3}{4}''$ (6 to 12 cm). Hepatomegaly (liver enlargement) may accompany many immune disorders, such as hemolytic anemia.

Then palpate the abdomen to detect enlarged organs and tenderness. An enlarged liver that feels smooth and tender suggests hepatitis; one that feels hard and nodular suggests a neoplasm. Hepatomegaly may occur in immune disorders that cause congestion by blood cell overproduction or by excessive demand for cell destruction. Abdominal tenderness may result from infections, commonly seen in patients with immunodeficiency disorders.

Finally, inspect the anus, which should be pink and puckered without inflammation or breaks in the mucosal surface. Defer internal examination of the anus and rectal vault in the patient with a known or suspected platelet insufficiency (less than 50,000/mm^3) or granulocyte insufficiency (less than 1,000/mm^3). (For more information about these procedures, see Chapter 12, Gastrointestinal system.)

Urinary system. Obtain a urine specimen and evaluate its color, clarity, and odor. Normally, urine is clear and amber or straw-colored, and is slightly aromatic. It may look pink or bloody as a result of bladder capillary hemorrhages in a patient with a coagulation disorder. Cloudy, malodorous urine may result from a urinary tract infection.

Inspect the urinary meatus. In a patient with a WBC deficiency or immunodeficiency, the external genitalia may be focal points for inflammation. Discharge or bleeding related to infection also may occur. (For more information about this assessment, see Chapter 13, Urinary system.)

Nervous system. Evaluate the patient's level of consciousness and mental status. The patient should be alert, and respond appropriately to questions and directions. Impaired neurologic function may occur secondary to hypoxia or fever or from intracranial hemorrhage related to a coagulation defect. Thus, an anemic patient may be unable to concentrate or may become confused; this likelihood also increases for an elderly patient. Hemorrhage also compromises oxygen supply to nerve tissues, causing similar symptoms. Bleeding within the cranial vault may lead to disorientation, progressive loss of consciousness, changes in motor and sensory abilities, changes in pupillary responses, and seizures. (These responses depend on the hemorrhage site.)

Other neurologic effects may occur in a patient with an immune disorder. For example, a patient with SLE may exhibit altered mental activity, depression, or psychosis; one with rheumatoid arthritis may have peripheral neuropathies, such as numbness or tingling of fingers. (For more information about neurologic assessment procedures, see Chapter 16, Nervous system.)

Musculoskeletal system. Ask the patient to perform simple maneuvers, such as standing up, walking, and bending over. The patient should be able to perform these maneuvers effortlessly. Then test joint range of motion, particularly in the hand, wrist, and knee. Palpate the joints to assess for swelling, tenderness, and pain. Autoimmune disorders, such as SLE, rheumatoid arthritis, and hemarthrosis, can limit range of motion and cause joint enlargement.

If palpation reveals bone tenderness in the sternum, the cause may be bone marrow hyperactivity, a mechanism that compensates for oxygen-carrying deficits and is prevalent in anemias. Bone tenderness also may result from a leukemic or immunoproliferative disorder, such as plasma cell myeloma, that causes cell packing in the bone marrow. Skeletal pain also may stem from direct disease invasion of the bone marrow in some leukemias or immunoproliferative disorders, such as plasma cell myeloma. (For more information about musculoskeletal assessment, see Chapter 17, Musculoskeletal system.)

Inspection

The first step in regional lymph node assessment is to inspect for color changes and visible lymph node enlargement in areas where the patient reports "swollen glands" or "lumps." Then inspect all other nodal regions. To avoid missing any region, proceed from head to toe. Normally, lymph nodes cannot be seen. Visibly enlarged nodes suggest a current or previous inflammation. Nodes covered with red-streaked skin suggest acute lymphadenitis (lymph node inflammation).

Palpation

Use the pads of the index and middle fingers to palpate the patient's superficial lymph nodes in the head and neck and in the axillary, epitrochlear, inguinal, and popliteal areas. Apply gentle pressure and rotary motion to feel the underlying nodes without obscuring them by pressing them into deeper soft tissues. (For an illustration of this procedure, see *Palpating the lymph nodes.*) The number of nodes varies among patients.

If palpation reveals nodal enlargement or other abnormalities, note the following characteristics: location, size, shape, surface, consistency, symmetry, mobility, color, tenderness, temperature, pulsations, and vascularity of the node.

To describe node location, use such reference points as body axis and lines to pinpoint the site, or sketch the location, if appropriate. Then indicate nodal length, width, and depth in centimeters, and describe or sketch its shape. Describe its surface as smooth, nodular, or irregular. Identify the consistency of the node as hard, soft, firm, resilient, spongy, or cystic. Evaluate the symmetry of the node, comparing it with similar structures on the other side of the body. Describe the node's degree of mobility. If it is immobile, indicate whether it is fixed to overlying tissues, underlying tissues, or both. Note whether the tenderness was elicited by palpation, movement, or the rebound phenomenon (tenderness that occurs after pressure of the palpating fingers is released).

Describe any color change in overlying skin, such as pallor, erythema, or cyanosis. Note whether the site feels warm.

Abnormal findings

Enlarged lymph nodes may result from an increase in the number and size of lymphocytes and reticuloendothelial cells that normally line the node or from infiltration by cells not normally part of the structure (as in metastasized cancers). The clinical significance of a palpated node depends on its location, the patient's age (a child with swollen nodes may have a mild infection whereas nodal enlargement in an adult usually is more significant), and even the patient's working and living environment (exposure to chemicals, pollutants, animals, or insects).

Red streaks in the skin, palpable nodes, and lymphedema may indicate a lymphatic disorder. Enlarged nodes suggest current or recent inflammation. Tender nodes usually denote infection. In acute infection, nodes are large, tender, and discrete; in chronic infection, they become confluent (run together). Metastasized cancer usually affects nodes unilaterally, causing them to become discrete, nontender, firm or hard, and fixed. Generalized lymphadenopathy (involving three or more node groups) can indicate an autoimmune disorder (such as SLE), an

Palpating the lymph nodes

When assessing a patient for signs of an immune or blood disorder, the nurse should palpate the superficial lymph nodes of the head and neck and the axillary, epitrochlear, inguinal, and popliteal areas, using the pads of the index and middle fingers. Always palpate gently; begin with light pressure and gradually increase the pressure.

HEAD AND NECK NODES

Head and neck nodes are best palpated with the patient in a sitting position.

To palpate the submandibular, submental, anterior cervical, and occipital nodes, position the fingers as shown. Palpate over the mandibular surface and continue moving up and down the entire neck. Flex the head forward or to the side being examined. This relaxes the tissues and makes enlarged nodes more palpable. Reverse the hand position to palpate the opposite side.

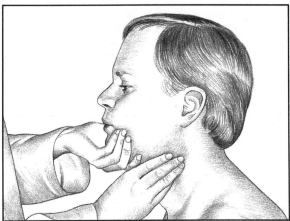

To palpate the preauricular, parotid, and mastoid nodes, place your fingertip pads on the mastoid surface. Continue to palpate, moving your fingertip pads anterior to the ear.

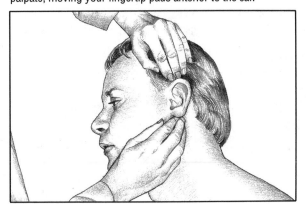

To palpate the posterior cervical nodes and spinal nerve chain, place the fingertip pads along the anterior surface of the trapezius muscle. Then move the fingertips toward the posterior surface of the sternocleidomastoid muscle.

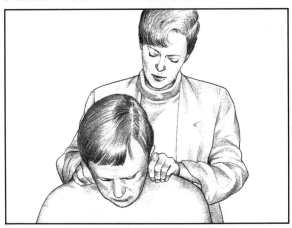

To palpate the supraclavicular nodes, encourage the patient to relax so the clavicles drop. To relax the soft tissues of the anterior neck, flex the patient's head slightly forward with your free hand. Then hook the left index finger over the clavicle lateral to the sternocleidomastoid muscle. Rotate the fingers deeply into this area to feel these nodes.

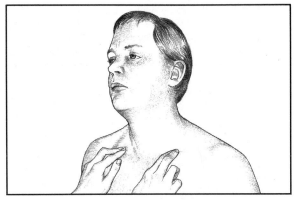

(continued)

Palpating the lymph nodes *(continued)*

AXILLARY AND EPITROCHLEAR NODES

Axillary and epitrochlear nodes are best palpated with the patient in a sitting position. Axillary nodes also may be palpated with the patient lying supine.

To palpate the axillary nodes, use the nondominant hand to support the patient's relaxed right arm, and put the other hand as high as possible in the patient's right axilla.

    Then palpate the axillary nodes, gently pressing the soft tissues against the chest wall and the muscles surrounding the axilla (the pectorals, latissimus dorsi, subscapular, and anterior serratus). Repeat this procedure for the left axilla.

To palpate the epitrochlear lymph nodes, place the fingertips in the depression above and posterior to the medial area of the elbow and palpate gently.

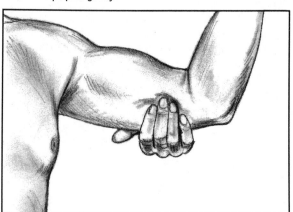

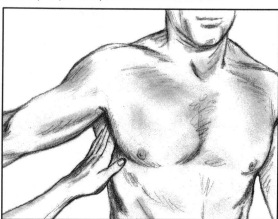

INGUINAL AND POPLITEAL NODES

Inguinal and popliteal nodes are best palpated with the patient lying supine. Popliteal nodes also may be assessed with the patient sitting or standing.

To palpate the inferior superficial inguinal (femoral) lymph nodes, gently press below the junction of the saphenous and femoral veins.

To palpate the superior superficial inguinal lymph nodes, press along the course of the saphenous veins from the inguinal area to the abdomen.

To palpate the popliteal nodes, press gently along the posterior muscles at the back of the knee.

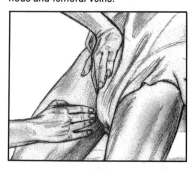

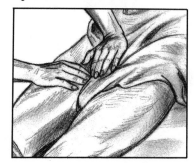

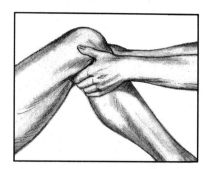

infection, or a neoplastic disorder. In SLE, nodal enlargement may be localized or generalized.

Developmental considerations

In a patient under age 12, lymph nodes commonly can be palpated. For instance, cervical and inguinal nodes, measuring from 1 to 3 cm (about an inch or less), may be felt. Moderate numbers of cool, firm, movable, and painless nodes indicate past infection.

In an elderly patient, immune system and blood-forming activities decline with age. Nodes also decrease in number and size with age, as lymphoid capabilities decline and fatty degeneration and fibrosis occur. This reduces the febrile response to infection.

Documentation
The following example shows how to document some normal physical assessment findings:

Height: 5′10″
Weight: 157 lb
Vital signs: Blood pressure 126/60, temperature 98.0° F (36.7° C), pulse 54 and regular, respirations 16 and regular.
Other findings: Oriented to person, place, and time. Eye examination normal. Skin color and integrity normal, without petechiae or ecchymoses. Other body systems normal, with recent pneumonia completely resolved. Lymph nodes not palpable.

The following example shows how to document some abnormal physical assessment findings:

Height: 5′1″
Weight: 96 lb
Vital signs: Blood pressure 140/90, temperature 99.2° F (37.3° C), pulse 120 and regular, respirations 28 and regular.
Other findings: Patient is alert but listless and lethargic. Buccal mucosa and palpebral conjunctivae are pale. Skin tone: pallor. Functional systolic murmur, grade 2, noted at aortic and pulmonic sites. Cervical nodes enlarged ¾″ (2 cm), nontender, and freely movable. Inguinal nodes present, ½″ (1 cm) across.

STUDY ACTIVITIES

Multiple choice

1. Which of the following are specialized immune system cells?
   A. Erythrocytes
   B. Lymphocytes
   C. Thrombocytes
   D. Leukocytes

2. When assessing a patient with a bleeding disorder, where is the nurse most likely to find petechiae?
   A. On the face
   B. At the waist
   C. On the chest
   D. On the back

3. To assess the preauricular lymph node, where should the nurse palpate?
   A. Behind the ear
   B. Behind the neck
   C. Under the mandible
   D. In front of the ear

4. Which lymph node may be palpated under the chin?
   A. Superficial cervical
   B. Submental
   C. Parotid
   D. Mastoid

5. As a patient grows older, what normally happens to the lymph nodes?
   A. They decrease in number and size.
   B. They increase in number and size.
   C. They decrease in number and increase in size.
   D. They increase in number and decrease in size.

Short answer

6. Describe how an immune system or blood disorder can affect the nervous system.

_____

_____

7. Identify four physical findings that suggest inflammation.

_____

_____

8. Jimmy Thurston, age 6, has what his mother calls a "lump" on his neck. On palpation, the nurse detects a nontender, movable, superficial cervical lymph node measuring 2 cm. Should the nurse be concerned about this finding? Why or why not?

_____

_____

9. Where should the nurse palpate to assess Jimmy's posterior cervical lymph nodes?

_____

_____

Fill in the blank

10. Exertional fatigue and weakness suggest _____.

11. A fever that recurs every few days may indicate _____; a

temperature that rises and falls within 24 hours suggests _____.

Matching related elements
Match the physical assessment finding on the left with its probable cause on the right.

12. ___	Plethora	**A.** Polycythemia
13. ___	Butterfly-shaped facial rash	**B.** Metastasized cancer
14. ___	Unilateral node enlargement and hardening	**C.** SLE

ANSWERS

Multiple choice
1. B. Lymphocytes and macrophages are the specialized cells of the immune system.
2. B. Petechiae are most likely to appear where clothing constricts circulation, such as at the waist and the wrists.
3. D. The nurse should palpate in front of the patient's ear to assess the preauricular lymph node.
4. B. The submental lymph node may be palpated under the chin.
5. A. Normally, lymph nodes decrease in number and size with age as lymphoid capabilities decline and fatty degeneration and fibrosis occur.

Short answer
6. Any disorder that causes intracranial bleeding can produce impaired neurologic function, such as disorientation, progressive loss of consciousness, changes in motor and sensory abilities, changes in pupillary responses, and seizures. Anemia may cause inability to concentrate or confusion. SLE may lead to altered mental activity, depression, or psychosis. Rheumatoid arthritis may cause peripheral neuropathies, such as numbness or tingling of the fingers.
7. Redness, swelling, tenderness, and heat are signs of inflammation. Also, pain accompanied by swelling, redness, or warmth typically suggests inflammation.
8. The nurse should not be concerned because such a cervical lymph node is typical in a child Jimmy's age. In a patient under age 12, lymph

nodes commonly can be palpated and measure 1 to 3 cm. Usually, they are nontender and movable. However, a change in the node should be reported.

9. The nurse should palpate the posterior cervical lymph nodes along the anterior surface of the trapezius muscle and the posterior surface of the sternocleidomastoid muscle.

Fill in the blank

10. anemia

11. Hodgkin's disease, infection

Matching related elements

12. A

13. C

14. B

CHAPTER 19

Endocrine system

OBJECTIVES

After studying this chapter, the reader should be able to:

1. Locate the endocrine glands.

2. Identify the hormone secreted by each endocrine gland, and describe its target structure and functions.

3. Describe the etiology, signs, symptoms, and treatments of common endocrine disorders.

4. Gather appropriate health history information for a patient with an endocrine disorder.

5. Differentiate between normal and abnormal endocrine system findings revealed by the physical assessment.

6. Demonstrate how to palpate the thyroid gland.

7. Demonstrate how to elicit Chvostek's sign and Trousseau's sign, and describe the significance of the findings.

8. Document endocrine system assessment findings appropriately.

OVERVIEW OF CONCEPTS

The endocrine system, together with the nervous system, regulates important body functions, including growth and development of body tissue, reproduction, energy production, metabolism, and the ability to adapt to stress. For this reason, endocrine dysfunction may affect virtually every body system and can profoundly influence a person's health and sense of well-being.

Such systemic signs and symptoms as fatigue and weakness, weight changes, abnormalities of sexual maturity or function, mental status changes, frequent urination (polyuria), or extreme thirst (polydipsia) should alert the nurse to the need for an endocrine system assessment. Although their relationship to the endocrine system may be less apparent, symptoms involving multiple body systems, such as headache, extreme hunger (polyphagia), nervousness, and depression, also may warrant a complete endocrine system assessment.

The endocrine system consists of three major components: glands, which are specialized cell clusters; hormones, which are chemical substances secreted by glands in response to nervous system stimulation; and receptors, which are protein macromolecules that determine the activity of a hormone at its target cell.

Endocrine glands release hormones into the bloodstream for transport to specific target sites. At each target site, hormones combine with specific receptors to trigger specific physiologic changes. (For more information on hormones, see *Endocrine glands and hormones*.)

Health history

The systemic effects of endocrine dysfunction typically are readily apparent and are related to the effects of hormone deficiency or excess. Sometimes, however, endocrine dysfunction manifests in nonspecific ways. Performing a careful body system review and assessing health and illness patterns, health promotion and protection patterns, and role and relationship patterns can provide valuable assessment information.

Health and illness patterns

Explore the patient's current, past, and family health status; the status of physiologic systems; and developmental considerations.

Current health status

Begin the interview by asking about the patient's current health status. Carefully document the chief complaint in the patient's own words, and use the *PQRST* method to elicit a complete description of the problem. (For a detailed explanation of this method, see *Symptom analysis*, page 15.) Common chief complaints associated with endocrine disorders include fatigue, weakness, weight changes, mental status changes, polyuria, polydipsia, and abnormalities of sexual maturity or function.

Do you feel tired, lethargic, or weak?
(RATIONALE: A decreased energy level may result from hypopituitarism, hypothyroidism, or an altered blood glucose level resulting from excessive or insufficient insulin.)

If you feel weak, is the weakness generalized or confined to a specific area or areas?
(RATIONALE: Generalized weakness occurs in various endocrine disorders, including diabetes mellitus, hyperparathyroidism, and Addison's disease. Endocrine disorders rarely cause weakness in a specific area.)

Do you feel any numbness or tingling in your arms or legs?
(RATIONALE: These sensations may indicate sensory peripheral neuropathy. Characterized by biochemical abnormalities and peripheral nerve degeneration, this abnormal condition is common in diabetes mellitus.)

Have you recently gained or lost weight unintentionally? If so, how much and over what time period?
(RATIONALE: Weight gain may result from hypothyroidism, syndrome of inappropriate antidiuretic hormone secretion [SIADH], or Cushing's syndrome. Weight loss may accompany panhypopituitarism, hyperthyroidism, Addison's disease, and hyperglycemia.)

Endocrine glands and hormones

The following chart summarizes the endocrine glands and hormones as well as the hormones's effects on target organs.

GLAND AND LOCATION	HORMONE SECRETED	TARGET ORGAN	HORMONE FUNCTION
Thyroid gland Directly below larynx, partially anterior to trachea	• Thyroxine (T_4) • Triiodothyronine (T_3) • Calcitonin	• All tissues • Bone, renal tubules	• Regulate metabolic processes • Lower ionized calcium level
Parathyroid glands Posterior surface of thyroid	• Parathyroid hormone (PTH)	• Gastrointestinal tract, bone, renal proximal tubules	• Regulate calcium and phosphorus levels
Adrenal glands Atop each kidney	*Adrenal medulla:* • Epinephrine • Norepinephrine	Adrenergic receptors in all tissues	• Control vasoconstriction
	Adrenal cortex: • Glucocorticoids, such as cortisol • Mineralocorticoids, such as aldosterone	• Renal distal tubules	• Metabolize carbohydrates, fats, and proteins; act as anti-inflammatory agents • Balance sodium, potassium, and water concentrations
Pancreas Posterior abdominal wall, in upper left quadrant behind stomach	• Glucagon • Insulin	• Throughout body • Liver, muscle, and adipose tissue	• Elevate blood glucose level • Lower blood glucose level
Testes (in males) Scrotum	• Testosterone	• Reproductive tract and other organs	• Maintain growth and development of reproductive organs; necessary for spermatogenesis
Ovaries (in females) Pelvis	• Estrogens (estrone and estradiol) • Progesterone	• Reproductive tract and other organs	• Maintain growth and development of reproductive organs
Thymus Superior mediastinum and lower part of neck	• Thymosin	• Lymphatic system and spleen	• Necessary early in life for normal immune system development
Anterior pituitary gland Sella turcica (at base of brain)	• Growth hormone (GH)	• Bones, muscles, organs	• Stimulate growth by increasing protein synthesis
	• Thyroid-stimulating hormone (TSH)	• Thyroid	• Stimulate thyroid to produce T_4 and T_3
	• Corticotropin (also known as ACTH)	• Adrenal cortex	• Stimulate secretion of all adrenocorticoids
	• Follicle-stimulating hormone (FSH)	• Ovaries and seminiferous ducts	• Promote development of ovaries, secretion of estrogen, and sperm maturation
	• Luteinizing hormone (LH)	• Ovaries	• Promote ovulation and secretion of progesterone

(continued)

Endocrine glands and hormones *(continued)*

GLAND AND LOCATION	HORMONE SECRETED	TARGET ORGAN	HORMONE FUNCTION
Anterior pituitary gland *(continued)*	• Prolactin	• Breasts, corpus luteum	• Maintain corpus luteum and progesterone secretion, promote breast milk secretion
Posterior pituitary gland Sella turcica (at base of brain)	• Oxytocin	• Uterus and breasts	• Stimulate uterine contractions and lactation
	• Antidiuretic hormone (ADH)	• Kidneys (collecting ducts and distal tubules)	• Promote water reabsorption

Have you recently experienced any behavior changes, such as nervousness or mood swings?
(RATIONALE: Endocrine disorders that alter levels of thyroid hormones, insulin, or corticosteroids can cause behavioral changes and emotional lability.)

Have you noticed an increase in the amount of urine you pass, or have you been feeling unusually thirsty lately?
(RATIONALE: Increased urination [polyuria] and increased thirst [polydipsia] are classic signs of diabetes mellitus and diabetes insipidus.)

Do you often feel hot or cold when other people in the same room are comfortable?
(RATIONALE: Heat intolerance commonly occurs with hyperthyroidism; cold intolerance, with hypothyroidism.)

Are you currently taking any prescription or over-the-counter drugs? If so, which ones and at what dosages?
(RATIONALE: Some drugs can mask or mimic symptoms of endocrine disorders.)

Past health status
Carefully assess the patient's past health status to help identify insidious and vague symptoms of endocrine dysfunction that otherwise may go unreported. Ask the following questions:

Have you ever experienced repeated fractures?
(RATIONALE: Repeated fractures in any area may be a sign of hyperparathyroidism.)

Have you ever had surgery? If so, when and what for? Did you have any complications afterward?
(RATIONALE: Surgery involving an endocrine gland may cause abnormal gland function. Stress from a surgical procedure can precipitate a crisis resulting from an underlying endocrine disorder.)

Have you ever had radiation treatment? If so, what for?
(RATIONALE: Radiation exposure can cause endocrine glands to atrophy, resulting in dysfunction.)

Have you ever had a brain infection, such as meningitis or encephalitis?
(RATIONALE: These infections can cause hypothalamic disturbances, which can disrupt the hypothalamic-pituitary-target gland axis.)

What was your growth pattern? Were you considered tall or short for your age? Did you have any growth spurts? If so, when and to what degree?
(RATIONALE: A slow growth rate could indicate hypopituitarism or hypothyroidism; a rapid growth rate, hyperpituitarism, hyperthyroidism, or gonadal hormone excess.)

Have you ever been diagnosed with an endocrine, or glandular, problem? If so, what was the problem, when was it diagnosed, and how has it been treated?
(RATIONALE: Most endocrine disorders are chronic, thus requiring lifelong treatment.)

Family health status

Because some endocrine disorders are inherited or have strong familial tendencies, ask the following question:

Does anyone in your family have diabetes mellitus, thyroid disease, or hypertension (high blood pressure)?
(RATIONALE: Diabetes mellitus [particularly Type II] and thyroid disease show familial tendencies. Pheochromocytoma, a rare tumor of the adrenal medulla that secretes excessive amounts of catecholamines and elevates blood pressure, may result from an autosomal dominant trait.)

Status of physiologic systems

Because endocrine dysfunction can produce signs and symptoms related to almost any body system, ask the following questions:

Have you noticed any changes in your skin, such as acne, increased or decreased oiliness or dryness, or changes in color?
(RATIONALE: Many endocrine problems produce cutaneous manifestations. For example, in adults, acne may result from Cushing's syndrome. Increased oiliness may reflect acromegaly or androgen excess. Dry, thick skin may result from hypothyroidism; scaly skin, from hypoparathyroidism. Patchy loss of pigmentation [vitiligo] is associated with hypothyroidism and Addison's disease. Purplish striae, especially on the abdomen and breasts, may indicate Cushing's syndrome.)

Do you bruise more easily than you used to?
(RATIONALE: Abnormal susceptibility to bruising may be associated with hypothyroidism or Cushing's syndrome.)

Have you noticed an increase in the size of your hands or feet? For instance, have you had to buy wider shoes or stop wearing your rings?
(RATIONALE: In adults, widening of hand and foot bones may result from acromegaly.)

Do your fingernails and toenails seem brittle? Have they thickened or separated from your fingers and toes?
(RATIONALE: Nail brittleness may result from hypoparathyroidism or hypothyroidism. Separation of the distal end of the nail from the nail bed [onycholysis] may occur in hyperthyroidism.)

Have you noticed any change in the amount and distribution of your body hair?
(RATIONALE: An overall decrease in hair growth may stem from hyperthyroidism. In males, decreased axillary and pubic hair growth commonly points to androgen deficiency. In females, excessive androgen levels can cause increased hair growth in a masculine pattern [hirsutism].)

Has your voice deepened or otherwise changed recently?
(RATIONALE: Vocal hoarseness can result from hypothyroidism. A deepened voice may indicate excess testosterone in females or excess growth hormone in both sexes.)

Do you ever have neck pain? Does your neck seem larger than normal? For instance, have you noticed that your shirts or blouses are tighter at the neck?
(RATIONALE: Neck pain may be related to thyroid inflammation [thyroiditis]; an enlarged neck, to thyroid hyperplasia [goiter] or adenoma.)

Are you having any vision problems, especially double vision (diplopia) or blurred vision?
(RATIONALE: Diplopia suggests a pituitary adenoma putting pressure on cranial nerves III, IV, or VI; or Graves' disease, a disorder commonly associated with hyperthyroidism. Blurred vision can be an early sign of hyperglycemia.)

Do your eyes burn or feel "gritty" when you close them?
(RATIONALE: Such sensations occur with exophthalmos [protruding eyeballs], a common manifestation of Graves' disease.)

Have you ever felt as though your heart were racing, even when you hadn't been exerting yourself?
(RATIONALE: Tachycardia [a heart rate above 100 beats/minute] may be associated with hyperthyroidism, diabetes insipidus, or Addison's disease.)

Have you ever been told you have high blood pressure?
(RATIONALE: Excessive catecholamine levels resulting from pheochromocytoma commonly cause episodic hypertension.)

Has your appetite increased or decreased recently?
(RATIONALE: Increased appetite [polyphagia] may indicate hyperthyroidism or diabetes mellitus. Decreased appetite [anorexia] frequently occurs in hypothyroidism and Addison's disease.)

Do you often experience constipation or frequent stools?
(RATIONALE: Constipation can result from hypopituitarism, hypothyroidism, decreased antidiuretic hormone [ADH], hyperparathyroidism, or pheochromocytoma. Frequent defecation is common in hyperthyroidism.)

Do you have less interest in people, things, and activities that once interested you? Do you ever feel depressed for no particular reason?
(RATIONALE: Apathy and depression may be related to hypopituitarism, hypothyroidism, hyperthyroidism, or increased or decreased levels of ADH, parathyroid hormone [PTH], glucocorticoids, or insulin.)

Do you have numbness or tingling around your mouth or in your hands or feet?
(RATIONALE: Paresthesias may result from diabetes-related sensory neuropathy.)

Have you ever had seizures? If so, what type and under what circumstances?
(RATIONALE: Seizures may be associated with hypopituitarism, hypothyroidism, hypoparathyroidism, Addison's disease, ADH excess, or hypoglycemia.)

Do you often have headaches? Do you ever have sudden, severe headaches that gradually go away?
(RATIONALE: Headaches may indicate pituitary problems or excessive catecholamine levels. Acute, severe headaches that resolve gradually may indicate pituitary hemorrhage or infarction.)

Developmental considerations for pediatric patients

When assessing a child, try to involve the child and a parent or guardian in the interview. With any patient who can understand and speak, invite that patient to participate in the interview, using age-appropriate terms. To help perform a thorough endocrine system assessment, ask the following questions:

Has the child's activity level changed? If so, please describe a typical day before this change occurred and a typical day now.
(RATIONALE: The answer to this question helps distinguish a quiet or hyperactive child from one with altered endocrine function.)

Have you ever been told that the child's growth and development rates are above or below normal?
(RATIONALE: Altered growth and development may indicate a disturbance in growth, thyroid, or gonadal hormone levels.)

Has the child recently lost weight and experienced excessive thirst, hunger, and urination?
(RATIONALE: These classic signs of Type I diabetes mellitus are common in children.)

Developmental considerations for pregnant patients
Keep in mind that some symptoms that arise during pregnancy (for example, mood changes and fatigue) also are symptoms of endocrine disorders. Use the following questions to help assess a pregnant patient's endocrine status:

Have you ever been told you had diabetes during this or a previous pregnancy?
(RATIONALE: Women who have had gestational diabetes mellitus [diabetes associated only with pregnancy] are at increased risk for Type II diabetes mellitus later in life.)

Have you ever given birth to an infant weighing more than 10 lb (4.5 kg)?
(RATIONALE: Delivery of a high-birth-weight infant may indicate a maternal predisposition to diabetes mellitus.)

Health promotion and protection patterns
Now ask questions to determine how the patient feels about and practices health care.

What types of exercise do you engage in? How regularly do you exercise? Have you had any difficulty exercising lately?
(RATIONALE: Weakness and fatigue related to endocrine dysfunction can decrease stamina. In a patient with diabetes mellitus, exercise patterns affect the timing and site of insulin injections [if required]. For example, insulin injected into the thigh before jogging is absorbed more rapidly because muscle motion increases blood flow.)

Have you been experiencing more stress lately? Can you talk about what may be causing this stress? Does your current problem seem to be related to this stress?
(RATIONALE: Stress can exacerbate diabetes mellitus and many other endocrine disorders. Also, treatment of certain endocrine disorders—such as diabetes mellitus, Addison's disease, and hypothyroidism—may require lifelong hormone replacement therapy and lifestyle changes [including activity restrictions and dietary changes], which may increase stress. Adapting to such lifestyle changes may be particularly difficult for an adolescent or an elderly patient.)

Can you afford your medications? Do you have health insurance?
(RATIONALE: Lifelong hormone replacement therapy for some endocrine disorders can be costly. A patient without adequate financial resources or health insurance coverage may have trouble affording certain treatments and may need referral to a social worker.)

What type of work do you do? What are your normal work or school hours? Do you have enough time for breaks and meals?
(RATIONALE: Scheduling of hormone replacement therapy attempts to mimic the body's natural rhythms. A patient with irregular sleep-wake cycles, such as a shift worker, may have problems adjusting to hormone therapy.)

Role and relationship patterns
Conclude with questions that assess the patient's self-perception and view of the social support system.

How do you perceive yourself? Do you think the problem you're experiencing will get better or worse? What bothers you most about your problem?
(RATIONALE: A patient with an endocrine disorder may have a poor self-image related to such effects as altered metabolism, increased susceptibility to and inability to cope with stress, and disfigurement or disability. Identifying the patient's concerns about self-image will aid in planning interventions that help the patient understand and cope with transient or permanent problems.)

Do you have family members or close friends that you can ask for help when you need it?
(RATIONALE: A patient receiving treatment for an endocrine disorder may need another person's help to administer prescribed medications, comply with lifestyle changes, or perform activities of daily living. For example, a patient with diabetes mellitus may need someone to inject glucagon to treat hypoglycemia or to help draw up and inject insulin correctly.)

Physical assessment
Physical assessment of a patient with a known or suspected endocrine problem must include a total body evaluation, focusing on the areas described in this section. It also must include a complete neurologic assessment because of the role the hypothalamus plays in regulating endocrine function through the pituitary gland. (For details on neurologic assessment, see Chapter 16, Nervous system.)

During the physical assessment for endocrine disorders, the nurse obtains most findings through inspection, augmented at some points by palpation and auscultation. Before beginning, gather a tape measure, a scale with a height-measuring device, a stethoscope, a watch with a second hand, a glass of water with a straw, a gown, and drapes. Make sure the examination room is warm and well-lit.

Vital signs, height, and weight
Start the assessment by measuring the patient's vital signs, height, and weight. Compare findings with the patient's baseline measurements, if available. (For more information on assessing vital signs, height, and weight, see Chapter 3, Physical assessment skills, and Chapter 5, Nutritional status.)

Abnormal findings

Vital sign changes may provide important clues to the presence and nature of an endocrine disorder. For example, hypertension develops in many endocrine disorders, particularly pheochromocytoma, Cushing's syndrome, and hyperthyroidism. Bradycardia (a heart rate below 60 beats/minute) occurs in hypothyroidism. Tachycardia can occur in hyperthyroidism and pheochromocytoma. (For details about the signs and symptoms of these disorders, see *Common endocrine disorders*.)

Weight gain unexplained by overeating or lack of exercise suggests Cushing's syndrome or hypothyroidism. In Cushing's syndrome, excessive cortisol secretion stimulates the appetite and frees glucose for fat synthesis, causing excessive fat deposition on the face, neck, trunk, and abdomen. In hypothyroidism, a decreased thyroxine level slows the metabolic rate and decreases nutrient use, leading to weight gain.

In children, a height consistently above or below normal for a sustained time could indicate increased or decreased growth hormone production by the anterior pituitary gland.

In hyperthyroidism, an increased metabolic rate can accelerate nutrient use and lead to weight loss.

Inspection

Next, perform a systematic inspection that begins with general appearance and then assesses all body areas described below.

General appearance. Assess the patient's overall physical appearance and mental and emotional status. Note such factors as overall affect, speech, level of consciousness and orientation, appropriateness and neatness of dress and grooming, and activity level. Evaluate general body development, including posture, build, proportionality of body parts, and body fat distribution. (For more information on how to perform a general survey, see Chapter 3, Physical assessment skills.)

Skin, hair, and nails. Assess the patient's overall skin color, and inspect the skin and mucous membranes for lesions and areas of increased, decreased, or absent pigmentation. Be sure to consider racial and ethnic variations. In a dark-skinned patient, color variations are best assessed in the sclerae, conjunctivae, mouth, nail beds, and palms. Also assess skin texture and hydration.

Inspect the patient's hair for amount, distribution, condition, and texture. Assess scalp and body hair, looking for patterns of abnormal growth or loss. Again, consider normal racial and ethnic—as well as sexual—differences in hair growth and texture. Then check the patient's fingernails for cracking, peeling, separation from the nail bed (onycholysis), and clubbing; check toenails for fungal infection, ingrown nails, discoloration, length, and thickness. (For more information on assessing these features and on normal findings, see Chapter 6, Skin, hair, and nails.)

Common endocrine disorders

The following chart helps the nurse detect and manage common endocrine disorders.

DISORDER	ETIOLOGY	SIGNS AND SYMPTOMS	DIAGNOSTIC TESTS	TREATMENTS
Pituitary gland				
Acromegaly (Growth hormone excess)	Pituitary adenoma	Enlarged hands, feet, tongue, and hat size; fatigue; increased sweating; headaches; voice changes; muscle weakness; joint pain; moist hands; parotid enlargement; visual field defects; decreased vision; goiter; hypertension	Growth hormone stimulation test, computed tomography, magnetic resonance imaging (MRI)	Radiation, surgery
Hypopituitarism (Deficiency of one or more pituitary hormones)	Congenital or acquired pituitary adenoma, postpartal pituitary infarction, trauma, pituitary surgery, inflammatory diseases	Vary with specific hormone deficiency; may include growth failure in children, fine wrinkling around eyes and mouth, increased sensitivity to insulin, amenorrhea, infertility, decreased libido, fatigue, weight loss, thinning and dryness of skin, bradycardia, hypotension	Growth hormone stimulation test, MRI	Hormone replacement
Parathyroid glands				
Hyperparathyroidism (Increased secretion of parathyroid hormone [PTH]), usually leading to hypercalcemia and hypophosphatemia)	Adenoma, benign neoplasm, malignant neoplasm (rare)	Mental status changes, cardiac irregularities, altered reflexes, muscle atrophy, pathologic fractures, peptic ulcer, nephrolithiasis	Serum calcium test, radioimmunoassay for PTH	Hydration, surgery (if indicated)
Hypoparathyroidism (Decreased PTH secretion, usually leading to hypocalcemia, vitamin D deficiency, or both)	Hereditary factors, thyroid surgery, hypomagnesemia, chronic renal failure	Muscle spasms, mental status changes, hair and skin changes, abdominal cramps, electrocardiogram (ECG) changes, papilledema, alopecia	Radioimmunoassay for PTH, serum calcium test, vitamin D metabolite test	Vitamin D, calcium, or calcitriol administration
Thyroid gland				
Hypothyroidism (Insufficient thyroid hormone secretion)	Autoimmune disorder, hypopituitarism, thyroid or pituitary surgery	Enlarged thyroid, fatigue, weight gain, slow cognition, depression, constipation, irregular menses, dry skin, slow deep tendon reflexes	Decreased serum triiodothyronine (T_3), serum thyroxine (T_4), and free T_4 levels; elevated TSH level	Oral thyroid hormone replacement

(continued)

Common endocrine disorders *(continued)*

DISORDER	ETIOLOGY	SIGNS AND SYMPTOMS	DIAGNOSTIC TESTS	TREATMENTS
Thyroid gland *(continued)*				
Hyperthyroidism (Excessive thyroid hormone secretion)	Adenoma, Graves' disease	Goiter, heat intolerance, sweating, weight loss, anxiety, palpitations, menstrual abnormalities, tachycardia, hypertension hyperactive reflexes, fine tremors	Elevated serum T_3 and T_4 levels, thyroid scan	Radioactive iodine, surgery
Cretinism (Severe congenital thyroid hormone deficiency)	Developmental defect	Hoarse cry, constipation, feeding problems, lack of growth, impaired mental development, short stature, protruding tongue, broad flat nose, widely set eyes	Thyroid-stimulating hormone test, serum T_4 test	Thyroid hormone replacement
Pancreas				
Diabetes mellitus (Absent or insufficient insulin production)	Autoimmune process that destroys insulin-producing beta cells of the pancreas; relative insufficiency of insulin production; inadequate target organ response	Fatigue, polyuria, nocturia, polyphagia, polydipsia, weight loss, irritability, vaginal yeast infection, underweight (in Type I diabetes), obesity (in Type II diabetes), skin infections, retinal abnormalities	Elevated plasma glucose and hemoglobin A1C levels	Insulin (Type I diabetes), oral hypoglycemic agents (Type II diabetes)
Adrenal glands				
Primary aldosteronism (Excessive secretion of aldosterone)	Adrenal adenoma	Headache, muscle weakness, fatigue, polyuria, increased diastolic pressure, ECG changes	Below normal serum potassium and sodium levels	Surgery (if indicated)
Addison's disease (Decreased cortisol and aldosterone secretion by adrenal cortex)	Autoimmune disorder, tuberculosis	Weakness, orthostatic hypotension, weight loss, diffuse brown hyperpigmentation, asthenia, decreased axillary and pubic hair	Above normal serum potassium level, below normal serum sodium and cortisol levels, reduced cortisol response on corticotropin stimulation test	Adrenocorticoid hormone replacement
Cushing's syndrome (Excessive cortisol secretion by adrenal cortex)	Adrenal adenoma, adrenal cancer, excessive pituitary corticotropin secretion (pituitary adenoma), exogenous steroid administration	Hirsutism, weakness, central obesity, ecchymosis, amenorrhea, deepened voice, moon face, buffalo hump, hypertension, cutaneous striae	Dexamethasone suppression test showing inadequate suppression	Surgery (if indicated), potassium and chloride replacement, mitotane administration

Common endocrine disorders (continued)

DISORDER	ETIOLOGY	SIGNS AND SYMPTOMS	DIAGNOSTIC TESTS	TREATMENTS
Adrenal glands (continued)				
Pheochromocytoma (Excessive catecholamine secretion by adrenal medulla)	Adenoma	Headache, palpitations, tachycardia, sweating, apprehension, hypertension	24-hour urine collection for catecholamines, vanillylmandelic acid, and metanephrine tests	Surgery

Head and neck. Assess the patient's face for overall color and for erythematous areas, especially in the cheeks. Note the facial expression—is it pained and anxious, dull and flat, or alert and interested? Note the shape and symmetry of the eyes and look for eyeball protrusion, incomplete eyelid closure, eyelid lag, and periorbital edema. Have the patient extend the tongue, and then inspect it for color, size, lesions, positioning, and tremors or unusual movements.

Standing in front of the patient, examine the neck first as the patient holds it straight, then slightly extends it, and finally while the patient swallows water. Check for neck symmetry and midline positioning and for symmetry of the trachea. (For more information on assessing these structures and on normal findings, see Chapter 7, Head and neck.)

Chest. Evaluate the overall size, shape, and symmetry of the patient's chest, noting any deformities. In females, assess the breasts for size, shape, symmetry, pigmentation (especially on the nipples and in skin creases), and nipple discharge (galactorrhea). In males, observe for bilateral or unilateral breast enlargement (gynecomastia) and nipple discharge. (For more information, see Chapter 11, Female and male breasts.)

Genitalia. Inspect the patient's external genitalia—particularly the testes and clitoris—for normal development. (For more information on assessing the genitalia and on normal findings, see Chapter 14, Female reproductive system, and Chapter 15, Male reproductive system.)

Extremities. Inspect the patient's arms and hands for tremors. To do so, have the patient hold both arms outstretched in front, with palms down and fingers separated. Note any muscle wasting, especially in the upper arms.

Next, inspect the legs for muscle development, symmetry, color, and hair distribution. Examine the feet for size, and note any lesions, corns, calluses, or marks made from socks or shoes. Inspect toes and the spaces between them for maceration and fissures. (For more information on assessing the extremities and on normal findings, see Chapter 17, Musculoskeletal system.)

Abnormal findings

Inspection may reveal abnormalities suggesting endocrine disease.

General appearance. Initial observation may identify the effects of a major endocrine disorder, such as hyperthyroidism or hypothyroidism, dwarfism, or acromegaly. Evaluation of the patient's overall affect, speech clarity and quality, and activity level may provide more insight. For example, a patient with hyperthyroidism may speak rapidly, perhaps incoherently at times; a patient with hypothyroidism may speak slowly, reflecting slow mentation; and one with myxedema may slur words and sound hoarse. In an adult male, a high-pitched voice may reflect hypogonadism; in an adult female, an abnormally deep voice suggests excessive androgen secretion related to Cushing's syndrome, acromegaly, congenital adrenal hyperplasia or tumor, polycystic ovaries, or an ovarian tumor.

Body development also may provide important clues to the presence and nature of an endocrine problem. In a patient with Cushing's syndrome, fat deposits typically concentrate in the face (moon face), neck, interscapular area (buffalo hump), trunk, and pelvic girdle.

Even the patient's clothing may provide clues to an endocrine problem. For instance, inappropriately heavy clothing in warm weather may indicate cold sensitivity resulting from hypothyroidism, whereas lack of outer garments in cold weather may indicate heat intolerance resulting from hyperthyroidism.

Skin, hair, and nails. Addison's disease typically causes hyperpigmentation of the joints, genitalia, buccal mucosa, palmar creases, recent scars, and sun-exposed body areas. Gray-brown pigmentation of the neck and axillae (acanthosis nigricans) may occur in a patient with polycystic ovaries, growth hormone excess, or Cushing's syndrome. Panhypopituitarism commonly causes an overall decrease in skin pigmentation.

Dry, coarse, rough, and scaly skin can indicate hypothyroidism or hypoparathyroidism. Coarse, leathery, moist skin and enlarged sweat glands are common in acromegaly. Warm, moist, tissue-thin skin may point to hyperthyroidism. In an adult, Cushing's syndrome or androgen excess frequently causes acne. Purple striae, typically on the abdomen, and bruises (ecchymoses) are common signs of Cushing's syndrome. Dry mucous membranes and poor skin turgor may indicate dehydration, perhaps secondary to diabetes mellitus.

Coarse, dry, brittle hair may be associated with hypothyroidism; fine, silky, thinly distributed hair, with hyperthyroidism. In an adult female, excessive facial, chest, abdominal, or pubic hair (hirsutism) may point to growth hormone or androgen excess. Hair loss or thinning in the axillae, pubic area, and outer third of the eyebrows may indicate hypopituitarism, hypothyroidism, or hypogonadism.

Thick, brittle nails suggest hypothyroidism; thin, brittle nails, hyperthyroidism. Increased nail pigmentation occurs in Addison's disease.

Head and neck. Eyeball protrusion (exophthalmos), eyelid lag, and incomplete eyelid closure (usually bilateral) are associated with Graves' disease, a common cause of hyperthyroidism. Increased tongue size may indicate hypothyroidism or acromegaly; in acromegaly, the enlarged tongue also may appear furrowed. A fine, rhythmic tremor of the tongue may occur in hyperthyroidism; fine, fascicular (twitching) tremors, in hyperparathyroidism. A mass at the base of the neck may represent an enlarged thyroid.

Chest. In an adult male, gynecomastia may be related to hypogonadism, hypothyroidism, estrogen excess from an adrenal tumor, or Cushing's syndrome. (However, keep in mind that transient gynecomastia may develop during puberty.) In a nonlactating female, nipple discharge could indicate prolactin or estrogen excess. Breast (areolar) hyperpigmentation may accompany excess corticotropin production, as in Cushing's disease or an corticotropin-secreting pituitary tumor.

Genitalia. In an adult male, abnormally small testes suggest hypogonadism. In an adult female, an enlarged clitoris may indicate masculinization. Recurring vaginitis may result from uncontrolled diabetes mellitus.

Extremities. Muscle atrophy in the arms and legs may occur in Cushing's syndrome, hypothyroidism, or hyperthyroidism. A fine, rhythmic tremor of the extremities also may result from hyperthyroidism. Abnormally large fingers and hands may indicate acromegaly; finger clubbing may be associated with thyroid abnormalities. In the lower legs, dependent redness or bluish coloration and absence of hair may indicate vascular insufficiency related to diabetes mellitus.

Palpation

Follow the guidelines below when assessing the thyroid gland. Usually, the thyroid is not palpable, but the isthmus (the center portion connecting the two lobes of the thyroid) may be felt. However, in a patient with an extremely thin neck, a normal thyroid may be seen or felt. An enlarged thyroid may feel well-defined and finely lobulated. Thyroid nodules feel like a knot, protuberance, or swelling; a firm, fixed nodule may be a tumor. Do not confuse thick neck musculature with an enlarged thyroid or goiter.

Attempt to elicit Chvostek's sign and Trousseau's sign in a patient with suspected hypocalcemia (abnormally low blood calcium level) related to deficient or ineffective PTH secretion caused by hypoparathyroidism or surgical removal of the parathyroid glands. To elicit Chvostek's sign, tap the facial nerve in front of the ear with a finger; if the facial muscles contract toward the ear, the test is positive for hypocalcemia. To elicit Trousseau's sign, place a blood pressure cuff on the patient's arm and inflate it above the patient's systolic pressure. In a positive test, which indicates hypocalcemia or hypomagnesemia, the patient exhibits carpal spasm (ventral contraction of the thumb and digits) within 3 minutes.

Auscultation

The nurse should auscultate the thyroid gland after palpating it. In a patient with an enlarged thyroid, auscultation may detect systolic bruits. Such bruits, caused by vibrations produced by accelerated blood flow through the thyroid arteries, may indicate hyperthyroidism. To auscultate for bruits, place the bell of the stethoscope over one of the lateral lobes of the thyroid, then listen carefully for a low, soft, rushing sound. To ensure that tracheal sounds do not obscure any bruits, have the patient hold the breath during auscultation. To distinguish a bruit from a venous hum, listen for the rushing sound, then gently occlude the jugular vein with the fingers on the side being auscultated and listen again. A venous hum (produced by blood flow of the jugular vein) disappears during venous compression; a bruit does not.

Developmental considerations for pediatric patients

When assessing a child's body development, keep in mind that the normal growth rate averages roughly 3″ (7.6 cm) per year from ages 1 to 7, and 2″ (5 cm) per year from ages 8 to 15. Hypopituitary dwarfism related to growth hormone deficiency usually becomes apparent at about age 2. Thyroid hormone deficiency in infants (cretinism) is characterized by a stocky build.

To evaluate a child's body proportions, have the child stand with arms outstretched to the left and right. Then measure the span between the tips of the middle fingers on both hands. Normally, this distance approximates the child's height. Short arms and legs may indicate gonadal dysfunction. Keep in mind that normal body proportions in children differ from those in adults, in whom the distance from the top of the head to the pubis and from the pubis to the bottom of the feet is approximately equal. In contrast, the distance from the top of the head to the pubis at birth normally is about 70% of overall height; at age 2, 60% of overall height; and at age 10, 52% of overall height.

Developmental considerations for elderly patients

A person normally loses about 3″ in height by age 70. For this reason, an elderly patient's arm span typically exceeds the height. When assessing an elderly patient, also keep in mind that dry, thin skin, slower responses and reflexes, and decreased body temperature may be normal physiologic effects of aging rather than signs of an endocrine disorder.

Documentation The following sample illustrates the proper way to document some normal physical assessment findings related to the endocrine system. Be sure to record pertinent positive findings first.
Weight: 150 lb
Height: 5′7″

Vital signs: Temperature 98.6° F, pulse 72 and regular, respirations 18 and regular, blood pressure 130/70.

Other findings: Patient is a well-developed, healthy male who appears to be his stated age of 35. Oriented to person, place, and time; speech clear. No visible abnormalities in skin, hair, nails, or facial characteristics. Neck supple, trachea midline. Thyroid palpable: firm, smooth, freely movable, and nontender. Breasts symmetrical, nipples everted. Abdomen slightly rounded, with no scars or striae. Upper extremities strong; no tremors noted. Lower extremities strong, with normal color and hair distribution.

The following example shows how to document some abnormal assessment findings:

Weight: 164 lb

Height: 5′2″

Vital signs: Temperature 96.8° F, pulse 52 and regular, respirations 14 and deep, blood pressure, 130/70.

Other findings: Patient is a well-developed male who appears older than his stated age of 52. Lethargic; oriented to person, place, and time. Speech slow and hoarse; skin and hair, dry and coarse; nails, thick and brittle. Nonpitting edema present on lower extremities. Thyroid palpable: firm, fixed, pea-sized nodule in left lobe.

STUDY ACTIVITIES

Short answer

1. Josephine Turner, age 31, reports that she's been experiencing fatigue and heat intolerance and has gained 10 lb in the last 3 months. Which endocrine disorder should the nurse suspect?

_____

_____

2. What are the four major disorders of the adrenal gland?

_____

_____

3. Identify at least eight assessment findings that suggest hyperthyroidism.

_____

_____

_____

4. Define the functions of luteinizing hormone (LH), oxytocin, ADH, and PTH.

_____

_____

5. Describe how to elicit Chvostek's sign and Trousseau's sign, and state the significance of a positive test for each sign.

_____

_____

6. During a complete body systems review, the nurse should inquire about which eye symptoms related to endocrine disorders?

_____

_____

Matching related elements

Match the endocrine gland on the left with the associated hormone on the right.

7. ___ Thyroid   **A.** Insulin

8. ___ Adrenal gland   **B.** Testosterone
     (medulla)

9. ___ Pancreas   **C.** Epinephrine

10. ___ Testes   **D.** ADH

11. ___ Pituitary gland   **E.** Thyroxine (T₄)
     (anterior)

12. ___ Pituitary gland   **F.** Thyroid-stimulating hormone
     (posterior)

13. ___ Adrenal gland   **G.** Aldosterone
     (cortex)

Fill in the blank

14. The adrenal glands are located atop the _____.

15. The _____ lies across the posterior abdominal wall, in the upper left quadrant behind the stomach.

16. The _____ gland is located at the base of the brain.

ANSWERS

Short answer

1. The nurse should suspect hypothyroidism, which commonly causes fatigue, heat intolerance, and weight gain.

2. The four major disorders of the adrenal gland are primary aldosteronism, Addison's disease, Cushing's syndrome, and pheochromocytoma.

3. In a patient with hyperthyroidism, assessment may reveal palpitations; sweating; weight loss; decreased attention span; heat intolerance; overall decrease in hair growth; diplopia; increased appetite; frequent defecation; rapid growth; anxiety; apathy; depression; restlessness; insomnia; pallor; onycholysis; hypertension; tachycardia; rapid, perhaps incoherent speech; warm, moist, tissue-thin skin; fine, silky, thinly distributed hair; thin, brittle nails; exophthalmos, eyelid lag, and incomplete eyelid closure; a fine, rhythmic tremor of the tongue or extremities; muscle atrophy in the arms and legs; and systolic bruits auscultated over the thyroid gland.

4. LH promotes ovulation and secretion of progesterone; oxytocin stimulates uterine contractions and lactation; ADH promotes water reabsorption; and PTH regulates calcium and phosphorus levels.

5. To elicit Chvostek's sign, the nurse taps the facial nerve in front of the ear with a finger; in a positive test, which indicates hypocalcemia, facial muscles contract toward the ear. To elicit Trousseau's sign, the nurse places a blood pressure cuff on the patient's arm and inflates it above the patient's systolic pressure. In a positive test, which indicates hypocalcemia or hypomagnesemia, the patient exhibits carpal spasm (ventral contraction of the thumb and digits) within 3 minutes.

6. When conducting a review of body systems, the nurse should ask the patient about changes in vision, such as double or blurred vision. Diplopia suggests a pituitary adenoma putting pressure on cranial nerves III, IV, or VI, or Graves' disease. Blurred vision can be an early sign of hyperglycemia.

Matching related elements
7. E
8. C
9. A
10. B
11. F
12. D
13. G

Fill in the blank
14. Kidneys
15. Pancreas
16. Pituitary

Selected References

Assessment. Nurse's Reference Library. Springhouse, PA: Springhouse Corp, 1986.

Beck, C.K., et al. "Cognitive impairment in the elderly." *Nursing Clinics of North America*, 28(2):335-47, 1993.

Bowers, A., and Thompson, J. *Clinical Manual of Health Assessment* (4th ed.). St. Louis: Mosby Inc., 1992.

Carpenito, L.J. *Nursing Diagnosis: Application to Clinical Practice* (5th ed.). Philadelphia: J.B. Lippincott, 1993.

Carroll-Johnson, R.M., ed. *Classification of Nursing Diagnoses: Proceedings of the Ninth Conference/NANDA.* Philadelphia: J.B. Lippincott, 1991.

Catherman, A. "Biopsychosocial nursing assessment: A way to enhance care plans." *Journal of Psychosocial Nursing and Mental Health Services,* 28(6), 31-35, 1990.

Clark, C. *Wellness Nursing: Concepts, Theory, Research, and Practice.* New York: Wiley & Sons, 1986.

Clevenger, F. "Interviewing the elderly client." *Advancing Clinical Care,* 5(6), 26-27, 1990.

DeGowin, E., and DeGowin, R. *Bedside Diagnostic Examination* (5th ed.). New York: Macmillan, 1987.

DeWitt, S. "Nursing assessment of the skin and dermatologic lesions." *Nursing Clinics of North America,* 25(1): 235-245, 1990.

Diagnostic Test Implications. Clinical Skillbuilders Series. Springhouse, PA.: Springhouse Corp, 1991.

Donnelly, E. "Family health assessment." *Home Healthcare Nurse,* 11(2):30-37, 1993.

Dunlap, W., and Sands, D. "Development of a set of instruments to assess independent living skills." *Journal of Rehabilitation,* 53(1):58-62, 1987.

Emra, K., and Herrera, C. "When your patient tells you he can't sleep." *RN,* 52(9):79-80, 82, 84, 1989.

Fischbach, F.T. *A Manual of Laboratory and Diagnostic Tests* (4th ed.) Philadelphia: Lippincott, 1992.

Giger, J., and Davidhizar, R. "Transcultural nursing assessment: A method for advancing nursing practice." *International Nursing Review,* 37(1):199-202, 1990.

Gordon, M. *Nursing Diagnosis: Process and Application* (2nd ed.). New York: McGraw-Hill, 1987.

Grimes, J., and Burns, E. *Health Assessment in Nursing Practice* (3rd ed.). Boston: Jones and Bartlett, 1992.

Hamaqui, E., Krasnopolsky-Levine, E., and Lefkowitz, R. "Nutritional support in an AIDS patient." *Nutrition in Clinical Practice,* 5(2):63-67, 1990.

Hill, L., and Smith, N. *Self-Care Nursing: Promotion of Health* (2nd ed.). East Norwalk, CT: Appleton & Lange, 1989.

Hollerbach, A., and Sneed, N. "Accuracy of radical pulse assessment by length of counting interval." *Heart & Lung,* 19(3):258-264, 1990.

Jackson, L.E. "Understanding, eliciting, and negotiating clients' multicultural health beliefs." *Nurse Practitioner, 18(4):30-32, 37-38, 41-43, 1993.*

Kelly, J.H., and Lehman, L. "Assessment of anxiety, depression, and suspiciousness in the home care setting." *Home Healthcare Nurse,* 11(2):16-20, 1993.

Kernicki, J.G. "Differentiating chest pain: Advanced assessment techniques." *Dimensions in Critical Care Nursing*, 12(2):66-76, 1993.

Kim, M.J., et al., (eds). *Pocket Guide to Nursing Diagnoses* (4th ed.). St. Louis: Mosby Inc., 1991.

Lunney, M. "Accuracy of nursing diagnoses: Concept development." *Nursing Diagnosis,* 1(1):12-17, 1990.

McConnell, E.A. "What's wrong with this patient? Assessing severe abdominal pain." *Nursing90,* 20(6):76-79, 1990.

Malasanos, L., et al. *Health Assessment* (4th ed.). St. Louis: Mosby Inc., 1990.

Malick, M., and Almasy, B. "Assessment and Evaluation—Life work tasks." In H. Hopkins and H. Smith (eds.), *Willard and Spackman's Occupational Therapy* (7th ed.). Philadelphia: J.B. Lippincott, 1988.

Melillo, K.D. "Interpretation of abnormal laboratory values in older adults." *Journal of Gerontological Nursing,* 19(1):39-45, 1993.

Mezey, M.D. *Health Assessment of the Older Individual.* New York: Springer, 1993.

Pender, N. *Health Promotion in Nursing Practice* (2nd ed.). Norwalk, CT: Appleton & Lange, 1987.

Report of the United States Preventive Task Force. *Guide to Clinical Preventive Practice.* Baltimore: Williams & Wilkins, 1989.

Rothenburger, R. "Transcultural nursing: Overcoming obstacles to effective communication." *AORN Journal,* 51(5):1349-1350, 1352, 1354+, 1990.

Scholz, J. "Cultural expressions affecting patient care." *Dimensions in Oncology Nursing,* 4(1):16-26, 1990.

Sherman, J., and Fields, S. *Guide to Patient Evaluation* (5th ed.). New York: Elsevier, 1987.

Smith, C.E. "Assesssment under pressure: When your patient says, 'My chest hurts'." *Nursing91,* 21(11):66-70, 1991.

Stotts, N., and Washington, D. "Nutrition: A critical component of wound healing." *AACN Clinical Issues in Critical Care Nursing,* 1(3):585-594, 1990.

Sundeen, S., Stuart, G., Rankin, E., and Cohen, S. *Nurse-Client Interaction: Implementing the Nursing Process* (4th ed.). St. Louis: Mosby Inc., 1989.

Swartz, M. *Textbook of Physical Diagnosis.* Philadelphia: Saunders, 1989.

Vessey, J.A., and Richardson, B.L. "A holistic approach to symptom assessment and intervention." *Holistic Nurse Practitioner,* 7(2):13-21, 1993.

Whitney, E., and Hamilton, E. *Understanding Nutrition* (5th ed.). St. Paul, MN: West Publishing, 1990.

Yura, H., and Walsh, M. *The Nursing Process* (5th ed.). East Norwalk, CT: Appleton & Lange, 1988.

Zimmer, E. "The nursing health history: A powerful tool." *Advancing Clinical Care,* 5(3): 31-32, 1990.

Index

i refers to an illustration; t refers to a table

i refers to an illustration; t refers to a table

i refers to an illustration; t refers to a table

i refers to an illustration; t refers to a table

i refers to an illustration; t refers to a table